The Anthropology of
Health and Healing

The Anthropology of Health and Healing

Mari Womack

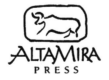

ALTAMIRA
PRESS

A division of

ROWMAN & LITTLEFIELD PUBLISHERS, INC.
Lanham • New York • Toronto • Plymouth, UK

Published by AltaMira Press
A division of Rowman & Littlefield Publishers, Inc.
A wholly owned subsidiary of The Rowman & Littlefield Publishing Group, Inc.
4501 Forbes Boulevard, Suite 200, Lanham, Maryland 20706
http://www.altamirapress.com

Estover Road,
Plymouth PL6 7PY
United Kingdom

British Library Cataloguing in Publication Information Available

Library of Congress Cataloging-in-Publication Data

Womack, Mari.
  The anthropology of health and healing/Mari Womack.
    p. cm.
  Includes bibliographical references and index.
  ISBN 978-0-7591-1043-4 (cloth: alk. paper) — ISBN 978-0-7591-1044-1
(pbk.   ) — ISBN 978-0-7591-1861-4 (electronic)
  1. Medical anthropology.   2. Public health—Anthropological aspects.   3. Human
body—Social aspects.   I. Title.
  GN296.W645 2010
  306.4'61—dc22

                                                                            2009040400

Printed in the United States of America

To my mother, Clara Rita Van Gennip Nall;
my brother, Edward Nall; and the excellent staff
at the UCLA Medical Center

Contents

Preface

A Tribute to My Teachers

My mother's dream was to become a nurse. In her day, however, ladies did not pursue careers. To her credit, the squashing of Mom's professional ambition failed to squash her spirit. Her grandfather was a circuit judge, who taught my mother to drive a car early in the 20th century. Mom drove her grandfather on his rounds in the southeast Missouri countryside. As her life unfolded, Mom's professional aspirations and driving skills became a great asset to her family and neighbors.

Mom's interest in all aspects of medicine led her to read books on medical theory and practice and to hone her skills by nursing me and my four siblings through our childhood illnesses. She consistently displayed the caring, compassionate efficiency that is the mark of a good nurse. She never wrung her hands, wailed or bemoaned a cruel fate that might have caused our complaints. Instead, she monitored us carefully and treated us with techniques that reduced our fevers and improved our ability to fight off our minor complaints. My mother had that ineffable quality known as "bedside manner." She understood both the biochemistry and the psychosocial chemistry of health and illness.

When our condition surpassed her skills, such as when I sprained my shoulder trying to emulate my brother James' acrobatic ability, Mom bundled us up and drove us to a doctor. Her ability to calmly discuss our condition with the doctor, as well as her ability to understand and follow through on recommended treatments, earned her the respect of the doctor and almost certainly helped us to recover from the slings and arrows of outrageous childhood fortune.

As she and her friends aged, my mother monitored their blood pressure and drove her friends to appointments with their doctors. When our grandmother, Mom's mother, developed melanoma late in life, Mom nursed her through that final illness. Mom's solicitous concern occasionally irritated that fiercely independent woman. Based on my own studies of psychology and health, I now realize that Grandma's irritation was directed toward her own weakening condition rather than to Mom's nursing.

Mom and my sister Nell nurtured Dad when he was diagnosed with lung cancer, and we all took turns maintaining a 24-hour-a-day vigil at his hospital bedside as he neared death. The vigil and assigned shifts were efficiently organized by Mom, so that two family members would be at his bedside at all times. As we kept watch, we entertained ourselves by reminiscing about our childhood. I'll never forget the night my sister Nell and I compared our memories of Dad and discovered that we had viewed him from entirely different perspectives. We both gained new insight into our family dynamic. And I'll never forget how we giggled that night as we compared notes on our childhood adventures.

Nell later nursed Mom when her health began to deteriorate. In a repeat of history, Mom was sometimes irritated by Nell's ministrations. Mom much preferred nursing to being nursed.

My turn came when my brother Ed was diagnosed with cancer. While tending Ed's needs through that 14-month battle, I was guided by memories of our mother's strong but compassionate nursing style. I discovered firsthand how hard it is to remain calm and compassionate while tending a critically ill patient linked to us through love. When nursing someone through an illness of that type, we must contend with our own grief as well as with the pain and grief of the patient.

Fortunately, I had learned from my mother that the patient is the pilot for that final journey. We are the flight attendants. Suffering from a debilitating illness impairs the autonomy of the individual undergoing treatment. Any attempt to control the course of the illness or treatment further undermines the autonomy of the patient. As caretakers, the best that we can do is serve the drinks, fluff the pillows, and maintain a positive but realistic atmosphere. During Ed's last days in the hospital, he carefully examined his own wasted body and asked, "Mari, am I healthy?"

I fleetingly considered lying to him about his condition, then said, "No, but we're doing the best we can." He seemed satisfied with that answer.

The anthropological approach to health and healing is ultimately about the totality of the human experience, its psychological, biological, cultural, and social dimensions. The social dimensions of health and healing include the political and the personal, the economic and the emotional aspects of being human. Anthropology is holistic and cross-cultural. Every aspect of the human experience is relevant to understanding the maintenance of health and the treatment of illness.

My mother was my first instructor in medical anthropology. As I followed her on her "rounds" among our relatives and neighbors, I learned that the practice of medicine is both a science and an art. My professional interest in the biology, psychology, sociology, and culture of health and illness developed when I was an undergraduate psychology major at UCLA. I had long been interested in the Western philosophical tradition that posits an antithesis between the mind and the body. Since I was wedded to the idea that all phenomena are either logically or experimentally verifiable, I could not comprehend how a "mind" could exist independently from a body.

In an effort to explore the conundrum of the Western model of the mind-body dichotomy, I directed my studies toward a specialization in physiological psychology. When I realized I preferred field research to laboratory research, I transferred into the UCLA Department of Anthropology. My formal education in anthropology coincided with the emergence of medical anthropology. Though I was not her student, Susan Scrimshaw's work in developing the medical anthropology specialization greatly influenced my thinking about the relationship between mind and body, health and illness, individual and society. My specific niche focuses on the interface among cognition, physiology, and behavior, where most of my research is concentrated.

My formal research in this area was conducted under the auspices of the UCLA Department of Anthropology. My undergraduate research, funded by a University of California President's Grant, focused on the relationship between academic success and social commitments among women students with children at UCLA. Based on that study—which included a statistical survey, survey questionnaires, and individual interviews—I concluded that lifestyle and social commitments of women students with children negatively affected their academic success, as measured by grade point average. On the other hand, marriage and being a parent enhanced male academic success, as indicated by the same measure.

Research for my master's thesis focused on faith healing among a Spiritualist group in an impoverished community in the greater Los Angeles area. In this study, I learned that faith healing through laying on of hands reinforced the solidarity of the group at the same time that philosophical values introduced factionalism. Thus, the rituals promoted solidarity, while disagreement over philosophical models promoted friction within the group. Ultimately, the differing philosophical models caused the group to fission after the departure of the charismatic founding father of the religious group.

My dissertation research weaved together threads of interests that had inspired me since my childhood: my mother's empathetic relationship with her "patients"; my academically inspired interest in the interrelationships among cognition, behavior, our experience of our bodies, and the psychological basis of our social relationships. My professional history provided me with an opportunity to conduct research on these interrelationships. As a professional writer, I was assigned to research and write an article on the rituals that professional and high-level amateur athletes used to prepare for the extreme stress of competition. At first, I was somewhat intimidated by this research because I knew that rituals are forms of communication based on symbols. Symbols are words, images, or behaviors that convey multiple levels of meaning. Because some of these meanings are unconscious, symbols evoke powerful emotions. As a female—an inherently powerful symbol for males—I was concerned about invading predominantly male territory.

To my surprise, most athletes were eager to talk about their rituals to me. This appeared to be related to two conceptual and social realities: (1) as a female, I was an outsider, so I could safely discuss their rituals with them; and (2) a number of the athletes expressed their frustration at sports fans and journalists who considered their rituals to be "primitive" behavior. The public attitude toward athletes' rituals is a product of the Western mind-body dichotomy, which seems to posit the idea that athletes are an inferior species. Even sports psychologists at the time of my study considered ritual preparation for athletic competition to be "superstition." In part as a result of my study (Womack 1992), sports psychologists have come to recognize that ritual preparation for a highly stressful events provides health and concentration benefits similar to those of meditation.

Research does not occur in a vacuum, and my more recent research for this book has been greatly enhanced by my participation in the Mind, Medicine and Culture seminar based in the UCLA Department of Anthropology. This provided me with the opportunity to interact with well-known scholars in medical anthropology and related disciplines, as well as with graduate students who hold the key to the future of medical anthropology. The vigorous discussions and the opportunity to interact with those specializing in various aspects of medicine and medical anthropology have helped me convert an idea into a reality: the writing and publication of *The Anthropology of Health and Healing*. It would have been impossible to accomplish the transition from idea to achievement on my own. Among the faculty whose insights especially guided my approach are Allen Johnson, Carole Browner, Douglas Hollan, Linda Garro, Thomas Weisner, and Jason Throop. Graduate students in the seminars also contributed greatly to my ideas on the value of medical anthropology

My three research assistants —Celso D. Jaquez, Kevin Huynh and Meena Abdelmalak—helped me sort out the vast quantity of data required to pull this book together. Jaquez and Huynh also participated in my medical anthropology class, the first to be taught at El Camino College, a two-year college serving demographically diverse communities, ranging from the affluent city of Manhattan Beach to the inner-city community of Compton.

My colleagues in the Behavioral and Social Sciences Division at El Camino College have taught me a great deal about the importance of collegiality in academic research. Dean Gloria Miranda has greatly supported my work, both through direct encouragement and by being one of the most skilled administrators I have encountered. She makes things happen! She greatly facilitated the development of a course in medical anthropology, and she gave me the honor of teaching it. Students in my medical anthropology classes tend to be medical professionals themselves, and their feedback has guided me in writing this book. I share an office suite with my anthropological colleagues Rodolfo Otero and Marianne Waters, with whom I am privileged to have stimulating discussions about anthropology.

A great advantage of my affiliation with ECC's Behavioral and Social Sciences Division is that I get to interact on a daily basis with colleagues in the related disciplines of psychology, sociology, and child development. We have all been strongly supported by the administrative staff: Barbara Grover, Beverly Knapp, Maria Cortez, and Michael Chung. One day, when I expressed my pleasure at being a part of such a positive group, Dean Miranda replied, "We like what we are doing." As I shall note in this book, being happy and enjoying our work is the best thing we can do for our health.

I have been fortunate in my teachers, both within my own family and in my formal training. Chief among my academic advisers are members of my PhD committee. Allen Johnson, my dissertation chair, guided me in research theory and methods. Douglass Price-Williams, whose affiliations include both the UCLA Department of Anthropology and the UCLA Neuropsychiatric Institute, fostered my interest in the cognitive basis of symbols. In working with him, I honed my understanding of the role of the unconscious in shaping cognition and behavior.

This understanding was increased through my participation in the Muse group, conducted by Douglass Price-Williams and Rosslyn Gaines of the UCLA Neuropsychiatric Institute. This group explored the dreams of artists, writers, and other creative people. Jacques Maquet, in the UCLA Department of Anthropology, and Ralph Turner, in the UCLA Department of Sociology, helped me extend my understanding of symbols into the realm of social relationships. Victor Turner's work on symbols among the Ndembu of Africa greatly influenced my own research. He was also the first to recognize the importance of my research on professional and high-level athletes' use of ritual to control the stress of competition.

Christopher Donnan's contribution to research on Peruvian shamanism, both through archaeology and his encouragement of ethnography on the subject, stimulated my interest in the healing aspects of symbols. This is belated but well-deserved acknowledgement of Chris' contribution to my intellectual development. Our discussions of sporting symbols and the symbolism of The Epic of Gilgamesh contributed significantly to research for my book *Sport as Symbol: Images of the Athlete in Art, Literature and Song*.

Rosalie Robertson asked me to write *The Anthropology of Health and Healing*, thus forcing me to move the book to the top of my writing agenda. Alan McClare urged me across the finish line and greatly contributed to the value of this book by forcing me to focus on a survey of medical anthropology rather than my own fascination with behavior, cognition, and symbols.

My biological children and my children through marriage—Laura Womack and her husband Richard Williams, Greg Womack, and Jeff Womack, along with his wife Michelle Womack, have improved my research in what is now called medical anthropology by recognizing the importance of my work, and even more, by contributing their own knowledge. Their offspring, a total of seven, have enriched my life and research through their existence and the development of their own talents.

These are only a few of the teachers who have participated in the development of my holistic perspective in researching and writing *The Anthropology of Health and Healing*. I could never have woven this intellectual tapestry together without the influence of Lex Hixon, a noted scholar on the world's religions. By instructing me in the religious traditions of Vedantic Hinduism, Tibetan Buddhism, Zen Buddhism, and Islamic Sufism, Lex taught me that there are aspects of the human experience that cannot be observed or quantified. The subjective and experiential aspects of illness, health, and healing may well be among them.

Most of all, I thank all those superb scholars from current and past centuries, without whom this book could not have been written.

Introduction

The Anthropology of Health and Healing

The anthropological approach to health and healing draws researchers into a variety of intellectual and experiential territories. Lessons learned in the classroom or the laboratory take on new urgency when applied in the field to human beings in crisis. The traditional method of cultural anthropology is **ethnography**, the analysis of particular cultures. The focus of anthropology is on learning from the people we study, rather than expecting that the people we study confirm our predictions. Ethnography allows us to consider all aspects of a particular medical situation. Epidemics, for example, are social as well as biological. This was dramatically demonstrated in the 1960s by Robert Glasse and Shirley Lindenbaum, who were able to link the devastating neurological disorder of kuru to the pattern of cannibalism among the Fore of New Guinea.

Though ethnography plays an essential role in understanding the **etiology** (cause) and **prognosis** (predicted outcome) of disease and epidemics, aid organizations and health care planners require statistics, budgets, and time frames when deciding which programs to fund and administer. In describing her work of bringing a stable food supply to villagers in Malawi in Africa, Sonia Patten notes: "Medical anthropology is difficult to define because it covers such a variety of research and practical programming. In the broadest sense, it can be defined as the study of patterns of human health in a variety of cultural and environmental contests" (2003:406). The definition of medical anthropology provided by the Society for Medical Anthropology is as follows:

Medical Anthropology is a subfield of anthropology that draws upon social, cultural, biological, and linguistic anthropology to better understand those factors which influence health and well being (broadly defined), the experience and distribution of illness, the prevention and treatment of sickness, healing processes, the social relations of therapy management, and the cultural importance and utilization of pluralistic medical systems.[1]

This definition of medical anthropology draws on traditional anthropological research among small communities as well as research in large-scale societies. It is both theoretical and applied, as the following description indicates.

> The discipline of medical anthropology draws upon many different theoretical approaches. It is as attentive to popular health culture as bioscientific epidemiology, and the social construction of knowledge and politics of science as scientific discovery and hypothesis testing. Medical anthropologists examine how the health of individuals, larger social formations, and the environment are affected by interrelationships between humans and other species; cultural norms and social institutions; micro and macro politics; and forces of globalization as each of these affects local worlds.[2]

The Society for Medical Anthropology supplies a list of topics that may be studied by medical anthropologists. This is not framed as "how to" but as an indicator and range of topics to be researched by medical anthropologists:

- Health ramifications of ecological "adaptation and maladaptation"
- Popular health culture and domestic health care practices
- Local interpretations of bodily processes
- Changing body projects and valued bodily attributes
- Perceptions of risk, vulnerability, and responsibility for illness and health care
- Risk and protective dimensions of human behavior, cultural norms, and social institutions
- Preventative health and harm reduction practices
- The experience of illness and the social relations of sickness
- The range of factors driving health, nutrition, and health care transitions
- Ethnomedicine, pluralistic healing modalities, and healing processes
- The social organization of clinical interactions
- The cultural and historical conditions shaping medical practices and policies
- Medical practices in the context of modernity, colonial, and postcolonial social formations
- The use and interpretation of pharmaceuticals and forms of biotechnology
- The commercialization and commodification of health and medicine
- Disease distribution and health disparity
- Differential use and availability of government and private health care resources
- The political economy of health care provision
- The political ecology of infectious and vector-borne diseases, chronic diseases, states of malnutrition, and violence
- The possibilities for a critically engaged yet clinically relevant application of anthropology

This list illustrates the **holistic** approach of anthropology. Medical anthropology does not focus on any single aspect of human experience. It considers all factors in human social, psychological, and biological life that may help us to understand the unique experience of individuals and groups.

Throughout its history, American anthropology has veered between the poles of academic anthropology, which focuses on the "purity" of research for its own sake,[3] and **applied anthropology**, which uses the discipline's analytical models and research methods to address human problems. Medical anthropology unites these two strands of anthropological history. Medical anthropologists can analyze the social and cultural contexts within which health and illness are defined and experienced and indigenous explanations for the etiology of illness, as well as the social and cultural dynamics of diagnosis and treatment. They can also advise on and administer programs in public policy and health care delivery systems. Most medical anthropologists pursue both academic and applied branches of the discipline, sometimes at different stages in their careers.

Anthropology and Medicine

At about the same time anthropologists began to search for careers outside the academy, medical schools were looking for ways to humanize the practice of medicine. From the partnership between medical schools and anthropologists emerged the contemporary field of medical anthropology as treated holistically in *The Anthropology of Health and Healing*. This book distinguishes between psychological and physical health and disorder, but does not consider these aspects of the human experience to be oppositions. Rather, it proceeds from the premise that psychological and physical health and disorder are interrelated phenomena.

The Anthropology of Health and Healing is also based on the idea that health and illness are components of a larger social, experiential, and explanatory complex. It draws on the ethnographic literature for examples to illustrate the complex "chemistry" that defines and addresses health and illness.

The approach of *The Anthropology of Health and Healing* is interdisciplinary. From the beginning I had planned to incorporate findings from disciplines whose concepts and research can contribute to a holistic medical anthropology. This approach is informed by my own interdisciplinary background, which incorporates physiological psychology with cultural anthropology. I have observed that different academic disciplines often study the same phenomena and come to the same conclusions, but present their data in different formats and in different arenas. Thus, we may all be saying the same things but talking to different audiences. My own research interests are integrative, bringing together cognition, physiology, behavior, and social context.

The Anthropology of Health and Healing covers many of the issues physicians Emeran Mayer[4] and Clifford B. Saper[5] address in their publication of the proceedings of a Mind-Brain-Body Medicine symposium held in March of 1998. Like *The Anthropology of Health and Healing,* that volume considers the interaction of mind and body with respect to health and healing, the emergence of integrative medicine, similarities and differences between Western medicine and other forms of healing practices, the neurobiology of stress, and the role of early environmental factors relating to maintenance of health and treatment of disease. Unlike *The Anthropology of Health and Healing,* as the title of the Mayer-Saper publication indicates, *Progress in Brain Research,* Volume 122 (Elsevier Science BV 2000) takes a medical approach and focuses on the neurobiology of the various healing factors, whereas *The*

Anthropology of Health and Healing approaches the issues from an anthropological perspective, which includes input from the four anthropological subfields: cultural anthropology, physical anthropology, linguistics, and archaeology.

Medical Practice and Power Relationships

The Anthropology of Health and Healing considers the numerous factors that influence the maintenance of health and the treatment of illness. The importance of the anthropological contribution to the definition and practice of medicine was brought home to me when I was diagnosed with high blood pressure during a particularly stressful time. I had undertaken the medical foray because of concern about my allergies. After a cursory examination, the physician's assistant who was assigned to the case repeatedly berated me for what she seemed to consider my negligence in failing to control my blood pressure. "You could have a stroke," she informed me as she was taking my blood pressure. "You could have brain damage."

I tried to explain to her that I had broken my foot and ankle in a fall at a time when I was teaching an overload of classes and trying to complete two books for publication. I also tried to explain that breaking my foot and ankle had interrupted my customary practice of brisk walking along the beach for at least an hour a day, a practice that would have reduced stress and hypertension. Drawing on my own area of specialization in stress management through behavioral means, I tried to explain that my hypertension was situational rather than medical. I also tried to explain that the stressful conditions leading to my hypertension would soon end because the semester was almost over, the most demanding of my books had gone to press, the two fractures that impaired my ability to walk and drive safely on the Los Angeles freeways was almost entirely healed, and in any event, I would soon be leaving on a long-anticipated vacation to visit my daughter and her husband in Singapore.

"I'm not interested in any of that," she replied. "I'm only interested in medicine." This statement convinced me that she didn't understand medicine because medicine involves taking a medical history. Instead of evaluating my medical history, or even looking at my charts, the woman added, "I don't want you getting on that plane until we lower your blood pressure." She indicated that she would be accomplishing that goal by prescribing hypertension medicine, which can be dangerous for one who has family and personal histories of food, skin, and respiratory allergies. Also, once begun, hypertension medication requires a long and careful period of withdrawal. Though I am typically careful to follow medical advice, in this case I was **noncompliant**. The "brain damage" my medical caretaker attempted to thrust upon me as a diagnosis was insignificant compared to the "brain damage," including increased level of stress, she had already inflicted on me as an incompetent medical care professional. Her own dire prediction of a stroke could have, in fact, induced a stroke.

First, foremost, and always, the patient's goals for treatment take priority over those of the health care professional. The physician is obligated by law and ethical practice in the United States to explain the implications of diagnosis and treatment. In this case, the medical care professional did not consider it necessary to mention the side effects of the medication she was preparing to prescribe. She did not consider social context, such as the fact that my hypertension was situational. The probability in this case was that my hypertension was likely to be reduced after my cast was removed and I was able to join my daughter and her husband on a holiday.

The patient is not obligated by law to follow the physician's recommendation. The informed consent laws were originally designed to protect the patient, but in practice, they typically protect the health care professional from legal liability. They do not protect the patient's health in the event a health care professional gives bad advice. Further, the practitioner should not assume the goals of the practitioner and the goals of the patient are the same. The doctor prescribes; the patient decides.

The physician or health care professional cannot possibly know all the factors that enter into the health care equation. The patient has a life that is almost entirely outside the domain of the medical practitioner. I was trying to provide the health care professional in this case with a medical history. She did not understand that a medical history is required when evaluating treatment for hypertension. I was not engaging in idle conversation, as she apparently assumed. Her casual dismissal of my attempts to provide context led me to withdraw from participating in the doctor-patient dialogue. Further, I lost confidence in her medical competence. She did not seem to be aware of basic considerations that I, as one who has conducted research on stress, took for granted. This loss of confidence virtually canceled any benefits of the patient-physician exchange; however, it did increase my interest in writing this book on medical anthropology.

Medical Anthropology: A Holistic Approach

The Anthropology of Health and Healing is based on the idea that the way in which health and illness are defined—as well as concepts of the self and the human body—shapes the process of diagnosis and treatment and has profound effects on medical outcomes. In it, I hope to synthesize the various studies that have shaped the long tradition within which the practice of medicine and the discipline of medical anthropology have developed.

Part I, "The Psychobiology of Health and Healing," provides an overview of the biological, social, psychological, and cognitive issues related to maintaining health and promoting healing. Part II, "Maintaining Health and Healing the Whole Person," focuses on the developmental and lifestyle issues that promote health and influence medical practice. Part III, "Models of Diagnosis and Treatment," considers treatment options—including Western biomedicine, Asian forms of healing, and other traditional healing systems—framed within their social and cultural context. It also considers the emerging field of integrative medicine, as defined by the National Institutes of Health. Part IV, "Contemporary Issues in Health and Healing," examines the role of medical anthropology in epidemiology and in the use of medicines and other interventions, as well as in public policy in designing health and healing programs.

Science and Healing

Medical anthropology falls under the purview of science. Anthropology is the study of human beings and our closest relatives, the nonhuman primates, which include chimpanzees, bonobos, gorillas, and rhesus monkeys, among many other species.

As a discipline, anthropology comprises four subfields: **physical anthropology**, which includes the study of nonhuman primates, human ecology and physiology, genetics and evolution; **linguistics**, the study of language and communication; **archaeology**, the study of human groups as represented in their material remains, including their physical remains, their **artifacts**, and their use of environmental resources; and **cultural anthropology**, which focuses on the study of contemporary groups, including their social relationships, means of communication, beliefs and customs, as well as the way in which they define themselves and their use of environmental resources.

Anthropologists have been studying healing practices and beliefs for more than 100 years, using the four-subfield approach that permits us to consider all contingencies that might affect the health of a particular population, as well as the practices of healing within that population. Anthropological research is **cross-cultural**, which allows us to explore similarities and differences within and among groups of people.

Anthropologists try to take the **insider perspective** in studying groups who live under conditions unlike our own. In medical anthropology, this allows researchers to design healing programs that respect the aspirations of the people they study and that provide an effective synthesis between traditional practices and medical practices proved to be effective in Western biomedicine. Anthropologists also take the position of **cultural relativism**, which means that we do not make value judgments about the beliefs and practices of the people we study. Not only does this approach permit anthropologists to gain access to groups who might otherwise be unwilling to admit outsiders, it also allows anthropologists to learn from the people whose healing practices have proved effective for perhaps more than the approximately 100,000 years of human existence. As the anthropologist Rodolfo Otero has noted, our bodies are the way they are because our ancestors survived. Had the healing beliefs and practices of groups in many parts of the world not contributed to the survival of those groups, the human species would have died out long ago.

The world has changed considerably within the last 100 years. Its population has nearly quadrupled, increasing from 1.9 billion in 1900 to almost 7 billion in 2009. This has placed strains on the environment that affect the lifestyle and health of human populations. It also provides an environment in which new diseases develop and thrive. International travel and commerce transmit those new diseases more rapidly than ever before. These changing conditions provide new challenges for maintenance of health and the practice of medicine. *The Anthropology of Health and Healing* is designed to consider factors relevant for sustaining health and to explore means by which healing practices can help promote the health and well-being of human populations.

The Marriage of Medicine and Anthropology

Medicine and anthropology have long marched side by side without being formally introduced. Both are sciences, and they study overlapping phenomena. One of the many things they have in common is that both focus on the study of human beings. A number of scientists in the two fields have independently come to believe that humans can best be understood holistically as biological, sociocultural, cognitive, and behavioral animals. Both medical researchers and anthropologists have studied healing techniques for more than 100 years.

So what has kept the two disciplines apart?

One thing that delayed the marriage was that they approached their common pursuit of understanding the human animal from different cultural perspectives. Western medicine has emphasized the biological aspects of the human body, while being aware that behavior of the patient and the physician plays an important role in healing and maintaining health. Anthropologists have focused on studying human behavior and cognition, while understanding that both were made possible by the unique capacities of the human body.

In the past few decades, the paths of the two disciplines have proved to be convergent rather than divergent, and the U.S. National Institutes of Health has signaled its approval. A number of scholars in the disciplines of medicine and anthropology are now engaged in integrating their rich stores of information about the human animal.

The Anthropology of Health and Healing celebrates the marriage of two traditions that have much to offer the world. As author of *The Anthropology of Health and Healing*, I anticipate that the offspring of this marriage, medical anthropology, has the potential to improve the lives and health of people in all parts of the world.

I

THE PSYCHOBIOLOGY OF HEALTH AND HEALING

A wise man should consider that health is the greatest of human blessings, and learn how by his own thought to derive benefit from his illnesses.

—Hippocrates, *Regimen in Health, Book IX*

Health is typically something we take for granted unless illness befalls us. Then we are likely to consult a medical practitioner in hopes of being healed. The book you are holding in your hands takes the position that health is a process that should be practiced every day; however, the practice of health differs widely from one culture to another. Part I of *The Anthropology of Health and Healing* explores issues of health and illness within their biological, social, and psychological context, focusing on the cultural models that shape health and healing practices cross-culturally.

Chapter 1, "Models of the Body, the Self and the Human Experience," examines the role of culture in shaping the way we view our own bodies and the bodies of others. Nowhere on earth do humans permit the body to exist in a natural state. Understanding the socialization of the body is important for situating this often unruly organism in social and cultural space.

Chapter 2, "Constructing Gender: The Body in Social Context," describes the process whereby human groups impose cultural categories onto the biological organism, the body. It also examines the economic, political, and conceptual bases that underlie the imposition of particular gender categories in human groups.

Chapter 3, "The Biology of Psychology and the Psychology of Biology," examines the intricate relationship between the way we think and feel, as well as the way our body functions. The inability to understand the role psychology plays in our biological well-being can have serious negative consequences for our health.

Chapter 4, "Metaphor, Labeling Theory, and the Placebo Effect," focuses on the importance of diagnosis in experiencing and treating illness by giving a disorder a name. Diagnosis—giving a disorder a name—shapes the course of treatment for the medical practitioner. For a patient, diagnosis shapes a lifestyle trajectory. Ambitions and plans may be put aside, priorities in social relationships may be changed and the daily routine is, almost certainly, rearranged.

1

Models of the Body, the Self, and the Human Experience

CASE STUDY
The Human Body as Universe: A Dogon World View

Dogon horticulturalists of Mali and Burkina Faso, in Africa, view the female body as a template for the design of the earth.[1] God's sexual intercourse with the feminine earth resulted in the birth of the Nommo, bisexual water gods,[2] the personified life force of the world present in all forms of water. The primary crop for Dogon has traditionally been millet, which can be stored in granaries. The granary is an important symbol for those who cultivate storable crops. The Dogon granary represents the universe in the form of an upturned basket, with the circular base of the granary representing the sun and the square roof representing the sky. The granary also symbolically represents the female body. A round jar placed in the center of the granary's bottom level represents the womb. The earth, the granary, and the upturned basket are all symbols of female generativity, which stores life in the womb. According to Dogon myth, God created humans by forming a womb and a male sex organ from clay. The original female and male humans, twins, arose from the lumps of earth. The ideal birth should produce twins, a female and a male, to balance the human species. However, since twin births are not always possible, the Spirit gave all humans two souls, one female and one male. A woman's male soul is in her clitoris; a man's female soul is in his foreskin. Since human life will not support two natures, the Dogon say, males must be circumcised and a female's clitoris must be excised. According to Dogon belief, circumcision of males and excision of females frees them from the instability of having two opposing natures. A Dogon male interviewed by Marcel Griaule stated, "The uncircumcised . . . think of nothing but disorder and nuisance" (1965:155). According to the Dogon, circumcision restores the unity of a person's soul as being either male or female, but not both.

11

As is the case with other world views, the Dogon **cosmology** reflects their particular experience of being human. In all societies, the body as physical entity is subject to interpretation both by the person possessing the body and by persons observing the body. The medical anthropologist Byron J. Good notes, "The body is subject, the very grounds of subjectivity or experience in the world, and the body as 'physical object' cannot be neatly distinguished from 'states of consciousness.' Consciousness itself is inseparable from the conscious body" (1994:116).

Humans are both biological and social entities, and in all societies, the body is viewed as raw material that must be tamed through **socialization**. The human child must be taught to regulate its biological processes in conformity to social expectations. In all societies, as well, concepts of the body are translated into definitions of health and illness, and are incorporated into procedures aimed at maintaining and restoring health.

The Body in Western Tradition

In Western **biomedicine**, the body is viewed primarily as a physical object, one that may be subject to physically caused illness and can be treated according to scientifically tested procedures. Good describes what he calls biomedicine's "folk epistemology" of disease: "Disease is located in the body as physical object or physiological state, and whatever the subjective state of individual minds of physicians and patients, medical knowledge consists of an objective[3] representation of the diseased body" (1994:116).

Good proposes what he calls an "anthropological alternative" to the biomedical view. As he frames it, the body is subjectively experienced: "For the person who is sick, as for the clinician, the disease is experienced as present in the body. But for the sufferer, the body is not simply a physical object or physiological state but an essential part of the self. . . . The diseased body . . . is a disordered agent of experience" (1994:116).

The Western tradition of medicine inclines toward a view of the body as object and of the various body organs as unrelated objects. For example, we may treat "heart disease," "colon cancer," and other conditions as being unique to a particular organ. In fact, the human body is an organism, a complex structure of interrelated parts that interact with each other. One limitation of Western medicine is that it has not yet reached the sophistication of some other medical systems, which treat the body as an organism rather than an organ. Some medical systems, which will be discussed in Part III of this book, also treat the biological, and individual, organism as part of a larger organism, the interacting community. Humans, like most other primates, are social animals.

The human animal is not a microcosm. Our well-being is dependent on the well-being of those close to us. This awareness is part of the great heritage that medical anthropology has to give to the world. Health and illness are not unique to individuals. They are part of the social fabric that binds us all together.

In recent years, biomedicine in the United States has become increasingly subject to externally imposed guidelines required by insurance companies and by the courts. A physician who deviates from these guidelines, even if such deviation benefits the patient, may be subject to censure or legal action. Medical practitioners and medical institutions can only protect themselves from censure or legal action by strict adherence to these externally imposed guidelines. Subjective knowledge and experience are not protected by law. Thus, it is not only the culture of medicine, but the culture of law, that determines medical practice in the United States.

The body both defines our experience of selfhood and, in illness, metaphorically represents our disjuncture with the world around us. In all societies, disease is viewed as chaotic and potentially disruptive to the social order. Therefore, healing addresses the restoration of the social order as well as the restoration of health. In Western medical tradition, healing is typically viewed as a process imposed on a patient by a medical practitioner who has greater intellectual and social power. In fact, healing results from a process engaging both the subjective experience of the patient and the trained experience of the medical practitioner. Whereas patients experience their bodies subjectively, medical practitioners draw on both their professional training and their subjective experience of their own bodies. Medical practitioners, like their patients, experience illness and hope for health. They are also subject to the bodily processes inherent in the life cycle.

The human body exists in social, physical, psychological, conceptual, and cultural space. It is bound by conventions, preconceptions, and expectations. Small wonder that this biological entity, the human body, is an important symbol in all human groups.

The Body as Physical Object

In its most basic form, the human body is primarily a sack of fluids. But what a sack of fluids! The intricate **biochemical** interactions within the human body—especially in the brain—produce a uniquely experienced universe, one that permits books to be written and the design of heavy metal objects, such as airplanes, that can fly through the air.

The body, as well as concepts regarding the body, comprises a fascinating component of the human experience. Though the body appears to the Western mind as a self-contained organism, it does not function independently of its environment. The body exchanges molecules with its surroundings through **respiration** and **alimentation**; however, its interaction with the environment is not limited to these functions. The body is affected by heat, cold, gravity, and other environmental factors.

Our hearts pump blood through our **arteries** to the rest of the body, but do not suck it back in. Returning blood to our hearts is a function performed by gravity and our muscles, which squeeze our blood vessels when we move. Movement helps counteract the effects of gravity, which pulls our bodily fluids to our lower extremities when we stand. That is why fluids, such as blood and **lymph**, pool in our feet when we sit or stand for extended periods. When blood is motionless for long periods of time, it can form **clots** or air bubbles. Prolonged sitting or standing also reduces movement of fluids through the **lymphatic system**. The lymphatic system is important for human health because it removes excess fluids from body tissues. It also absorbs **fatty acids** and moves them to the **circulatory system**. In addition, the lymphatic system produces **immune cells**, thus promoting our body's ability to ward off diseases.

Important bodily functions such as alimentation and elimination are affected by a combination of gravity and motion. Aided by gravity, the alimentary canal transports and absorbs nutrients. Movement assists this process. Walking, especially, is important because it flexes muscles in the abdomen, which contains the longest part of the alimentary tract.

The Body as Symbol

Despite its biological importance, we do not experience this physical entity—our body—only on **empirical** terms. The human body is encircled by **symbols**[4] and metaphor. For example, English speakers have extended the term "head" to refer to heads of state and the head of the company. The term "head" can even be used to refer to that eminently functional object, the toilet, especially when on board a ship. We can also get to the "heart" of a matter or lend a "hand." Conversely, we can describe both the anus and an obnoxious person as an "ass." We can "strong arm" a proposal through a committee or "lend an ear" to an acquaintance who is undergoing a rough time.

Since our most immediate experience is that of our own bodies, it is not surprising that the body gives rise to **metaphor**, symbolic comparisons between imagery that can be experienced through our senses and concepts that can only be experienced through symbols and language. In their book, *Metaphors We Live By*, George Lakoff and Mark Johnson link our experience of the world to the way we experience our bodies in space. These linguists note that, in English, use of the term "up" is associated with positive factors, while "down" is negative: "These spatial orientations arise from the fact that we have bodies of the sort we have and that they function as they do in our physical environment" (Lakoff and Johnson 1980:14).

We can feel "up" when we are having a good day or "down" when things aren't going well. We can look "back" in time or present a good "front." We can look up to the "head" of an organization or look "down" on someone who is "beneath" us in social space. In his book *Culture and the Human Body: An Anthropological Perspective*, John W. Burton notes that metaphors of the body can be extended to society as a whole: "The economy is 'healthy'; newspaper editors write about the 'pulse' of local life; major 'arteries' leading into cities can become clogged, and so on" (2001:29).

TAMING THE BODY

The process by which this bag of chemical reactions, the human body, acquires the means to produce poetry and nuclear weapons is complex. As a purely physical entity, the human body is often unruly. It makes unacceptable noises and produces offensive excretions. In all societies, the human body is tamed. It is brought under the control of the social forces that define appropriate behavior, as well as appropriate ingestions and secretions.

The body is also subject to much ornamentation and alteration. It is the most widely decorated canvas for which there is cross-cultural evidence. Though we cannot document the origins of body decoration, some form has probably existed for at least 35,000 years. Pleistocene foragers decorated the walls of their caves and carved representations of female figures, so it is likely they decorated that most universal of canvases, the human body.

Though the human body is a biological entity, it is universally expected to conform to social expectations. Typically, modifications of the human body are aimed at bringing it into alignment with social expectations. Modification of the body transforms it from a biological entity into a social entity capable of forming stable relationships and taking on responsibilities toward others.

Burton joins a host of philosophers and other scholars in trying to explain how the human body, a biological entity, could acquire the cultural significance that would cause humans to carve it into a social entity, to in effect, inscribe our initials on it through circumcision and other forms of surgery. Burton and others have noted that humans, unlike other animals, subject their bodies to social control through **circumcision, scarification, tattooing,** and other forms of bodily "decoration." Cross-culturally, both male and female bodies may be decorated in ways that communicate cultural values.

The Painted Body

In his book *Behind the Mask: On Sexual Demons, Sacred Mothers, Transvestites, Gangsters and Other Japanese Cultural Heroes,*[5] Ian Buruma notes that many idealized hero types are reflected in Japanese literature, film, art, theater, and comics. He adds that the Japanese aesthetic frames humans within an Asian concept of nature: "Love of nature is generally regarded as the basis of Japanese aesthetics. In China and Japan . . . man blends with nature; there is no dichotomy, such as exists in the West, where man is inclined to oppose the forces of nature. . . . [In Asian art] Natural scenery is not simply a backdrop for depicting man . . . man is part of the natural scene" (1984:64).

Buruma notes that this aesthetic is based in both the Shinto and Buddhist view that nature is sacred. However, nature has a dual aspect. She is a fertile mother, but she can unleash destruction on human life through "devastating earthquakes, murderous typhoons and floods. Like woman, that other mysterious force liable to erupt in frightful passions, nature must be tamed, or at least controlled" (1984:65). Buruma provides the example of the geisha, whose natural beauty must be tamed by converting her into a totally social being. Through makeup and dress, her individuality is subsumed under face paint and clothing that reduce her social persona to that of a doll.

Painting is an important part of body decoration. Painting of the face, especially, is widespread, though it varies from culture to culture and within cultures. Among Tiwi of Australia, face and body painting are traditionally closely associated with ritual transitions and ritual protection. Both females and males paint their faces and bodies to observe socially significant occasions. On the fifth day after a woman gave birth, she brought the child to her husband's fire, but he could not then touch the child: "The baby is covered with charcoal, and the mother is painted with a red stripe down the center of her body, both front and back. The lower half of her face, from the bridge of her nose downward, is painted black, while the upper half is painted red" (Goodale 1994[1971]:27). A girl who had just finished her first menses was painted with a red stripe down the front of her body. This was said to symbolize a snake.[6]

Messengers were painted red or red, white, and black, depending on the nature of the message. Battles were announced by a messenger painted all three colors. A death was announced by a messenger painted in red. Upon learning of a death, those involved in the mourning ceremony quickly painted themselves, using any paint that was at hand. The paint was renewed daily, and once the preliminary mourning dances had begun, the painting became "much more elaborate and in various designs" (Goodale 1994[1971]:263). People who were relatives of the deceased typically smeared white or yellow paint over their bodies. Others painted their faces and bodies in colors and patterns appropriate to their role in the mortuary ceremony.

In the *kulama* ceremony [yam ceremony], in which men and women were initiated as adults, men dipped their hands in white clay paint and patted the paint on their hair. They then held their paint-covered hands up to the sun, so they would not be killed by the *tarni*, spirits that cause illness. They then placed white paint around their eyes so they would have good eyesight when they grew old.

The *kulama* ceremony, described by Goodale, lasted four days. On the morning of the third day, the men who were being initiated completely covered themselves with red ochre mixed with water. They also painted their children. Later that day, they painted their hair, face, and bodies in elaborate designs using white, yellow, black, and red pigments.

The Tattooed Body

Among Samoans, both men and women were traditionally tattooed in an extremely painful and costly procedure, using sharpened bone or teeth in the form of combs, which were hammered into the initiate's skin. Then black dye was inserted into the wounds. The process took place in stages over many weeks and was attended by a high degree of ritual. Males were more extensively and densely tattooed than females. Males were typically tattooed from above their navels to their knees, and that entire portion of the body was covered in dark geometric designs.

The density and extent of the tattoo was both a mark of a man's status and a contributor to his status because of the courage needed to endure the great pain such tattooing required. In her book *Coming of Age in Samoa*, Margaret Mead writes that men arranged their *lava lava*, which is like a sarong, so their tattoos would show above and below the garment. This is a public, visual demonstration of male courage and status. Women played a role in the tattooing ceremony. They sang to the men as they were tattooed, comparing the pain of being tattooed to the pain of childbirth.

Tattooing was a required puberty rite for adolescent males. The tattooing of women was much less ritualized and extensive. More recently, females may undergo the pain of tattooing to express their pride in their Samoan heritage. A seventeen-year-old girl, Harmony Anita Matago, told *Samoa News* she was getting a malu (traditional female tattoo) from a master tattoo artist: "Getting a 'malu' . . . is an honor and a privilege every young Samoan woman should be really proud of. . . . It would also serve as my identity as a young Samoan woman when I leave for school off island."[7]

For Samoans, tattoos traditionally marked status, which included the ability to undergo the pain of acquiring a tattoo. Though status was traditionally bestowed by birth, acquiring a tattoo affirmed the legitimacy of the **ascribed status**, the status bestowed by birth. Undergoing the pain of acquiring a tattoo conferred **achieved status**, status that is attained by one's skills or qualities. As Samoa became more Americanized, the achieved status of tattooing became less important in marking status, whereas the ascribed status of birth maintained a Samoan's high rank.

As Matago's decision to undergo tattooing indicates, modern Samoan identity may involve the choice of returning to traditional Samoan practices, including tattooing. This is not unusual in societies that have undergone culture change introduced from outside. Change may initially be welcomed as a novelty. Eventually, the people recognize that, although the incursive culture offers some advantages, their traditional culture continues to be important to them. This process often gives rise to what the anthropologist Anthony F. C. Wallace calls **revitalization movements**. Wallace defines revitalization movements as "any conscious, organized effort by members of a society to construct a more satisfying culture" (1966:30).

Revitalization movements are typically described by the people involved as being aimed at restoring cultural traditions. In fact, these movements coordinate a synthesis of the old and new. Matago's decision to get a *malu* is an individual choice rather than a collective action; however, revitalization movements and the decision to retain an important symbol of her culture serve the same purpose. In Matago's case, the *malu* integrates her two identities, as a Samoan and as a modern educated woman. She has wedded traditional Samoan values related to tattooing with the value of obtaining an education that equips her for high status in a technological world.

THE REBELLIOUS BODY

Whereas contemporary Samoan tattooing practices integrate the traditional organism of the kin-based social group into a changed social context, contemporary American tattooing practices appear to represent a form of rebellion against an industrialized and mechanized universe. Tattooing has traditionally been considered a form of rebellion in the United States. Parents may forbid their children to get tattoos. Advice columnists caution against it. In the minds of many Americans, tattooing is associated with rebellious subcultures, such as bikers, teenagers, and Hollywood film stars.

There are subcultures in the United States and other countries in which tattooing is a mark of social unity among defiant subcultures. In the Philippines and other parts of Asia, members of gangs or tongs may be extensively tattooed on parts of the body that will be hidden by business suits or other street clothes.[8] These practices afford a kind of dual identity, in which the individual's body reserves a private identity for members of the "club," but presents a conforming identity to the society as a whole when the body is covered by clothing.

Personal Tattoos

Since there is not a tattooing tradition common to all or most Americans, designing custom tattoos for individuals has become a growing industry in the United States. Many tattoo designers market their wares on the Internet. At the time of this writing, the website Tattoo Designs & Symbols[9] surveyed tattoo design websites and posted a monthly compilation of the most popular tattoos. Tattoos include "tribal designs," which appeared to be based on Maori art of New Zealand. In fact, a number of tattoo websites extol their "Maori" tattoos.

A number of the symbols mentioned on the site are associated with power, including Thor's hammer, bears, dragons, knights, crowns, and the sun. Even more prevalent are symbols relating to aspiration and transcendence, including stars, angels, wings, the Phoenix, and butterflies. Modern industrial societies are organized around conformity to routine, and tattoo designs chosen by individuals may reflect a desire to transcend the routine and powerlessness of industrialized society.

It is remarkable that none on the list of most popular tattoo designs is associated with urban or industrial life, since people who are able to "surf the 'net'" for tattoo images are clearly from industrialized and mechanized societies. Art of the late nineteenth century and much of the twentieth century glorified mechanistic images that celebrated industrialization. In 1932, Lewis Mumford wrote of U.S. aesthetics: "We value the positive results of science, disciplined thinking, coherent organization, collective enterprise, and that happy impersonality which is one of the highest fruits of personal development" (cited in Lynes 1980:147–48).

Mumford celebrates industrialist art as a triumph of American ingenuity and the free enterprise system. He ignores the fact that most art celebrating the machine was produced in Europe. Some of the most prominent artists were from Germany, where the Bauhaus School flourished from 1919 to 1933, when Nazis forced it to close.

The Decline of "Happy Impersonality" and the Rise of Impermanence

The glory of the machine appears to have eroded after the novelty faded. The current generation of tattoo clients may have become disenchanted with the "happy impersonality" of the machine age. The only tattoo images surveyed for this book that could come close to machine imagery fall into the category "friendship/family," which includes symbols that represent group affiliations, rather than loyalty to machines and industrialization as a way of life.

Not surprisingly, the "friendship/family" category ranks third on the "most popular" tattoo designs, since affiliation with a sympathetic group is often difficult in urban industrial environments. Industrialization weakens organic human bonds in favor of such rewards as money, job titles, power, or fame. Relationships can be reinforced by inking in the name of a significant other deemed to be permanent in an individual's life. We can ink in our names on marriage licenses, credit card contracts, and job applications. Tattooing is a symbolic way of making permanent on one's body a relationship one considers permanent in one's life. Or a relationship one would like to be permanent.

Changing Affiliations

A 2007 article on the Internet edition of *The New York Times* noted that a new industry in the United States consists of removing no-longer-relevant tattoos. According to a 2003 Harris Interactive poll, 17 percent of people who had acquired tattoos regretted it. In many cases, the tattoos people regretted acquiring represented an earlier stage of their lives. A woman cited in *The New York Times* article opted to remove the name of a former fiancé from her wrist, stating that she had learned an important lesson: "I'm not going to get a tattoo of another guy's name until I get married."[10]

This woman's experience is a poignant reminder of the fragility of social bonds in an industrialized society. Promises, like engagements, can be broken. Workers can be fired. Contracts can be voided. Sentences can be commuted. The most compelling image of the woman willing to get another tattoo when she got married is that she assumed that marriage offered a guarantee of permanency.

In an urban industrialized society, marriage is as fragile as many other social bonds.[11] Samoan tattoos reinforce the link to traditions and permanency. The symbolism of American tattoos may well represent nostalgia for a less mechanistic society, reaching out for personal power, a yearning for affiliation with a supportive group or a quest for permanency that no longer exists. Overwhelmingly, the most popular tattoo images listed on the Tattoo Designs & Symbols website evoked associations with the past, or with fantasy and transcendence.

MEDICINE AND THE BODY AS MACHINE

A number of scholars have suggested that the metaphor of the human body as a machine has found its way into the practice of Western medicine, in which the body is treated as a collection of parts. For example, Robbie E. Davis-Floyd (1993) describes medical childbirth practices in the United States as being based on a technocratic model. She writes:

> The experience of childbirth is unique for every woman, and yet in the United States childbirth is treated in a highly standardized way. No matter how long or short, how easy or hard their labors, the vast majority of American women are hooked up to an electronic fetal monitor and IV (intravenously administered fluids and/or medication), are encouraged to use pain-relieving drugs, receive an episiotomy (a surgical incision in the vagina to widen the birth outlet in order to prevent tearing) at the moment of birth, and are separated from their babies shortly after birth. Most women also receive doses of the synthetic hormone pitocin to speed their labors, and they give birth flat on their backs. Nearly one-quarter of babies are delivered by Cesarean section. (2005:449)

Though the body is experienced as being particular to oneself, it exists in social space. Thus, our concepts of our own bodies are greatly shaped by cultural definitions and controlled by social priorities.

The Body Politic and the Subjugated Body

Body metaphors can be extended into the social realm, and this is not always a benign process. In stratified societies, heads of the political body can subjugate others by using their power of coercion. These "heads of state" can send "foot soldiers" into battle. Differences in social power over the human body are illustrated in Alfred Lord Tennyson's poem, "The Charge of the Light Brigade," which recounts a devastating setback to the British Light Cavalry on October 15, 1854. The Crimean

War, which lasted from 1853 to 1856, was fought between Russia and the Western allies—including the Ottoman Empire, Britain, France, and Sardinia—over control of Palestinian lands.

The Battle of Balaklava pitted a heavily overmatched cluster of British regiments against a Russian army that had taken up positions on both sides and at the end of a valley in the eastern part of the Ukraine. The result of the uneven encounter is described in "The Charge of the Light Brigade." The British mounted cavalry was demolished by the Russian army. Lord Tennyson extolled the valor of the English cavalry who rode to their deaths. The French Marshall in the Crimea had a different view. He is quoted as saying of the British effort, *"C'est magnifique, mais ce n'est pas la guerre"* (It is magnificent, but it is not war.").

The Russian commander N. Ushakov described the charge in more technical terms. Noting that the British had occupied the battle scene before the Russians arrived, he questioned why the British had not secured the valley themselves, especially since they were supported by a large French battalion. He added, "Another circumstance allowed by the allies was that the Traktir bridge was not destroyed and our troops' crossing of the aqueduct was completely unopposed. Tearing down the bridge and building batteries on the northwest slopes of the Fedyukhin Heights would have made our undertaking very doubtful."[12]

The Light Brigade was largely composed of the aristocracy. They were subjugated by their own sense of honor. The members of the Light Brigade had no choice but to obey their command, even if they knew the charge was a mistake.

As is characteristic of virtually all military commanders, the Russian commander Ushakov attributed the Russian victory to their own expertise: "It must be understood that the main reasons for our success were the precise execution by unit commanders of skillful directives based on experience, and the confidence of the troops in the proficiency of their beloved commander and the dispositions he arranged."[13]

The Body as Political Symbol

In his book *Discipline and Punish*, Michel Foucault describes the body as a *mise-en-scène* in which forms of government can act out their control over the bodies of subjects. He compares concepts of the body reflected in punishment policies of the French ancien régime with those of the Enlightenment. The term "ancien régime" designates the social and political system established in France under the Valois and Bourbon lineages (fourteenth to eighteenth centuries).

Foucault argues that the ancien régime used rigorous punishment, including torture, to assert its control over the bodies of its subjects. He describes the public torture of one individual who was torn apart by various means for a crime that was puerile compared to the punishment. As the prisoner called out to the heavens blessing those who conducted and witnessed the punishment, the forces of "law" continued to try pulling his body apart. Most of these means failed, thus subjecting the prisoner to greater pain. Though Foucault does not make this point, the human body—held together by sinew and bone—withstood for some time the efforts of the state to dismantle it.

Foucault adds that the stated goals of the Enlightenment were to develop a system of punishment applicable to all. It was envisioned as a more democratic form of punishment, aimed at applying punishments suitable to the crime. Still, Foucault notes, systems of punishment serve the needs of the state, rather than the needs of individuals. He adds that centers of control in society need criminals for the purpose of demonstrating their control over the bodies of lawbreakers.

Controlling the Body of Scientific Knowledge

In medicine, those who control the body of scientific knowledge can extend that control to the bodies of patients, or in the case of European colonialism, to the bodies of entire groups of people. Anthropologists have noted that body metaphors historically have been used to reinforce other forms of social power. Anthropologist Jean Comaroff suggests that nineteenth-century European colonialists seeking access to African resources used medical terminology as a means of justifying their control over the "dark continent" and the black body. That metaphor links the state to the prevailing color of its occupants. Comaroff notes that this metaphor extended to concepts of health and disease. In her article "The Diseased Heart of Africa: Medicine, Colonialism, and the Black Body" Comaroff notes, "Medicine held a special place in the imagination that colonized nineteenth-century Africa" (1993:305).

Medicine provided a model for regulating relationships between the colonizers and the colonized, between the "civil" and the "unruly": "As an object of European speculation, 'Africans' personified suffering and degeneracy, their environment a hothouse of fever and affliction" (Comaroff 1993:305-306).

According to Comaroff, the European invasion of Africa was symbolically equated with European medical procedures. Europeans "linked the advance of reason in the interior of the dark continent with the biological thrust into the dim recesses of the human person" (Comaroff 1993:306). The economic and political thrust of colonialism was linked to medical and religious models, as Europeans became committed to "saving" and "healing" inhabitants of "the dark continent": "Early evangelists in South Africa saw social and political obstacles to their 'human imperialism' as natural contagions, responsive to medical control. As their philanthropic dreams hardened into colonial realities, the black body became ever more specifically associated with degradation, disease, and contagion" (1993:306). Comaroff suggests that the conquest of Africa became framed as a medical rescue effort, defined in European concepts of health:

> The frontiers of "civilization" were the margins of a European sense of health as social and bodily order, and the first sustained probe into the ailing heart of Africa was a "mission to the suffering." It followed that the savage natives were the very embodiment of dirt and disorder, their moral affliction all of a piece with their physical degradation and their "pestiferous" surroundings. (1993:306)

The early colonialists drew on medical terminology to define their subjugation of the people and resources of Africa as a rescue mission: "The early soldiers of Christendom were also the cutting edge of colonialism, and when they tried to domesticate the realities of the 'dark' interior, they drew heavily on the iconography and practice of healing" (Comaroff 1993:306). Thus, the politics of conquest were "civilized" by the metaphor of liberation. In framing the conquest of Africa as a medical discourse, rather than as a political and economic discourse, missionary healers resisted the control of newly formed agencies of public health. Comaroff writes:

> By the turn of the [20th century] their [European] talk of civilizing Africa had given way to a practical concern with the hygiene of black populations—and to the project of taming a native workforce. Here, as elsewhere in the colonized world, persons were disciplined and communities redistributed in the name of sanitation and the control of disease. For as blacks became an essential element in the white industrial world, medicine was called upon to regulate their challenging physical presence. (1993:306)

Missionaries defined Africa as a sick organism in need of healing. Robert Moffat, father-in-law of David Livingstone and a pioneer of the London Missionary Society (LMS) among the Tswana, presented this position to a large and admiring public in London: "Africa still lies in her blood. She wants . . . all the machinery we possess, for ameliorating her wretched condition. Shall we, with a remedy that may safely be applied, neglect to heal her wounds? Shall we, on whom the lamp of life shines, refuse to disperse her darkness?" (Moffat 1842:616).

In retrospect, we may question Moffat's attempts to save Africa during the same era that England was neglecting its own urban poor. A short time later, Herbert Spencer was decrying free schools and public health programs of all kinds in England as an erosion of his idea of the "survival of the fittest" ([1876]1896:233). This cannot be credited to cynicism. Spencer genuinely believed that England's urban poor endangered the social evolution of the human species. He advised that doctors and nurses not be certified because certification of medical personnel kept unfit members of the species alive. Spencer believed that the human species was "evolving" toward perfection. Thus, impoverished and diseased individuals lowered the "fitness" of the entire human "race." Spencer was attempting to adapt Darwin's concept of **natural selection**, which states that species evolve in the process of adapting to a particular environment, to Spencer's own view of moral superiority.

Spencer had apparently learned no lessons from the experiences of English colonists in India a few decades earlier, when large numbers of English elites died in a cholera epidemic spread to them from the streets by the servants they hired to clean their houses and tend their children, as well as to cook and serve their food.

Moffat's appeal to the English public served the needs of colonial administrators. Moffat genuinely believed, or convinced himself, that it was the "white man's burden"[14] to "save" Africans. Though their beliefs were no doubt genuine, these beliefs justified their own sense of superiority and their exportation of colonial wealth to Europe. Comaroff writes: "Thus did the metaphors of healing justify 'humane imperialism,' making of it an heroic response rather than an enterprise of political and economic self-interest. . . . The early evangelists conceived of themselves as restorers both of body and spirit, bearers not only of salvation, but of a healing civilization" (1993:313–314). Comaroff concludes, "[Medicine] gave the validity of science to the humanitarian claims of colonialism" (1993:324).

Though Comaroff deals with nineteenth-century justification of the colonization of Africa through medical terminology, colonialism continues today. Early in the twenty-first century, I sat in an evangelical church in Seattle, Washington, and heard a minister deliver a quote attributed to American General Douglas MacArthur: "Send in the missionaries and you won't need to send in the armies." Both armies and ideologues prevail by defining the "enemy" as inferior and in need of "rescue." The medical idiom can justify invasion and subjugation of other cultures by framing them as a rescue effort.

Conformity and the Body Politic

In her book *National Past-Times: Narrative, Representation, and Power in Modern China*, Ann Anagnost describes imagery of the body in Zhang Yimou's film *Hong gao liang* (*Red Sorghum*) as exalting the festive excess of peasant culture, which she writes, "aims to recoup the image of a prepoliticized, spontaneous body, still 'intact' after the onslaught from the political rituals of the socialist party-state" (1997:98). Anagnost uses the film as a starting point from which to examine the Chinese government's use of festive rituals to produce docile political subjects that project the party-state as the unified voice of the "people as one." She notes that this imagery "conceals the internal fragmentation and diversity not only of 'the people' but also within the organization of the [Communist] party" (1997:98).

Though we typically view the body as existing in objective reality, it is bound about with cultural models and social expectations. Anagnost addresses subjectivity in Chinese representations both "at the level of individual bodies and at that of the body politic" (1997:98). She cites an example of the power of the state to designate "law-abiding households" (those that conform to the model provided by the state) as a means of exacting conformity.

A certain Zhou Yixian was a diviner who went from village to village to read horoscopes, a practice that was regarded by the Chinese government as a "feudal superstition." He gave up the practice in hopes of winning a red and gold plaque awarded to "law-abiding households," but he was passed over when these awards were given out. Zhou Yixian complained to the local party secretary, who told him he was passed over because of his previous divining activity. Zhou Yixian protested this ruling on the basis that he had "corrected" the behavior the party deemed unacceptable.

A neighbor advised Zhou Yixian to stop arguing with the party secretary because there was no monetary grant involved in the award, and "It doesn't matter whether you have a plaque or not." Zhou Yixian became even angrier, saying, "If there had been an award of ten or so yuan, then I wouldn't have said anything. It would have reflected badly on the issue of my reputation. But if it is simply a matter of qualifying for this status, then I must contend for it!" (1997:99–100)

Anagnost collected a number of stories of this kind appearing in newspapers during her research in China in the 1990s. She describes the recounting of the bestowal of honors in the stories as a "representation of a contemporary political ritual" (1997:100). Though Anagnost does not draw on this analogy, the story of Zhou Yixian is a kind of hero myth, in which Zhou, the main character in the myth, has followed a path of "error," as defined by the Chinese government. When he acknowledges the "error" of his ways, he displays his heroic character by claiming his prize because of honor rather than monetary reward.

Anagnost suggests that "contemporary political rituals," as exemplified in the story of Zhou Yixian, illustrate the power of the state to elevate status by naming:

"The bestowal of status honors, through the issuing of ritual markers and public processions, demonstrates the power of the state to define discursive positions in political culture through its classificatory strategies, its power to name, to sort persons into the hierarchically arranged categories of a moral order" (1997:100). She adds, "This categorical exclusion of individuals from the social body isolates them in a state of extreme moral, as well as political ambiguity" (1997:101).

It was not the red and gold plaque that led Zhou Yixian to seek recognition as a "law-abiding householder." Nor was it a matter of monetary reward. Instead, he sought the award to avoid becoming a **pariah**, a category that would have deprived him of the rewards of being an accepted member of an orderly society.

Discipline and Punish: An Egalitarian Solution

The ability to "discipline and punish," to draw on Foucault's model of the power of the state, is characteristic of all social groups. Each of us has some degree of power to bestow on or withhold approval from our fellows. In most cases, however, we do not have the power to inflict punishment upon another person's physical body.

In societies such as that of the traditional Netsilik, who live above the Arctic Circle, populations were small and environmental conditions were harsh. People relied on each other for survival. Thus, bodies of individuals were valuable. As is the case in all societies, grievances arose, but "the formalized techniques for peacemaking . . . were positive in the sense that usually they brought conflict in the open and resolved it in a definitive manner. These techniques were fist fights, drum duels, and approved execution" (Balikci 1970:185). In the case of fist fights and song duels, the object was to resolve conflicts and preserve life. Asen Balikci writes: "Any man could challenge another to a fist fight for any reason. . . . Opponents stood without guard and took turns, the context continuing until one of the fighters had had enough and gave up" (1970:189).

The outcome appeared to resolve the hostilities. As one informant told Balikci, "After the fight, it is all over; it was as if they had never fought before" (1970:189).

Men who held grudges against each other could resolve the issue through song duels. Each man secretly composed a song insulting his opponent and taught it to his wife. Each wife sang her husband's song in turn, while the men drummed and danced. The winner of the song duel was decided by the audience, not on the basis of what Americans or Europeans might consider justice, but on the basis of who wrote and performed the most entertaining song. Thus, a potentially disruptive quarrel was tamed through humor and entertainment, converting a negative situation into a resolution that enhanced the solidarity of the group.

In the case of the Netsilik, no individual was allowed to exert control over the body of another, except when extreme behavior threatened the security of the entire community. As Foucault notes, in hierarchical societies—where there are extreme differences in status—those in positions of authority can reinforce their status by exerting control over bodies of lower-status individuals.

In the practice of medicine, whether Western biomedicine or otherwise, the body can become disputed territory. The medical practitioner is operating from a position of power due to her or his expertise and experience, but the stakes are higher for the patient. A mistake by the practitioner can cost the patient her or his life or health.

The practice of medicine, therefore, implies a negotiation of realms of power. Ideally, the medical practitioner and the patient should establish a partnership, but for many reasons addressed throughout this book, this is extremely difficult to do.

CONCEPTS OF THE BODY, ILLNESS, AND POWER

A number of anthropologists have noted that cultural concepts of the body and illness are related to definitions of power in other realms. In her book *The Woman in the Body* (2001), Emily Martin suggests that the American concept of PMS (premenstrual syndrome) is actually a paradigm for the negotiation of power. She adds that the PMS concept has rewards both for women and for the industrial workplace, which labels the reduction of work energy characteristic of PMS as an illness.

Anthropologists have noted that pollution taboos, which require menstruating women to seclude themselves in menstrual huts and to avoid men and children, also permit women to escape from the duties of being a wife and mother. During the time of seclusion, cowives and other females are obligated to assume the menstruating woman's duties. One famous photo taken by an anthropologist shows a television antennae protruding from a menstrual hut. Similarly, some anthropologists say, PMS concepts in the United States permit women to escape excessive demands placed on them both in the workplace and in the home.

Alma Gottlieb affirms the physical basis for PMS, but notes that symptoms of PMS are culturally constructed. Gottlieb observes that PMS sufferers are predominantly married women and that their symptoms are in opposition to mainstream Western assumptions that women should be "nice" and "quiet," compassionate and self-effacing. Women are expected to maintain the home as "a sanctuary to which men can escape after being polluted by the symbolic dirt of the workaday world" (Gottlieb 1993:55).

Gottlieb suggests that the opposition of being "nice" throughout most of the month and of being "irritable" and "hostile" during PMS results in a bifurcated model of femininity, in which the "normal" personality of submissiveness is favored over the "illness" and aggressiveness of PMS. Gottlieb notes that defining PMS as an uncontrollable biological phenomenon permits women to voice their complaints at a time when they know their complaints will not be taken seriously:

> Many American women have not found a voice with which to speak such complaints and at the same time retain their feminine allure. They save their complaints for that "time of the month" when they are in effect permitted to voice them yet by means of hormones do not have to claim responsibility for such negative feelings. In knowing when their complaints will not be taken seriously yet voicing them precisely during such a time, perhaps women are punishing themselves for their critical thoughts. (Gottlieb 1993:57)

Gottlieb adds, "As long as American society recreates its unrealistic expectations of the female personality, it is inevitable that there will be a PMS, or something playing its role" (1993:58). There is a downside to linking mood and behavior to the menstrual cycle. Gottlieb notes that defining PMS as resulting from biological processes producing uncontrollable urges reduces personal volition and denies women authorship of their own states of mind. She concludes, "As women in con-temporary America struggle to find their voices, it is to be hoped that they will be able to reclaim their bodies as vehicles for the creation of their own metaphors, rather than autonomous forces causing them to suffer and needing to be drugged" (1993:48).

The contemporary concept of menstruation as a "disease" flies in the face of science. Menstruation would have to be selected for as a condition of the survival of the human species. As Gottlieb suggests, the contemporary metaphor of menstruation as an "illness" suggests that there are factors in contemporary society that require women to be defined as unable to function like "normal people" (men?) during menstrua-tion. Though based in biology, the contemporary concept of PMS could well be a form of feminine rebellion in which women reject the cultural mandate that they should be "nice."

Concepts of the Body and a Chinese AIDS Epidemic

Most contemporary writings linking body metaphors to social power and defini-tions of health address gender relationships; however, anthropologists have noted that body metaphors are also used to reinforce other forms of social power. The medical anthropologist Kathleen Erwin writes: "Beginning in the early 1990s—and accompanying the acceleration of capitalist-oriented economic reforms that fol-lowed the 1989 Tian'ammen massacre—military units, cash-strapped provincial health bureaus, and other entities created business ventures to procure and resell blood for both urban and international markets" (2006:139–140).

For-profit efforts to obtain blood for resale targeted impoverished rural village-dwellers. Many donors gave blood twice a week and some gave almost daily.

> The blood was not tested for HIV and, in many cases, was not tested for any blood-borne viruses. To save money and increase donation frequency, many blood collection centers pooled the blood by type and used plasmapheresis to separate plasma from whole blood. Donors were reinjected, in some cases with pooled blood, or in other cases with reused needles and other unsanitized equipment. (Erwin 2006:140)[15]

The nascent attempt to inject capitalism into medicine had disastrous conse-quences. It triggered an AIDS epidemic that has reached deep into the heart of China. Henan Province, on which Kathleen Erwin's analysis centers, is both histor-ically important and has great potential for a lucrative tourist industry. Henan Province is considered the cradle of Chinese civilization. Its archaeological treasures date back to the 6,000-year-old Yangshao culture and the 5,000-year-old Dahe cul-ture. Luoyang city, in Henan, has been the capital of nine dynasties, beginning with the Eastern Zhou Dynasty of 770 to 221 BC. The city is home to art treasures, includ-ing Tang three-glaze horses and the Longmen Grottoes, famous for the treasure trove of Chinese Buddhist statues sculpted when Luoyang was the capital of the Northern Wei Dynasty (386–534 CE). Henan Province is also the location of the Shaolin Monastery, famed as the birthplace of Chan (Zen) Buddhism and the Kung Fu tra-dition of the martial arts.

In 1996, the Chinese government closed its state-run blood banks and, in 1998, outlawed for-profit blood centers. The Chinese government also began to promote voluntary blood donation and agreed to provide free or low-cost drugs to those infected by HIV through illegal blood procurement. This does not adequately address the problem of the possibly 1 million Chinese who contracted HIV through the blood procurement program. Erwin reports that HIV-infected parents are seeking adoptive parents for their children who will inevitably be orphaned by AIDS.[16]

Erwin notes that blood procurement is viewed as a benign process in North America and Europe, but she adds that this view obscures the "social and economic relations embedded in blood procurement. In attempting to unmask these relations, I am initiating a critical inquiry into what is at stake in this circulation of blood as a commodity, as a potential 'gift,' and as an essence of vitality and life itself" (2006:141). She adds:

> This article is entitled "The Circulatory System" to emphasize that, just as blood circulates through the physical body in systematic and highly structured biological pathways, so is blood donation a highly structured practice in which blood circulates systematically through the social body. . . . blood—like the physical body itself—serves as a metaphor through which meanings about society and the self are constantly created and exchanged. (2006:142)

Along with other scholars, Erwin notes that sale of body parts, such as kidneys, reflect social inequities. Nancy Scheper-Hughes (2000) observes that body parts inevitably travel from the bodies of the poor to the rich, the brown and black to the white, the Third World to the First World, and from women to men.

In Traditional Chinese Medicine (TCM), Erwin notes, blood is considered an essential life force similar to *chi* (*qi*) in that both affect physical vitality and character. They are both considered essential for health and well-being; however, they differ in that "*qi* flows freely within the body and across its boundaries" (Erwin 2006:145). In fact, qi that is blocked is considered to be a cause of illness. On the other hand, "blood must be retained within [the body]": (Erwin 2006:145). Loss of blood through injury, menstruation, childbirth, or blood donation is believed to lead to a loss of vitality.

Erwin notes that blood is associated with the feminine (*yin*), whereas *qi* is masculine (*yang*). A woman nurtures her fetus through blood and ensures the blood health of other members of the family through food and nurturance. Thus, blood donation is more consistent with the feminine role in Chinese society, and "many Chinese men are reluctant to part with their blood" (2006:146). Sixty percent of blood donors in Henan Province were women between the ages of fifteen and fifty-five, and more women than men are infected with HIV from contaminated blood.

In philosophical terms, *yin* and *yang* are female and male energies that must be balanced at all levels of the universe. Heaven (*yang*) and earth (*yin*) must be balanced to ensure the smooth functioning of the universe. On the political level, the Chinese emperor traditionally was expected to balance the relationship between heaven and earth. On the individual level, health rests on the balance of *yin* and *yang* energies in the bodies of both females and males.

The conditions of blood donations in which young females give blood to support their families (typically the families of their husbands) is not due to Chinese philosophy, but to the economic reality that young Chinese women contribute to the wealth of their husbands' families, rather than to their own well-being or to the well-being of their own lineages. Historically, the economic contribution of in-marrying women to the well-being of the patrilineal household is not due to philosophical traditions but to the economics of the patrilineal inheritance system.

In contemporary Chinese society, once the HIV contamination of commercially sold blood became widely known, the Chinese government attempted to eradicate blood selling in favor of "altruistic" blood donation like those of Western models. Though voluntary blood donation is favored by the United Nations and transfusion experts as the best way to ensure a safe blood supply, Erwin notes that economic and cultural factors mediate against the effectiveness of voluntary blood donation. Even in the United States, where blood donation is exalted, many people sell their blood for economic reasons. Though China's urban economy has flourished, Erwin writes, the rural economy in central China has slid deeper into poverty, making blood selling an economic necessity for most families.

The Chinese government outlawed blood selling in 1998, but donation is still far from voluntary. University students in Shanghai are required to donate blood at least once as a condition of graduation, and state-owned work units provide cash bonuses and paid time off to workers who donate blood. The tradition of voluntary or altruistic blood donation developed in the United States during World War II, when many civilians were encouraged to donate blood as a contribution to the war effort. Erwin notes that, in spite of its altruistic origins in the United States, only 8 percent of the U.S. population are blood donors, and those who do donate blood receive incentives such as T-shirts and time off work. Donors may also gain self-esteem or social status, as well as free or low-cost blood for themselves or their families.

Erwin suggests that voluntary blood donation is not supported by the Chinese model of balanced reciprocity: "Gift giving produces reciprocal obligation in the context of building social relationships," in which "the roles of giver and recipient [are] continually exchanged" (2006:150). Voluntary blood donors do not receive anything in return. Therefore, no social relationship is furthered. Even further, Erwin notes, "voluntary donation actually does nothing to minimize the commercialization of blood":

> As it circulates outside the body of the donor, through the middlemen who procure and distribute it via local and global capitalist biomedical institutions, to the final consumer, blood becomes an increasingly value-added-commodity, which is supplied to the recipient at a substantial cost. Nonrenumerated donation masks the true costs of blood, which become absorbed by donors. (2006:151)

In the process of donation, whether for economic or altruistic motivation, body parts and blood become commodities in broader systems of exchange. Erwin writes, "What is at stake, fundamentally, is the social contract that binds not just individuals, but also the inalienable parts of humans that flow through other circulatory systems" (2006:153).

2

Constructing Gender

The Body in Social Context

Revisiting Yurok Menstrual Taboos

The anthropologist Thomas Buckley was treated to a new take on menstruation taboos when he was invited to eat dinner at the home of an American Indian friend. The friend explained that he would be cooking dinner because his Yurok wife was "on her moontime" (menstruating). The wife would cook her own food and eat by herself. This modern couple had not built a separate menstrual shelter for her, but they had set aside a special room for her use during her "moontime." They had also allocated space in the kitchen for her food, as well as for the cooking and eating utensils she used during her moontime. The couple adapted the wife's menstrual seclusion to modern times in other ways. When her husband and the anthropologist arrived, the wife joined them and entered into their conversation. This proved beneficial for the anthropologist's understanding of menstrual taboos. The anthropologist was naturally curious about the reason for continuing to observe these taboos. The wife told him that "as a foster child in non-Indian homes she had been taught that menstruation is 'bad and shameful' and that through it 'women are being punished'" (Buckley 1993:134). When she returned to live among the Yurok, her grandmother and aunts taught her that the menstrual shelter is "like the men's sweathouse" (1993:135). It's where you "go into yourself and make yourself stronger" (1993:135): "A menstruating woman should isolate herself because this is the time when she is at the height of her powers. Thus the time should not be wasted in mundane tasks and social distractions, nor should one's concentration be broken by concerns with the opposite sex" (1993:135). The wife was told by her grandmother and aunts that her time in the menstrual shelter should be spent "in concentrated meditation" to find out her purpose in life and to accumulate spiritual energy. She was told that all her actions should be "fully conscious and intentional": "You should feel all of your body exactly as it is, and pay attention" (1993:135).

At first, Buckley considered the wife's views on **menstrual seclusion** to result from modernization. He notes that anthropologists' descriptions of **menstrual taboos** in the world's cultures are uniformly negative. Women were described as **polluting** and, therefore, dangerous to men and their enterprises. Buckley notes that these reports were written by males based on information gained from male informants. A point missed in these reports is that, though menstruating women are viewed as being polluting to men, men are viewed as being polluting to women.[1]

Elizabeth Faithorn notes that men, as well as women, have the capacity "to endanger others through improper control of their own powerful substances, particularly semen" (1975:131). She adds, "not only may men and women endanger each other, they may also threaten or contaminate others of the same sex, or even themselves" (1975:132). Based on her research in New Guinea, Faithorn adds that the main source of friction between husbands and wives relates to their social and economic roles.

Separating the Sexes: Ritual Complementarity

Yurok live near the Klamath River close to the California-Oregon border, where the early anthropologist A. L. Kroeber conducted much of his fieldwork. A few weeks after his conversation with the Yurok woman, Buckley went to Bancroft Library at the University of California, Berkeley, where Kroeber's papers are kept. Among the papers, Buckley found notes on an interview Kroeber conducted with a Yurok woman, identified as "Weitchpec Susie" in his publications.

Kroeber did not use most of the descriptions and texts he collected from the woman, but Buckley learned from Kroeber's notes that the woman's descriptions of Yurok myths and ritual practices substantiated the idea that male training and female menstrual seclusion play complementary and equal roles in Yurok society: "There are . . . direct parallels in conception, ritualization, and goal orientation between male training and female menstrual practice" (Buckley 1993:138).

Among other parallels, both female menstrual practices and male training among Yurok involved the flow of blood. Women's blood flowed naturally through menstruation; men gashed their legs with flakes of white quartz. The flow of blood, whether occurring naturally or self-induced, was believed to carry away impurity. Both female and male **ritual** purifications included daily bathing in lakes sacred to their own sex, and in both cases, the rituals were aimed at attracting wealth (described by Buckley as spiritual advancement). Both female and male rituals were performed according to the monthly cycles of the moon. Female rituals were held during the full of the moon, and male rituals were held during the dark of the moon.

Among Sambia of New Guinea, as well as among Yurok, menstrual blood is considered to be beneficial for women but polluting and dangerous for men. Sambia consider two fluids, blood and semen, to be essential for life and gender. Sambia distinguish between circulatory blood and menstrual blood. All humans have circulatory blood, but only females have menstrual blood. Sambia also distinguish between reproductively competent humans, trees, and animals, which are fluid (wet) and those that are dry, which are either sexually immature or old and used up.

Females are naturally "wet" because they have plentiful circulatory and menstrual blood, as well as vaginal fluids. They also "ingest" semen through sexual intercourse. Sambia consider blood to be "cold," whereas semen is "hot." Sickness and plague are caused by active animated agents, such as spirit beings, which are attracted to heat and repelled by cold. Therefore, semen-possessing beings (males) are more subject to illness than blood-possessing beings (females):

> So men are prone to be ill and women healthy. Menstrual periods are compared to a periodic natural defense that rids female bodies of excess menstrual blood and any sickness that manages to penetrate them. Ironically, then, women bounce back from their periods with even greater vitality because of this natural function. The female capacity to create and discharge blood is thus perceived as a sign by the society of the structure and functioning of women's bodies, the fertile powers of birth-giving, procreative sexuality, and health, so men reckon this is why women typically out-live men. (Herdt 1987:77)

Whereas women are naturally fluid, and therefore more alive, according to Sambia, maleness must be generated socially through male puberty rites. The process of creating males occurs over a period of approximately fifteen years, in which male initiates socially acquire the procreative power that is acquired naturally by females as a result of their biological natures.

Sambia consider ingesting of semen to be the only means of acquiring this life-giving fluid. Semen is not believed to be produced naturally. Women "ingest" semen through sexual intercourse. Boys undergoing the first two stages of **initiation rites** ingest semen by performing fellatio on older initiates. Females are considered to be biologically complete by virtue of their birth, but males must be "made" through rituals undergone during their puberty rites. Gilbert Herdt writes, "maleness is cultural and bisexual, and femaleness is natural and heterosexual."

Separating the Sexes: Nature and Nurture

Among the Sambia, as in many other cultures, it is believed that the female body is a natural product, whereas the male body must be socially constructed. Though Sambia belief may be an extreme version of this view, the association of the female body with nature and the male body with culture underlies the private/public distinction that is virtually a universal category in assigning gender. The anthropologist Sherry Ortner (1975) argues that, since the purpose of culture is to subjugate nature, the association of women with nature relegates them to second-class status. More recently, the question has arisen as to who and what defines women as second class.

The view that the role of culture is to subjugate nature is not characteristic of many other traditions. Nor is the idea that females represent nature necessarily associated with the idea that females are inferior to males. In traditional Shinto beliefs of Japan, for example, the Japanese landscape was created by the gods Izanami and Izanagi through procreation. The sun, Amaterasu, is one of their offspring, a female child so beautiful she was elevated to the heavens. The divine origin of the female sun god Amaterasu is still enshrined in the Japanese emblem of the sun on the national flag and in the practice of giving decorative packages of perfect oranges as a high-status gift. The name Japan, or Nippon, means "the origin of the sun."

The association of females with nature and males with culture may reflect the essential role of female child-bearing, without which no group could survive. Ultimately, the natural and cultural roles of both females and males are essential to group survival. Cultural models that denigrate the biological and cultural roles of females may, in fact, reflect the reality that female fecundity is a vital part of group survival and that the relationship between mother and son has great social power. Anthropologists have suggested that the purpose of harsh male puberty rituals, which are pervasive cross-culturally, are aimed at severing the close mother-son bond so that male children can transfer their loyalty from their mothers to the all-male group.

Philosophers, poets, and scholars have noted that vigorous protests often mask secret doubts. Rena Lederman notes that, among the Mendi of New Guinea, **clan** leaders deliver speeches to assert the importance of male clan exchanges over individual economic exchanges. Both women and men participate in **balanced reciprocity**, which establishes partnerships based on exchanging goods of equal value. Clan exchanges enhance the status of "big men," who promote their own social position in competition with exchange partnerships based on balanced reciprocity. "Big men" must argue against individual exchange partnerships, which may be engaged in by both men and women to further their own cause, which is enhancing their own status:

> Collective "clan" identities and concerns are not taken-for-granted or ritualized inevitabilities in Mendi; they need to be argued for. They do not take precedence over "personal" identities and involvements. The value and priority sometimes accorded to male collectivity is not an objective fact but rather a relative weighting. It cannot be understood without a simultaneous appreciation of what it is an argument *against*. (Lederman 1993:215)

Mendi individuals, whether female or male, do not have to be harangued into participating in balanced reciprocity, which is an individual choice. Though women are barred from the more "prestigious" clan exchange, which favors the male clan head, they are free to participate in the more personally rewarding individual exchange. Men must choose between the higher status clan exchanges that benefit the clan leader and the lower status exchanges based on balanced reciprocity, which benefit themselves.

Exuding Femininity and Defining Masculinity

Creek Indians originated along river valleys in the southeastern part of the United States but were later relocated to Oklahoma. According to the Creek **world view**, female is a "watery cosmological domain that generates all life" (Rector Bell 1993:28). Each morning, grandfather sun emerges from this watery fundament cleansed and purified, to order the generative and undifferentiated mass into ordered existence. Amelia Rector Bell writes: "A symbol of male definitional power, the sun passes through and separates from the water in rays of light each morning. This mythical metaphor encapsulates the Creek ideology of the separation of gender: human social ordering requires light and heat obtained by and through the male capacity to differentiate from the mother" (1993:28).

Integration of females and separation of males is illustrated in the Corn-Mother myth. Rector Bell writes: "Corn-Mother is the paradigmatic Creek mother, who feeds her children from corn that grows on her legs and is scraped off daily. She contains the germ of life within her. In the myths, male children, when old enough to see her secretly scraping corn from her legs, are horrified and kill her. They flee their home and live as warriors hunting in the forest" (1993:28).

The Corn-Mother myth provides a model for Creek life in general. Creek are **matrilineal**, so a woman remains with her clan throughout her life. A man is a member of his mother's clan until he marries, when he changes his primary affiliation to that of his wife. Thus, a male must be prepared for the sundering of his relationship with his mother, and by extension, with his mother's clan. To some extent, the Corn-Mother myth is true of us all. We must all leave the mother's body and chart our way through the forest of social relationships. The womb that nurtures us also expels us.

The construction of socially appropriate roles requires both biology (sex) and culture (gender). **Gender** refers to the social status and cultural expectations accorded to females and males; **sex** refers to their biological differences. Since, cross-culturally, males are associated with "culture" whereas females are associated with "nature," the male body is more likely than the female body to "need" reconstruction. Thus, the male body undergoes more extreme biological and social alteration cross-culturally.

Separating the Sexes: The Biological Basis

In terms of physiology, males and females are more similar than cultural categories of gender would suggest. All **embryos** have "growth buds" that can develop into either female or male organs. If the embryo has XY sex chromosomes, the bud of the **gonads** begins to develop into testicles at about the sixth week of embryonic development. If the embryo has the XX chromosomes, the buds will begin to differentiate into ovaries at about the twelfth week after conception, when it has become a **fetus**. Both male and female embryos produce all the hormones that differentiate sexual characteristics, including **estrogen**, **progesterone**, and **androgens**. "The proportion of hormones varies between men and women and between individuals within each sex group and over the life cycle. Testicles produce more androgen than estrogen, and ovaries produce more estrogen than androgen" (Stockard and Johnson 1993:18–19).

All fetuses possess the *wolffian* structures and the *mullerian* structures. At around the third to fourth month after conception, the *wolffian* structures begin to develop as the *seminal vesicles*, the basis of internal male **genitalia**. Hormones produced by the testicles prevent the *mullerian* structures from developing into female genitalia. If the testicles do not develop and male hormones are not produced, female internal genitalia develop.

The necessity of producing male hormones during early fetal life has led some biologists to suggest that mammals are essentially female. It is more likely that both male and female fetuses are awash in female hormones produced by the mother, so that male hormones are necessary for overcoming the prevalence of maternal female hormones. In the absence of male hormones produced by the testicles, fetuses will develop female genitalia. Roger Gorski, an expert on sexual differentiation and a neurobiologist at the University of California, Los Angeles, notes that "the brain is inherently female and to develop as male it must be exposed to masculinizing hormones."[2]

Whereas internal genitalia develop from different structures, external genitalia develop from the same fetal structure. The presence of hormones determines whether this structure becomes male external genitalia or female external genitalia. If hormones secreted by the **testicles** are present, the preliminary genital tubercle develops into a penis and a scrotum. The scrotum holds the testicles when they descend. If hormones produced by the testicles are absent, the tubercle remains small and becomes the **clitoris**. In addition, the two folds of skin that form the **scrotum** in males becomes in females the **labia minora**, which encloses the vagina and urethra, but separates their functions. The vagina opens to the uterus, whereas the urethra opens to the bladder.

Throughout our life cycle, there is overlap between the sexes, though differences are accentuated by the production of hormones. "Our bodies are constantly changing from the day we are born until the day we die. Puberty is the period of time when children begin to mature biologically, psychologically, socially, and cognitively. Girls start to grow into women and boys into men."[3]

Females at puberty produce more estrogen and progesterone than androgen. Males produce more androgen than estrogen and progesterone. These account for differences between the sexes beginning at **puberty**. Males develop deeper voices, greater body and facial hair, and greater upper body strength, among other characteristics. The defining characteristic of puberty for females is **menarche**, the onset of menstruation. This is accompanied by breast development and other changes in body shape. With aging, females produce less estrogen and progesterone, which reduces the importance of these hormones in masking male characteristics. Males produce less androgen, which reduces its influence in masking female characteristics.

Though the importance of biology in marking differences between the sexes cannot be refuted, many differences between the sexes are imposed by culture. Opposition of the sexes is imposed culturally by naming customs, socialization, dress, hair styles, and other forms of distinguishing gender.

Separating the Sexes: Socialization Public and Private

Emile Durkheim (1965) suggested that society is the invisible force that governs our view of the universe, which gives rise to our religions and our concepts of gods, heroes, demons, and ancestors. Pierre Bourdieu (1977) describes our conceptual experience of the universe as a dialectical relationship between the body and the environment, a relationship that grows out of a child's social relationships. The child acquires a sense of these relationships by mimicking the behaviors of the people he or she observes.

Socially appropriate actions are also acquired through what Bourdieu (1977) calls the "structural exercises" society provides for the teaching of culture: riddles, games, sports, and forms of "let's pretend." Through these observations and games, the child acquires a structural model of the social universe, not through discourse, but through practicing the actions of others.[4] Bourdieu suggests that, through the learning process of observation and practice, the child acquires a spatial model of the universe experienced on multiple levels. The following example is based on Bourdieu's fieldwork in Algeria during the Algerian war of independence from France (1954-1962).

> The opposition between the sacred of the right hand and the sacred of the left hand, between *nif* and *haram*, between man, invested with protective, fecundating virtues, and woman, at once sacred and charged with maleficent forces, and, correlatively, between religion (male) and magic (female), is reproduced in the spatial division between male space, with the place of assembly, the market, or the fields, and female space, the house and its garden, the retreats of *haram*. (1977:89)

According to Bourdieu, an alternate form of the Arabic term *haram* refers to the harem, a sacred female space. Bourdieu uses the term *nif* to refer to "point of honor," in the sense of a man defending his honor, and the term *haram*, to that which is sacred, which Bourdieu defines as the most vulnerable part of the group.

As noted earlier referring to the Creek Corn-Mother myth, males are expelled from the female body and must disengage themselves from the company of females. The linguistic usage of a contrast between *nif* and *haram* or *harem* suggests a contrast between contested (public) space and the safety of the womb, as well as parallels among the safety of the womb, the sacred space of the *haram*, and the female space of the harem.

Bourdieu notes that males must procure suitable wives for themselves, their sons, and, perhaps, their grandsons in competition with other males. Thus, they are at a disadvantage in marriage negotiations. Further, males must, as a point of honor, defend the female *haram* or *harem*. Males must demonstrate their power in public places. Female power is covert, unspoken, and often confined to private spaces.

For Bourdieu, movements of the body reflect the negotiation of social space organized around "the division of sexual work and the sexual division of work, and hence in the work of biological and social reproduction" (1977:91). According to Bourdieu, orientation of the male body is *centrifugal*, in that it moves outwardly into "the fields or market, toward the production and circulation of goods," whereas the orientation of the female body is *centripetal*, inwardly toward the accumulation and consumption of the products of work" (1977:92). Bourdieu views this as the projection of body metaphors into social and cosmic space, metaphors that have been acquired through the negotiation of behaviors during the process of socialization.

Since Bourdieu's fieldwork took place in a society centered on the marketplace, it is only natural that he considered the marketplace the center of social life. If we look to societies that have no marketplace, such as the traditional !Kung of Africa's Kalahari Desert, we discover a different form of gender relationships. Women provide most of the food, so the economy centers on their productive potential. Males provide a luxury, meat, through their hunting prowess. Though meat is a better source of protein than vegetable materials, it is a less reliable source of nutrients. Thus, meat provided by males is prestigious, whereas the daily nutrients provided by females are taken for granted.

A pioneer in feminist anthropology, Louise Lamphere, notes that even in societies considered to be "male-dominated," women occupy important social roles. Drawing on Cynthia Nelson's article "Public and Private Politics: Women in the Middle Eastern World" (1974), Lamphere notes;

Because they are born into one patrilineal group and marry into another, women are important structural links between social groups and often act as mediators. Because there are segregated social worlds, all-female institutions are important for enforcing social norms: Women fill powerful ritual roles as sorceresses, healers, and mediums; women are important sources of information for their male kin; and women act as "information brokers," mediating social relations within both the family and the larger society. (2005:88)

As Rena Lederman has suggested (1986, 1993), males may assert the greater importance of their role simply because they are dependent on the social, economic, and socializing function of women.

Cultural categories of masculinity and femininity obscure the complexity of human relationships because they ignore the range of diversity that characterizes real human beings. As the French anthropologist Claude Lévi-Strauss has noted, humans conceptually order the world in binary oppositions in an attempt to impose order onto a potentially unruly universe.

Sex and gender are particularly unruly categories, and nature is especially reluctant to be subdued. Public protestations of male power may, as Rena Lederman suggests, arise from attempts of socially powerful males to gain the allegiance of males who might prefer to follow private inclinations. In the film *Onka's Big Moka*, the aspiring "big man" Onka tried to persuade other men to "stop playing" under their wife's aprons so they could contribute to the male clan exchange he was organizing. This suggests that ordinary males would rather "play" under their wife's aprons than support clan exchanges that do not directly benefit them. Rather, these exchanges support men who desire public power over other men.

Separating the Sexes: The Economic Basis

Status relationships based on gender are inevitable within all families, as within all human groups. The sex of offspring becomes especially important when ownership of property, wealth, and/or social position are involved. Among English nobility or royalty, titles and most forms of property are passed down through the male line; that is, patrilineally. If, for example, Prince Charles survives Queen Elizabeth, his mother, he will inherit the throne and all of Elizabeth's great wealth.

Historically, King Henry VIII's attempts to find marital happiness were political, rather than sexual or romantic. As monarch, he could have had his choice of ladies of the realm. His quest was aimed at producing a legitimate male heir. When no legitimate male heir was apparent, Elizabeth I inherited the throne, along with its attendant power and wealth.

Now that the sex of a fetus can be determined with some exactness, a family can choose to abort an unwanted fetus. Traditionally, in India, a female fetus was more likely than a male fetus to be aborted. This is because inheritance in most parts of India is **patrilineal**, residence after marriage is **patrilocal**, and **dowry** is provided by the bride's family to the groom's family. Since status and property are inherited through the male line, a son can continue the lineage and retain family resources, whereas a daughter cannot. Thus, a family that has only daughters can lose their land to a distant relative who has sons.

Anthropologist Barbara Miller checked sex ratio figures for juveniles under ten years of age in districts in the Northwest Provinces of India for 1871 during

British occupation and estimated that "It would not be unreasonable to assume that one-fourth of the population preserved only half of the daughters born to them, while the other three fourths of the population had balanced sex ratios among their offspring."

The British described the practice as due to "pride and purse," in that the pride of upper caste and tribal families led them to kill a daughter rather than surrender her to a more dominant group. "Purse" referred to providing a daughter with dowry at the time of her marriage. Miller notes that "most groups that practiced infanticide did have the custom of giving large dowries with daughters" (1993:426[1987]). However, the rural Jats, a landed peasant caste, were also characterized by high male-to-female sex ratios even though they acquired wives through brideprice or bridewealth, in which they were compensated for their daughter's contribution to the husband's family. One would expect that families who would receive brideprice for their daughters would preserve them, though this was not the case among the Jats.

Typically, in a patrilocal/patrilineal system, when a daughter marries, she goes to live with her husband's family, she bears children to continue his lineage, and her work contributes to the wealth of his family. Thus, a woman contributes to the well-being of her husband's family and takes wealth from her own family. Her family bears the expense of raising her, but her husband and his family benefit from her fertility and labor. Thus, the inheritance pattern of most of India has favored families who had sons over families who had daughters. Miller notes:

> Sons are economic assets: they are needed for farming, and for income through remittances if they leave the village. Sons play important roles in local power struggles over rights to land and water. Sons stay with the family after their marriage and thus maintain the parents in their old age; daughters marry out and cannot contribute to the maintenance of their natal households. Sons bring in dowries with their brides; daughters drain family wealth with their required dowries and the constant flow of gifts to their family of marriage after the wedding. Sons, among Hindus, are also needed to perform rituals which protect the family after the death of the father; daughters cannot perform such rituals. (1993:427[1987])

Since Miller's writing, the picture in India has begun to change, as the economic base shifts from predominantly agriculture to technology, especially computer technology. A December 2007 article in *The New York Times* illustrates the implications of this economic shift.[5] As a literate person in India, G. P. Sawant was a professional letter writer who played an important role in the lives of people who were not themselves literate, or who did not possess the skills necessary to communicate with officials or with members of their family from whom they were separated. As India became important in the telecommunications boom, mobile phones replaced traditional letter writers. Sawant's business could no longer support his family.

Due to the traditional solidarity of the Indian family, Sawant was not thrown into poverty by the dramatic national economic change. Some members of his family, including a daughter, Suchitra, have benefited financially from the telecommunications boom. Sawant continues to be respected for the role he played in facilitating other people's lives, but he is glad the telecommunications economy has benefitted India as a whole. The new economic prosperity of Sawant's family is based on his skills as a letter writer. He used his proceeds to send all four of his children to private schools. His son and two of his daughters are now employed at professional, prestigious, and profitable jobs that benefit the family as a whole. A third daughter is studying computers in college.

Further evidence that gender preferences are based in economics is provided by a shift in gender preferences in South Korea. In 1990, 116.5 boys were born for every 100 girls. This indicates that a decision to abort was based on gender bias against females, since more female babies are likely to be born than male babies where there is no selective pressure.[6] As of 2006, the ratio was 107.4 boys for every 100 girls, an indicator that the preference for males is decreasing. An October 2007 study by the World Bank suggested that South Korea is the first of several Asian countries to reverse the previous trend of preference for male babies.[7]

The trend toward industrialization in South Korea in the 1970s and 1980s eroded the preference for boys associated with patrilineal agricultural societies, since educated daughters can contribute as much to the economic well-being of their families, both natal and conjugal, as educated sons. Also, in societies that are shifting from an agricultural to an industrial economy, daughters educated and employed in the professions can make more favorable marriages, thus increasing their value to both families.

The case of the Nayar in the southern India state of Kerala may illustrate some economic factors that favor the preservation of daughters. The inheritance and residence pattern favored females because inheritance of status and access to resources was matrilineal (through the female line) and residence was matrilocal, so that a woman and her children continued to reside with her own family. A Nayar household typically consisted of members of the same matrilineage, which included three or more generations. Nayar were members of the warrior caste, so producing sons and daughters was equally important economically. Sons were warriors, and daughters were mothers of warriors. Thus, a woman contributed to the wealth of her own family, rather than to the wealth of males outside her lineage. Consequently, her status was high.

In the twentieth century, and previously under British rule, the power and wealth of Nayars were largely eroded through modernization and redistribution of land. Because Nayars were highly educated, they began to take professional jobs outside of India. Industrialization and wage labor jobs favor the **nuclear family** over the **extended family** because the nuclear family is more mobile and industries are better served by mobility among their workforce. As a result, the status of Nayar women was eroded, but remained higher than that of women in other parts of India because their education permitted them to contribute economically to their own families.

China: Opening the Door

China, like most of India, is a society based on agriculture, which requires a large and stable labor force. As a result, China shares with most of India a patrilineal inheritance pattern, extended family household formation, and patrilocal residence. As is the case in India, these shape the status of women and their desirability as offspring. In modern China, a different set of circumstances favors the desirability of male offspring. As in India, women are more valuable to their husband's family than to their own. A bride is said to "open the door" to the next generation of her husband's lineage.

A woman's status and power within her husband's family depends on her ability to produce sons that continue her husband's lineage. A new bride enters the family as an outsider, and consequently, has low status. If she is able to produce sons, her status in the family quickly rises. As the sons mature and bring their brides into the family compound, she becomes a "mother-in-law" who is able to exert a great deal of control over the household through her influence over her sons and their wives.

Because they are among the earliest agricultural societies, China and India have large populations compared to most other nations. China's institution of the one-child policy as a population control device exerts pressure on families with daughters.

One of my male students from Hong Kong, a sophisticated urban center, described to me a visit of his family to a rural relative in southern China. The rural family had two married sons. Under traditional circumstances, the older son would take precedence over the younger son. Concomitantly, the wife of the older son would outrank the wife of the younger son. In this case, the wife of the older son gave birth to a daughter, whereas the wife of the younger son gave birth to a son. The wife of the older son was treated like a servant. She and her daughter were relegated to the kitchen and expected to do all the chores. The wife of the younger son mingled with guests and was not required to do any chores.

In the absence of the one-child policy, the senior wife might have been able to restore her status by bearing a son. Because of the one-child policy, she had no chance of restoring her status unless her female child died. Since having a daughter reduces a woman's status in her husband's household and prevents the family from having a son, a female fetus is more likely than a male fetus to be aborted, and a baby girl is more likely than a baby boy to be abandoned or killed. The one-child policy has resulted in a change in the sex ratio. When the first generation of boys born since the one-child policy was instituted reached maturity, they faced a shortage of wives. There was no one to "open the door" for them.

Separation of the Sexes: A Survival Strategy

In all societies, kinship, including descent and marriage, involves the allocation of resources. If, as in some examples provided above, a son can inherit property whereas a daughter cannot, a son will inevitably be preferred over a daughter. In societies where there are no such rigid class distinctions but survival is tenuous, one sex is not likely to be favored over another.

Among the Siriono foragers of eastern Bolivia, there are no terms to distinguish one's female and male children (Holmberg 1969). Kin terms reflect kin relationships, so this may indicate that sons and daughters were equally valued. It is difficult to evaluate this exactly, since anthropological studies of kinship vary in accordance with the research interests of the anthropologist. This use of kin terms among the Siriono may also reflect the ungendered social status of children who have not yet attained the status of reproductive adults.

Among traditional Barabaig cattle herders of Tanzania, in Africa, children of both sexes are highly valued and treated equally during the first years of life. This may be due, in part, to the fact that both girls and boys can contribute to the economic well-being of the natal family. It is also due to the high rates of various forms of diseases that lead to sterility, miscarriage, and infant mortality, as well as deaths of children and adults:

> Birth rate among the Barabaig is limited by biological and cultural conditions. The presence of a wide variety of disease causing organisms in the physical environment imposes certain problems on the Barabaig that may or may not be amenable to cultural solutions, depending upon the magnitude of the problem and people's knowledge and ability to recognize a problem when it exists. (Klima 1970:45)

Due to high rates of disease, George Klima notes, "Among the Barabaig, replacing societal members is a question of being able to have children and to keep alive those that are born" (1970:45).

Among the Barabaig, pregnancy and childbirth are fraught with danger for mother and child. A pregnant woman is described by a term meaning "one with enemy" since the child she is carrying has the power to kill her and others. This is based in medical fact. A pregnant woman is especially subject to disease because of the energy required to sustain a pregnancy and childbirth.

Barabaig address this issue through taboos. For example, "No one is allowed to use a pregnant woman's drinking and cooking utensils" (Klima 1970:46). This is a valid medical procedure because it protects the woman and her fetus from parasites that may be transmitted to her by others. It may also protect others from parasites that invade the woman at a time when her immune system is most compromised. In purely medical terms, a fetus is an invading organism, since it carries the genetic coding of the father as well as the mother. Thus, the mother's immune system must suppress this information to allow the invading organism—the fetus—to develop.

Because of its procreative powers, the female body is hotly contested territory. The ability to control this territory is rigorously regulated in all societies. As the anthropologist Mary Douglas has written, all human groups structure the world in such a way that our experience can be sorted into neatly defined categories: "Culture, in the sense of the public, standardized values of a community, mediates the experience of individuals. It provides in advance some basic categories, a positive pattern in which ideas and values are tidily ordered. And above all, it has authority, since each is induced to assent because of the assent of others" (1966:38–39). Anything that does not fit tidily into the cultural order is likely to be viewed with suspicion.

Separating the Sexes: Male-Female Dominance Relationships

A number of anthropologists have remarked upon the sexual antagonism between women and men in New Guinea. The antagonism is largely structural in that women and men occupy separate realms. Men make war; women tend the gardens. Men increase their status by holding public feasts; women increase men's status by bearing their children and tending their pigs. Economically, males are dependent on females.

A pervasive pattern in traditional New Guinea society is that men attempt to prevail over women through public discourse and physical strength. Women prevail over men through the threat of menstrual pollution, and in some cases, negotiation of sorcery practices between males. Kenneth E. Read notes that Kahuku men of New Guinea sought wives from other clans of their own tribe or from among women of a friendly tribe as a means of avoiding threats from a hostile neighboring group: "The danger lay in a wife's opportunity to procure her husband's semen at the request of a sorcerer who wished to harm him, and she was more likely to receive the request if her kinsmen were among his traditional enemies" (1965:44).

One problem with accounts of traditional life in other cultures is that most of our understanding of these groups is based on accounts of male anthropologists talking to male informants. Roger Keesing notes that, among the Kwaio in the Solomon Islands near New Guinea, males tried to control their access to "women's knowledge," but he appealed directly to the women. The women's perspective, he discovered, "accords women a central place in social life" (Womack 1993:67):

> A woman, standing in the center of the clearing, the heart of a tiny Kwaio social universe, standing astride the generations, with the powers of life and death in her and her daughter's hands, creates and perpetuates order, maintains the boundaries the unseen spirits police. Feeding and teaching, canonically social and cultural acts, are key symbols of a woman's life. The cycles that connect mothers and daughters in these constructions women place on their lives and culture are as central as the cycles that connect men to their ancestors through patrifilial links, in male accounts. (1985:34)

In his book *'Elota's Story: The Life and Times of a Solomon Islands Big Man*, Keesing records the lament of a man whose wife and daughter had died. 'Elota's status was dependent on his wife and they had formed a close bond:

> It was here at 'Aifaafasu that I gave my first mortuary feast, in my father's memory. There were four hundred valuables at that feast, and forty pigs. I thought then about feast-giving—thought that it was not so hard. And after that I gave eighteen feasts. But Maerua [his dead wife] has left me now. For five years I've been in [mourning] dishevelment—I haven't eaten pork or any relishes, in mourning for her—because she had come to me, and we had labored together in the taro gardens, and worked to earn money together. And now I've mourned her for five years, hungry and disheveled. But now it is over. She who raised pigs for me is dead. I haven't wanted to eat pigs raised by anyone else, for these five years. (1983:4)

Elota's account reflects the complex relationships between New Guinea males and females. Males dominate the public realm by organizing pig feasts. If a man can accumulate enough pigs and other goods to give a pig feast, his status increases. The accumulation of these valuables depends on his ability to coax his kin—both consanguineal and affinal—to donate pigs and other valuables to his cause. The most important of these kin is his wife. Males own pigs, but they cannot tend them because that is woman's work. Thus, a man's status depends on his wife's skill at raising pigs.

THE SOCIAL CONTEXT OF GENITAL ALTERATION

Some form of genital alteration occurs in almost all societies studied by anthropologists. The most common form cross-culturally is practiced on males. Female genital alteration is less common, but it receives most attention in the United States.

The Biology and Culture of Female Genital Alteration

The term "circumcision" is used to describe a number of forms of genital alteration, which vary greatly in their invasiveness for both males and females. Daniel Gordon states that *sunna* (the Arabic term for "duty") is the form of female genital surgery that "most closely conforms to [circumcision] in males, involving removal of the clitoral prepuce (foreskin) by razor, knife or smoldering stone, depending upon where and by whom it is practiced" (2008:102). The use of the word "*sunna*" with reference to female genital surgery is rejected by most Muslim clergy since they oppose all forms of female genital surgery as a social custom, rather than as a religious practice.

The World Health Organization (1997) identifies four types of female genital alteration: Type I involves removal of the prepuce, the sensitive tip of the clitoris equivalent to the male foreskin, as well as part or all of the clitoris. The WHO refers to these practices as **clitoridectomy**. Type II, which the WHO calls **excision**, involves removal of the clitoris and parts or all of the labia minora. Type III, **infibulation**, involves excision, as well as cutting and stitching of most of the labia major, leaving a small opening for the passing of urine and menstrual blood. Type IV is a category reflecting various local customs, including removal of the labia minora only, scraping away tissue from around the vaginal opening "and posterior cuts from the vagina into the perineum" (Yount and Carrera 2006:182).

The variability of the practice of female genital alteration on the continent of Africa is due to two traditions. The less invasive form, which Daniel Gordon calls *sunna* but is also called clitoridectomy depending on who is using the term, and excision, which involves removal of the clitoris, developed among sub-Saharan African cattle herders. An intermediate form of female genital surgery involves excising the clitoris, as well as removing part of the labia minora, the inner part of the **vulva**, and sewing together the skin of the labia minora. This can be more problematic, since it allows the collection of fluids that may lead to infections.

An extreme form of female genital cutting is sometimes called infibulation or pharaonic circumcision, a form that is believed to have been introduced into Egypt and the Sudan by Egyptian pharaohs. This is supported by a Greek papyrus dating from 163, which mentions girls in Egypt undergoing circumcision. Evidence from mummies suggests that both clitoridectomy and infibulation were spread from Egypt to other areas by Arabic slave traders. Clitoridectomy is the female surgery typically practiced in sub-Saharan Africa. Infibulation is the form practiced in Egypt and the Sudan, as well as among some sub-Saharan African groups.

The term "infibulation" comes from the Latin "infibula," a clasp fitted through the labia majora of a woman to ensure her chastity. The term "infibulation" also refers to the ancient Roman practice of suturing the foreskin of the penis, a procedure performed to ensure the chastity of male slaves. The practice was aimed at preventing sexual intercourse, but did not prevent masturbation.

Though female genital surgery is linked to Islam in the public mind, the practice of female circumcision and infibulation developed independently from Islam. These practices became identified with Islam as Islam spread across Africa, and as the religion absorbed the local customs. Clitoridectomy and excision are practiced in a wide diagonal belt across Africa from Senegal and Mauritania to Cameroon in West Africa, across central Africa to Chad, and in East Africa from Tanzania to Ethiopia. After Sudan and Egypt, infibulation is most prevalent in Somalia, followed by Mali, Ethiopia, and Nigeria.

Genital alteration in general is not supported by the Qur'an, and is not practiced in 80 percent of the Islamic world, including Saudi Arabia, Jordan, Iran, Iraq, and Syria (Gordon 2008). Circumcision of males is not mentioned in the Qur'an, and such alteration of the human body appears to be contrary to teachings of the Qur'an, which describes the creations of God [Allah] as perfect. "Allah perfected everything He created" (32:7). An even stronger expression of this idea in the Qur'an views alterations of nature as defacements inspired by the devil (4:119). Sami A. Aldeeb Abu-Salieh at the Swiss Institute of Comparative Law, argues that genital surgery violates the Qur'an, which states, "Our Lord, You did not create all this in vain" (3:191). Thus, according to this view, mutilation of the body is forbidden by the Qur'an because it is a rejection of the world created by God (Allah).

Circumcision can appear to be justified by the *haditha*, the sayings of Muhammad; however, what Muhammad meant by *khafd* (reduction) is subject to interpretation of whether he was referring to *sunna* (duty) or *makrama* (embellishment). These have been interpreted by some as "duty" and reinterpreted as referring to circumcision. It seems likely, as with the case with most religions, that interpretations of this type are attempts to reconcile scripture with custom. Scripture has the virtue of being amenable to interpretation, and custom reflects people's reluctance to depart from their customary way of doing things.

The Western view is that female circumcision is imposed by patriarchy over the rights of women. In reality, female status, and its effect on male status, is negotiated within female social space. Ellen Gruenbaum notes, "Women in Sudan generally must derive their social status and economic security from their roles as wives and mothers" (1993:412[1982]). Though men may control the public realm of wealth and power, women control what is perhaps a more important realm, the availability of women for men to marry. Pharaonic circumcision, the most extreme form, is believed to certify a woman's status as virgin, and therefore, her desirability as a wife. It is not the personal preference of males, but their status in the group, which dictates the desirability of virginity. Proofs of virginity, including circumcision, are controlled by women.

Egyptian religious leaders have spoken out against the practice of Pharaonic circumcision. The Egyptian Ministry of Religious Affairs issued a booklet explaining why female circumcision is not an Islamic practice, and Grand Mufti Ali Gomaa declared female circumcision to be a *haram*, something prohibited by Islam. Grand Mufti Ali Gomaa holds a religious position established by the Egyptian government. Muhammad Sayyid Tantawy is the Grand Imam of Al-Azhar Mosque and Grand Sheikh of Al-Ashar University. He has been described as possibly the foremost Sunni Arab authority. His response to the incident was more muted, calling the practice "harmful." It remains to be seen whether government and religious authority can prevail against a custom supported by the economic value of female virginity in marriage practices.

Male Genital Surgery: The Pursuit of Pain and the Avoidance of Pleasure

In spite of the cross-cultural variability in genital surgery and similarities in the biology of the body, most Western observers view all female genital surgeries as "mutilations," but do not take a similarly stern view of male genital surgeries. The most common form of male genital surgery, far more common than female genital surgery, is circumcision, which involves cutting away of the foreskin. The degree to which the foreskin is cut away varies, depending on the cultural tradition and the skill of the circumciser.

A far more invasive form of male genital alteration is **subincision**, a form of surgery in which the underside of the penis is slit open. The operation, which is practiced by some groups of Australians, is described by Ashley Montague: "The initial cut is generally about an inch long, but this may subsequently be enlarged so that the incision extends from the **glans** to the root of the scrotum, in this way the whole of the under part of the penile urethra is laid open" (1975:312).

The anthropologist W. Lloyd Warner did not observe subincision in the Murngin, the group he studied in northeastern Arnheim Land in Australia, but was aware that the Gunabibi (or Kunapipi) ceremony took place in surrounding groups. Warner describes what may be a pattern for subincision in these groups: "Two men go out and stand in a river or pool to above their waists. One takes a sharp stone knife and splits the urethra of the other, either at the same time or later, the one who has been cut reciprocates by performing the same operation on his friend" (1958:445).

The practice as described by Warner differs from male circumcision, which is typically imposed by adult males on infants or boys. The ceremony described by Warner suggests a relationship of equals. Subincision is associated with the mother of fertility, Kunapipi or Gadjeri, who is the bestower of fertility for both females and males. It has been widely suggested that subincision is an attempt to obtain female fertility for males. This is supported by the association of subincision with the fertility goddess Kunapipi, who is considered the genatrix of the human race. In his book *Symbolic Wounds: Puberty Rites and the Envious Male*, the psychoanalyst Bruno Bettelheim (1954) attributed subincision and other male puberty rituals involving alteration of the penis to the male desire to acquire female fertility. Subincision, especially, has been described as the construction of a male vagina, which has the ability to bleed similarly to menstruation.

The debate over whether the extreme harshness of male puberty rites is due to acquiring feminine generative power or to cutting away of the feminine influence on males has never been settled among anthropologists. In fact, it may never be settled, and both explanations may have merit. In most parts of the world where male genital surgery is practiced, female generative power appears to be a given. In most of these cases, male generative power and concomitant social power must be earned.

One problem with theories about both male and female genital surgery is that they presume that cultural practices are based on what individuals want. This is hardly the case, especially when it involves extreme alteration of the body. Parents may not want to circumcise their offspring, but they may do so to prevent their children from becoming pariahs. Their offspring may not want to be circumcised, but they may consent to the operation to increase their status in the group. Individuals learn to want what society permits them to have, to paraphrase Ralph Waldo Emerson:

> Society everywhere is in conspiracy against the [personhood] of every one of its members. Society is a joint-stock company, in which the members agree, for the better securing of his bread to each shareholder, to surrender the liberty and culture of the eater. The virtue in most requests is conformity. Self-reliance is its aversion. It loves not realities and creators, but names and customs. (1968:148)

As Emerson suggests, social customs and cultural values are not about the preferences of individuals; instead, they are aimed at ensuring conformity to the dictates of the group.

Subduing Sexuality: The Victorian Approach

For both females and males, the most sensitive and responsive parts of the genitalia are similar, though they do not have similar functions. For females, the tip of the clitoris contains the most neurons for responding to stimulation. For males, the foreskin contains the most neurons for responding to stimulation. These are the areas most subject to genital surgery cross-culturally. Cross-culturally, males are more likely than females to undergo genital alteration.

In almost all societies in which circumcision is practiced, it is performed as a rite of passage, a sacred rite aimed at transforming the initiate physically, psychologically, socially, and spiritually from a biological child to a social adult. In Western tradition since the nineteenth century Victorian era, circumcision has been performed as a secular "hygienic" process. The secularization of circumcision is concurrent with the emergence of medicine as a dominant influence on health care. In both sacred and secular contexts, circumcision is viewed as a cleansing ceremony. Whereas sacred circumcision "cleanses" the spirit, secular circumcision "cleanses" the body.

The history of secular circumcision in the West suggests that it was aimed at reducing pleasure for both males and females. Secular male circumcision in the West dates from the Victorian era, when U.S. and British physicians viewed it as a form of moral sanitation. Circumcision was aimed at curbing male masturbation, which was considered the cause of health problems ranging from epilepsy and gout to curvature of the spine and kidney failure.

Circumcision, clitoridectomy and a variety of mechanical devices were developed in Europe during the second half of the nineteenth century as a means of preventing masturbation. Masturbation had been defined as a moral problem in the first half of the nineteenth century, but with the rise of the medical profession in the second half of the nineteenth century, masturbation became defined as a medical problem. To combat loss of semen in males through nocturnal emissions or masturbation, a number of mechanical devices were developed to prevent this possibility. These included genital cages, strait jackets, penis rings with sharp points on the inside, blistering agents, and acid solutions. Leeches were also applied to the genitals.

During the same era, circumcision was recommended as a "cure" for female masturbation. Females, considered to be frail creatures, were viewed as being even more endangered than males by masturbation, which was believed to cause such "female" disorders as insanity, hysteria, "nervousness," and epilepsy.[8] Circumcision contin- ued to be recommended as a "medical" treatment for women in the United States as late as 1968 in the popular Christian coming-of-age manual *On Becoming a Woman*, written by Harold Shryok and first published in 1951.[9]

According to Shryok, masturbation is to be avoided because it renders a girl stu- pid by sapping her "nervous energy," thus making her susceptible to mental and physical ailments. When a person's nervous energy is reduced, Shryok writes, "the entire body suffers": "The tissues lose part of their normal resistance to disease. Infections overtake the body more easily. There is an increased tendency to catch cold. There is a loss of that sparkle and bounce which is characteristic of the person in the pink of condition."

Shryok notes that masturbation among women may result from "an anatomical factor that sometimes causes irritation about the clitoris and thus encourages a manipulation of the delicate reproductive organ." The medical cure for this "disor- der," Shryok writes, is circumcision:

> Although such cases are not very common, evidence of irritation of these tissues is suf-
> ficient reason for a young woman to consult a Christian physician. Oftentimes the rem-
> edy for this situation consists of a minor surgical operation spoken of as *circumcision*.
> This operation is not hazardous and is much to be preferred to allow a condition of irri-
> tation to continue.

The "condition of irritation" mentioned by Shryok indicates sexual excitement. In both females and males, sexual arousal produces engorgement of blood to the rele- vant organ. In females, it is the clitoris; in males, it is the penis.

It is ironic that some practitioners of Western medicine send a dual message about female circumcision to the rest of the world. It is "female genital mutilation" if prac- ticed for social and religious purposes in other parts of the world, but it is a "minor surgical operation" if practiced in the United States as a means of reducing a woman's interest in sex. Dr. E. Harold Shryok taught at Loma Linda University School of Med- icine for forty-one years and wrote thirteen books. He also served as dean of the Sev- enth-day Adventist medical school from 1951 until 1954. The Alfred Shryok Hall at Loma Linda University is named after his father.[10]

The anthropologist Mark Gordon[11] notes that female genital alteration continues as a secular trend in the United States, among avant garde groups in Los Angeles. The practice is linked to tattoo parlors and tattooing. Women who seek tattoos may also seek surgical alteration of their prepuce, the tip of their clitoris. Gordon states that their reason for altering their clitoris is that it "looks cool." Thus, in the United States, female circumcision has "progressed" from an attempt to reduce female sex- ual pleasure by removing the offending nerve endings to enhancing sexual appeal by sculpting the clitoris into an art form.

CONSTRUCTING GENDER

The English anthropologist Mary Douglas (1966) wrote that people universally feel the need to impose order on a chaotic universe. The French anthropologist Claude

Lévi-Strauss wrote that people impose order on aspects of nature, on people's relationships with nature, and on relations between people in the form of **binary oppositions** (paired opposites).[12] Binary oppositions do not accurately portray how the universe actually is. Rather, they are constructions of our universe based on the need to impose order on unruly experience. This is true of sex and gender, as well as much of our other experiences.

As noted earlier in this chapter, external genitalia of females and males develop from the same fetal structure. Some people are born with ambiguous external genitalia, a phenomenon known as **intersexuality**. Individuals with ambiguous external genitalia are sometimes called *hermaphrodites*. An infant with the XX chromosome may exhibit external genitalia similar to those of a male, or an infant with the XY chromosome may exhibit external genitalia similar to those of a female. Traditionally, these "conditions" were treated by surgically altering the genitals to conform to the expected appearance of "normal" male or female genitalia. Morgan Holmes was the object of a surgical process called "clitoral recession," which removed most of her clitoris. In an article written for *Undercurrents*, published by Faculty of Environmental Studies at York University in Ontario, Canada, Holmes criticizes "the cultural imperative to surgically alter intersexual children's genitals":

> The medical definition of what female bodies do not have and must not have: a penis. Any body which does possess a penis must either be designated 'male' or surgically altered. . . . In the minds of doctors, bodies are for procreation and heterosexual penetrative sex. . . . I would have liked to have grown up in the body I was born with, to perhaps run rampant with a little physical gender terrorism instead of being restricted to this realm of paper and theory. Someone else made the decision of what and who I would always be before I even knew who and what I was.[13]

Holmes' master's thesis on the subject "Medical Politics and Cultural Imperatives: Intersexuality Beyond Pathology and Erasure" was filed in September 1994.[14]

The website oneindia lists organizations and support groups for intersexuals. It states, "Intersexuality is not a life threatening deformity. What intersexuals need most in their lives is support and acute counseling."[15] An article on the website entitled "Intersexuality: Preventions and Treatments," written by Dhanyasree M, notes that intersexuality can be prevented through early discovery, but cautions against facile solutions or coercing intersexuals into treatment:

> The treatment of an intersexual person should not be based on the external genitals but on a thorough analysis of the chromosomal gender. An intersexual should not choose female sexual roles based on the easy reconstructions[16] of female genitalia. In addition, other factors such as chromosomal, neural, hormonal, psychological, and behavioral factors can also influence gender identity and gender satisfaction than functioning external genitalia. Since intersexuality is a complex issue, its treatment also has short and long term consequences.

External genitalia do not necessarily determine gender, though there are attempts in most societies to coerce individuals into assuming a gender identity that matches their external genitalia. The form of external genitalia may not match either the DNA coding of the individual or the sexual characteristics of the internal genitalia. Even in "normal" individuals, there are great differences in the hormone balance of estrogen, progesterone, and testosterone, and the balance within individuals differs depending on calendrical cycles, life cycles, and activities. The monthly hormonal cycle of females has been well-studied, but the daily hormonal cycle of males is less well-known.

Acceptance of individual variation in sex and temperament differs widely from one society another. In a number of societies, variability in gender orientation may be accepted as being beneficial for the society as a whole.

HIJRAS OF INDIA

Most of what the Western world knows about hijras, biological males who fill the intermediate social category of "neither man nor woman," is due to the fieldwork of the anthropologist Serena Nanda. Most hijras are in northern India. Most of the hijras in the village Nanda studied have connections in Mumbai (formerly Bombay) on the northwestern coast of India. Nanda notes that "Whereas Westerners feel uncomfortable with the ambiguities and contradictions inherent in such in-between categories as transvestism, homosexuality, hermaphroditism, and transgenderism, and make strenuous attempts to resolve them, Hinduism not only accommodates such ambiguities, but also views them as meaningful and even powerful" (1999:20).

Hindu creation stories celebrate the unity of femininity and masculinity—whether united in one body or in sexual intercourse—as being an emanation of Brahman, the creative energy that underlies the universe. Nanda writes: "In Hindu mythology, ritual, and art—important vehicles for transmitting the Hindu world view—the power of the combined man/woman is a frequent and significant theme" (1999:20).

Brahman, the creative energy underlying the universe, is neither man nor woman, being complete within itself. This creative energy manifests itself in the interplay of masculinity and femininity in the world available to the senses. The world is itself the playful energy of Brahman. In Hindu belief, feminine energy is manifest; masculine energy is latent and must be aroused by feminine energy. Thus, the universe is feminine, represented by Mahamaya, the great illusion.

Though creation stories describe the universe as an ordered entity, this is not necessarily reflected in the lives of individuals or the interactions within or among groups. Conflict is essential to the drama, one meaning of the term "play." In Hinduism, the term for this unfolding of the universe is "lila" (play), which contains within itself multiple levels of meaning, in addition to "theater." The universe is a playful entity that never resolves into stasis. It is constantly enacting a play. These activities are assumed to provide amusement for the gods, who are themselves manifestations of Brahman.

Hijras are part of a gender category called *kothi*, which refers to men who "like to do women's work" (Reddy and Nanda 2005:280). Hijras are devotees of the goddess Bahuchara or Bedhraj Mata. In Hinduism, all female deities—and human females—are viewed as manifestations of Śakti, the female emanation of Brahman. Bahuchara Mata is a mother goddess. "Mata" is an honorific that literally means "mother."

Bahuchara acquired her status as the result of her heroic act as a young woman: "Bahuchara was a pretty, young maiden in a party of travelers passing through the forest in Gujarat. The party was attacked by thieves, and, fearing that they would outrage her modesty, Bahuchara drew her dagger and cut off her breast, offering it to the outlaws in place of her virtue" (Nanda 1999:25).

There is a great deal of ritual inversion and conversion in the story of Bahuchara, thus providing fertile ground for symbolic negotiation, as well as the "play" so favored by the gods. Bahuchara's sacrifice of her own potential to become a mother gave her the power to confer maternity onto childless women, who pray to her in hopes of bearing a child, especially a son. Her act of self-mutilation also made her patron of hijras. Many of them emasculate themselves in hopes of cutting away male "contamination" to acquire the spiritual power of being "neither man nor woman."

Emasculation and Social Rebirth

The series of rituals involved in **emasculation** is closely associated with female fertility and is symbolically linked to childbirth. Ideally, the emasculation is performed as a secret ritual by a hijra who is called a *dai ma* (midwife). The emasculation process is called a *nirvan* (rebirth), a term also applied to the individual undergoing the operation. The operation is preceded by a *puja* (ritual offering of food, flowers, and other desired items) to Bahuchara Mata, which is also a **divination** ceremony to ascertain whether the operation has her blessing. The hijra is asked to look at Mata's picture to see if she is smiling. If she is smiling, the operation will be performed; if she is not smiling, plans for the operation will be canceled.

If the operation is to proceed, the *nirvan* begins a period of ritual seclusion that lasts from several days to a month. The operation takes place at around 3 or 4 a.m., a time considered auspicious, and is often the time for marriage ceremonies. The only ones present are the *nirvan*, the dai ma,[17] her assistant and Mata, as represented by her picture. The dai ma and her assistant perform a puja for Mata and then wake the *nirvan*.

> The client's clothes and jewelry are removed; "they must be as naked as the day they were born." After being given a bath the client is ready for the operation. She is seated on a small stool and held from the back by the dai ma's assistant, who also crosses the client's hair over her face for her to bite on. The client's penis and scrotum are tightly tied with a string, so that a clean cut can be made. The client looks at the picture of Bhuchar and constantly repeats her name, Mata, Mata, Mata. (1999:27-28)

Nanda suggests that the chanting of Mata's name apparently produces a trancelike state, during which the dai ma quickly performs the operation, removing both the penis and the scrotum with two quick cuts. According to Nanda, hijras who had undergone the operation reported that they felt no pain, that it was "a small pinch" or "like an ant bite." The reduction of pain is likely due to the tight tying off of the penis and the testicles, as well as to the trancelike state of the client.

Nanda writes, "When the cut is made, the blood gushes out, and nothing is done to stem the flow" (1999:28). Hijras view the blood flow as beneficial because it is the "male part" draining away. The hour after the operation is considered critical for the newly emasculated hijra. During this time, the client's genitals are secretly placed in a pot by the dai ma's assistant and buried under a tree. After the surgery, the client begins a forty-day period of ritual seclusion, similar to that of women who have given birth.

During the period of ritual seclusion, hijras observe food and other prohibitions, are given ritual baths, and are provided with the same foods given to parturient women.

On the fortieth day, the hijra is dressed as a bride, adorned with elaborate jewelry and new clothing. Late at night, accompanied by a procession of hijras, she is taken to a body of water, where a puja is performed to Mata. Milk is then poured three times over the hijra's head and into the water. During her postoperative seclusion, the hijra had not been allowed to even see milk. In Hindu belief, milk is a sacred substance, especially *ghee*, the clarified butter that is made from milk. *Ghee* is often provided as an offering to the gods. The fact that milk is **taboo** for a hijra during her forty-day seclusion marks it as a time of **liminality**, when she has been severed from her previous identity and has not yet acquired a new identity (see Victor Turner 1967). According to Nanda, pouring of milk over the head of the *nirvan* and in the water "is the final act in the ritual. Only now is the nirvan free from the curse of impotence and reborn as a hijra, who can call on the Mata and act as a vehicle of her power" (1999:29).

The Ritual Role of Hijras

Though hijras could be said to embody the culturally affirmed ideal of masculine/feminine unity by combining a masculine body with a feminine identity, they occupy a marginal and dangerously ambiguous category in Hindu social life. Human reproduction requires two biologically unambiguous beings, a male and a female, to continue the lineage and consolidate the family holdings. Hijras cannot provide that service, though they provide services that foster the reproductive capacity of others. Among their ritual functions are conferring fertility onto male children and blessing marriages, which provide ritual validation of reproduction.

Nanda describes the performance of hijras at a ceremony aimed at conferring fertility, prosperity, and long life onto a male baby. The ceremony combined entertainment with ritual. Accompanied by a drummer and accordion player, "Tamasha, the leader of the group, twirled in a grotesque, sexually aggressive parody of feminine behavior, which caused all of the older ladies to laugh loudly and all of the younger women to giggle with embarrassment behind their hands" (1999:1). Tamasha and the other hijras then danced and sang both traditional folk music of the region and songs from popular films.

Then Tamasha took the infant Ram from his mother's arms and held him in her own. As she danced with him, she closely inspected his genitals. "Give money to bless this baby," she demanded of the baby's grandmother. Taking the proffered two-rupee note, Tamasha passed it over the baby's head in a ritualized gesture that is a blessing and that wards off evil spirits (1999:1–2).

The other hijras continued to dance as Tamasha performed this ritual, calling upon the Hindu goddess Parvati and Bahuchara Mata. Both are mother goddesses. Parvati is associated with fertility and devotion to her spouse Śiva, the destroyer of corruption. Together the divine couple represents fertility and marital bliss. Parvati is also ritually important as the mother of Ganesha, the elephant-headed god who removes and creates obstacles.

After returning the baby to his mother, Tamasha stuffed a pillow under her sari and, clowning, imitated "the slow, ungainly walk of a pregnant woman" (1999:2).[18]

She then "sang a traditional hijra song describing the time of a woman's pregnancy from beginning to childbirth" (1999:2). Tamasha's humorous descriptions of the stages of pregnancy are interspersed with blessings and greetings from the child in the womb to his paternal and maternal grandmothers:

> The kid says in the stomach, *dadi, dadi* [paternal grandmother].
> Little kid, may you be healthy and live long. (1999:2)
>
> . . .
> Seventh month, yes, yes,
> How will it be?
> I have difficulty walking. I cannot walk.
> I have difficulty sitting.
>
> . . .
> The little kid in the stomach says *nani, nani* [maternal grandmother].
> Little kid, may you be healthy and live long. (1999:3)

Tamashi's parody of pregnancy and feminine behavior permits women to laugh at their discomfort and at any resentment that might rise from their social roles and their importance in sustaining the status of males. The child's crying out to both grandmothers ritually recognizes the bond between the maternal and paternal lineages.

As an alternative gender, hijras transcend the traditional roles enforced on both females and males.[19] Hijras surrender their potential to produce **progeny**, an important duty for all Hindus, except for those who ritually opt out of their obligation to become householders, such as yogis and *sadhus* (wandering holy men). In the case of hijras, their inability to reproduce affirms the ability of other males to produce progeny. Nanda sums up her description of the hijra performance:

> In a final gesture, Tamasha passed her hands over the head of the infant Ram to bless him, giving to him what she herself does not possess: the power of creating new life, of having many sons, and of carrying on the continuity of his family. It is this role that defines their identity in relation to the world around them. (1999:3)

Berdache or "Two-Spirit"

The Amazon River of Brazil takes its name from Tupinamba Indians in northeastern Brazil, observed by the Portuguese explorer Pedro de Magalhães de Gandavo in 1576. Even today we can almost hear the awe in his voice as he describes these remarkable women:

> There are some Indian women who determine to remain chaste: these have no commerce with men in any manner, nor would they consent to it even if refusal meant death. They give up all the duties of women and imitate men, and follow men's pursuits as if they were not women. They wear the hair cut in the same way as the men, and go to war with bows and arrows and pursue game, always in company with men; each has a woman to serve her, to whom she says she is married, and they treat each other as man and wife.[20]

From a perspective of almost 450 years later, this description provides a counterpoint to the attitudes toward women common to the United States. Whereas U.S.

women who share attributes with men are viewed with derision, Spanish and Portuguese explorers of the seventeenth century viewed them with admiration.

A study conducted by the Oregon Health & Science University School of Medicine suggests that sexual diversity may be selected for, since it apparently has a biological basis. Conducting experiments on humans is difficult, since human psychology has many components, both biological and social. Researchers in the Oregon study focused on sheep, which do not have so many psychological and behavioral issues as humans. They noted that about 8 percent of domestic rams display mating preferences for other rams as sexual partners and that this seems to be unrelated to dominance or flock hierarchies.

Researchers in the Oregon study determined that a densely packed and irregularly shaped cluster of nerve cells in the hypothalamus of rams that preferred females was significantly larger and contained more neurons than in ewes or males that preferred males. The hypothalamus is the part of the brain that regulates sex hormone secretion, blood pressure, body temperature, water balance, and food intake. It also plays a role in regulating complex behaviors, such as sexual behaviors. The lead author of the study, Charles E. Roselli, professor of physiology and pharmacology, states that "Same-sex attraction is widespread across many different species."[21]

Studies among animals are not always generalizable to humans because humans are more complex psychologically and socially than any other animal. However, studies of animals, such as the Oregon study, cast light on human behavior, which is much more subject to complex socialization processes. Though the range of human motivations and personality is extensive, gender categories are necessarily limited, because they are organized around production and reproduction.

Among native peoples of the Americas, gender categories range from two to four: man-like-man; man-like-woman; woman-like-woman; and woman-like-man. Contemporary people in what is now the United States consider men to be more socially powerful than women. This ethnocentric view would lead one to think that women would seek the "more powerful" status of woman-like-man than men would seek the "less powerful" status of man-like-woman. In fact, the opposite is true. More native American societies have man-like-woman categories than have woman-like-man.

The term *berdache* has traditionally been used by anthropologists to refer to the man-like-woman gender category. It derives from the French term *bardache*. The term is offensive to some groups for a number of reasons, including the fact that the word means "male prostitute." Thus, the term implies that males are selling sex to other males. The indigenous concept refers to a male assuming a social role similar to—but not identical to—that of females. Further, the word "berdache" is a term used by colonial occupiers to describe customs prevalent in the Americas. Thus, it reflects differences in social power after European colonialists displaced native peoples of the Americas as the dominant power and were thus able to impose European values onto indigenous groups.

At the third annual intertribal Native American/First Nations gay and lesbian conference in Winnipeg, Canada, in 1990, the term "two-spirit" was adopted to refer to the gender categories of men-like-women and women-like-men on the basis that people in these categories have two spirits, rather than only one. Two-spirited people take on important social roles that, in some cases, may be shunned by others.

For example, in some groups, male-bodied two-spirits conducted death rituals, such as digging graves and preparing the deceased for burials. Thus, they ritually transcended the boundary between life and death.

In some groups, male two-spirits also did work characteristic of women, such as making quillwork and beadwork. Two-spirits in female bodies took on such typically male roles as warrior and hunter, as well as leadership roles. Both male-bodied and female-bodied two-spirits played important roles in spiritual matters, including vision quests and healing.

3

The Biology of Psychology and the Psychology of Biology

CASE STUDY
Stress and Behavior in High-Level Athletic Participation

To professional and high-level athletes, sport is not a game. It is life, limb, and lifestyle. High-level sports competition is one of the most stressful occupations one can pursue for a number of reasons. One of these is that an athlete must consistently perform at maximum levels under the critical scrutiny of individuals who could not possible perform at those levels. As one sport researcher put it, a professional foot-ball kicker can kick the ball farther than a horse could kick it. Athletes who cannot consistently perform at such high levels are subject to unemployment and ridicule. A neighbor who barely has the coordination to mow his lawn feels free to critique a professional athlete's performance in a game. In addition, a slump or injury can end an athletic career. One physician specializing in sport medicine told me athletes often ask him to "fix me up any way, so I can compete. I don't care if I die after-wards." Professional athletes customarily use rituals to prepare for the stress of sports competition. Prior to my research among professional and high level athletes, sport psychologists dismissed athlete's rituals as "superstition." Based on my interviews and observations of athletes, I concluded that athletes use rituals, or pre-game "rou-tines," to control stress, and that these rituals improve athletic performance. I write, "Ritual helps the player focus his [or her] attention on the task at hand. It can be used by the player to prevent anxiety or excessive environmental stimuli—such as the chanting of fans—from interrupting his [or her] concentration. . . . Ritual provides a means of coping with a high-risk, high-stress situation" (Womack 1992:200). Ritual also reduces anxiety by defining interpersonal relationships within the team and with people on the periphery of the team, such as management and the public. Since ath-letes respect each other's rituals, this repetitive, sequential behavior "can be used to reinforce a sense of individual worth under pressure for group conformity, without endangering the unity of the group. . . . Ritual directs individual motivations and needs toward achieving group goals" (Womack 1992:200). Ultimately, ritual aids athletic performance by providing a sense of control over factors that would otherwise disrupt his or her concentration.

My study of rituals of professional athletes analyzed the relationship among stress, ritual, and the performance of complex motor tasks. It links together the fields of physiological psychology and behavioral psychology, as well as anthropological studies of **shamanism**, which involves healing through rituals. The shamanic aspect of healing will be addressed in Chapter 11 of this book, "Calling on the Spirits: Shamans and Mediums." In this chapter, we will analyze the intricate relationship among cognition, behavior, and biology. In so doing, we will discuss what constitutes cognition, the biochemistry underlying cognitive processes, as well as the influence of behavior on the biochemistry of our brains and bodies.

WESTERN PHILOSOPHY AND
THE MIND-BODY DICHOTOMY

When I try to explain the interdependence of psychological and biological processes to my students, someone will inevitably say, "It's mind over matter." The concept of "mind over matter" stems from a Western philosophical tradition that postulates a battle between "matter" (the body) and "mind." The "mind" is often conceptualized as an ethereal substance that does not conform to scientific principles and that exists independently of the body. The term for this model is the **mind-body dichotomy**. The psychobiology of human health and illness is complex. It cannot be reduced to "mind over matter."

The distinction between the mind (ether or spirit) and the body (matter) can be traced to the Greek philosopher Plato, who formulated a model of the world as being based in ideal forms that are reflected in debased **corporeal** forms. In later Christian formulations, as expressed by the Apostle Paul, the body is the enemy of the soul. Drawing on sporting metaphor, Paul writes, "I do not box as one beating the air; but I pummel my body and subdue it, lest after preaching to others I myself should be disqualified." In the transition from Greek philosophy to Christian theology, concepts relating to the body also took a beating. Plato's concept of the ideal versus the corporeal becomes expressed as a war between the soul and the impulses of the flesh.

In medieval theology, the distinction between mind and body was even more clearly defined as a war between God and the carnal form of the human body. The word "carnal" refers to "flesh" and is associated with meat, as expressed in the word "carnivore." In theological terms, the word "carnal" is linked to consumption and enjoyment of bodily pleasures, such as eating, drinking, and sexuality. These activities—which are essential to the continuation of the human species—are condemned as "sinful." If eating, drinking, and sex are sinful, then human life in general is opposed to divine nature. This is a view characteristic of extreme forms of Christianity, and many Christians postpone sensory delights for what they expect will be divine delights in heaven. In terms of health and healing, stifling bodily pleasures is a sound plan for getting to heaven more quickly than by enjoying life on earth, since a healthy appreciation of pleasure is a prescription for preserving health.[1]

In the Calvinist and Puritanical traditions, the spiritual aspects of human experience are associated with God, which is conceptualized as the ideal of human perfection. This is often viewed as existing independently of the physical world. This binary opposition implies that the spiritual entity "God" and the carnal entity "human" occupy opposite ends of the spectrum. A view of the human body as an inferior product has negative implications for both the motives and means of maintaining health. The motive for avoiding death is often driven by the fear of the unknown (death) rather than the enjoyments of earthly pleasures such as a beautiful sunset, the smell of a newly mown field, or the laughter of a child chasing a butterfly.

Binary oppositions do not admit intermediate positions. They are powerful metaphors for explaining differences on multiple levels. To draw on a metaphor, binary oppositions are like Japanese steel. There is almost nothing stronger than a Japanese sword or the Japanese sushi knife. Had a Japanese samurai and a medieval European knight met in battle, the samurai could have cut the medieval knight in half through his armor. But, as a Japanese sushi chef explained to me, the sushi knife is brittle. Sushi knives slice easily through sinew and bone, but they break easily when put to the test of time.

The same is true of binary oppositions. They slice through confusing categories with disarming ease, but they are static, as the sushi knife is brittle. There must be room for negotiation. As Claude Lévi-Strauss notes, there must be negotiation between the two opposing categories through a third, intermediary principle. In Judaic theology, the opposition between G-d and man is resolved when G-d blew life into the nostrils of Adam. In Christian symbolism, God is both a father who is not susceptible to human corporeal frailty, and a son who unites the supposedly opposing realms of heaven and earth, spirit, and body.[2]

Biology, Psychology, or Both?

Though scientists have long rejected the theological model of the spiritual/carnal dichotomy, the opposition continues in the metaphor of "mind over matter" and the debate over whether health and illness are psychological or biological. This debate ignores the fact that emotions, which are experienced as psychological states, are essentially biochemical. This is not to suggest that biology determines psychology, rather that there is no clear-cut distinction between psychological states and biological processes. The biology and psychology of the human organism cannot be traced to a single cause. The whole is greater than the sum of its parts. In fact, it is the relationship among the parts that produces our experience of ourselves, of others, and of the surrounding universe. The **neurobiologist** Bruce D. Perry[3] describes the interrelationship among genetics, experience, and social interdependency:

> We now know more about our genes and more about the influence of experience on shaping biological systems [than] ever before. What do these advances tell us about the nature or nurture debate? Simply, they tell us that this is a foolish argument. Humans are the product of nature *and* nurture. Genes and experience are interdependent. (2002:80)

According to Perry, human behavior and the social context of behavior define the expression of potential that genes make possible:

> Genes are merely chemicals and without "experience"—with no context, no microenvironmental signals to guide their activation or deactivation—create nothing. And "experiences" without a genomic matrix cannot create, regulate or replicate life of any form. The complex process of creating a human being—and humanity—requires both. The amazing malleability and adaptability of humankind is allowed by our genetically-mediated capacity to perceive and respond to myriad environmental cues including the complex social-emotional milieu created when humans live together; and the organ most sensitive and responsive to the environment is the human brain. (2002:80)

The mind-body dichotomy characteristic of Western philosophy obscures our understanding of the intricate relationship between biology and psychology. Cognitive processes produce chemical changes in the body. Conversely, bodily states and movements can alter cognitive processes. My research among professional and high-level athletes focused on the means by which ritual, symbolic behavior, can bring unruly cognitive processes under control, thereby resulting in greater control over performance.

This examination of the mind-body dichotomy can be extended further to explain the metaphors we use to describe ourselves as "pathological" or "normal." This is not to suggest there is no such thing as **pathology** or illness, or that health and pathology are simply products of the human imagination. Rather, redefining the relationship between the human mind and body allows us to consider that negatively experienced physiological states (such as exhaustion, deprivation of food and water, succumbing to disease **pathogens**, and the onslaughts of old age) cannot be extricated from the more subjective experiences of loneliness, hopelessness, feelings of abandonment, and lack of self-confidence. Emotions often express themselves in physiological symptoms, and bodily experiences take a toll on the emotions.

This biology-versus-psychology debate ignores the fact that emotions, which are experienced as psychological states, are biochemical. There is a feedback loop between the way we feel emotionally and the way we experience our bodies as being "healthy" or "sick."

THE BIOLOGY OF THE BRAIN

Relative to body size, the human brain is larger than that of any other animal, and its complexity is greater than that of any computer yet devised. In fact, the brain is so complex it virtually defies attempts to categorize its components. Though **neurologists** agree in general on the **loci** of the brain's functions, there is still much to learn about their functions and components. The basic unit of the brain is the **neuron** or nerve cell. The brain and the spinal cord make up the central nervous system. The spinal cord is, in fact, a single long neuron extending from the brain to the base of the spine.

The neuron that comprises the spinal cord culminates at the top in a bulbous structure known as the **brain stem**. The brain stem controls bodily functions, such as breathing, heart rate, digestion, and movement. This part of the brain is similar to the reptilian brain and is sometimes referred to as such.

The **midbrain** has multiple functions. It relays information received from the peripheral nervous system (the nerves that measure sensory data and bodily functions) to the **cerebral cortex** and is involved with consciousness. The **thalamus** is important in regulating sleep and wakefulness. It also regulates arousal, including the level of awareness and activity. The thalamus could be compared to a switching station which mediates among the auditory, somatic, visceral, gustatory, and visual systems, but not the olfactory system.[4] The thalamus also plays an important role in the motor system. The **motor cortex** conveys sensory data through the thalamus to the **basal ganglia** and **cerebellum**, which are large collections of nuclei that modify movement on a minute-to-minute basis. "The output of the cerebellum is excitatory, while the basal ganglia are inhibitory. The balance between these two systems allows for smooth, coordinated movement."[5] The basal ganglia and cerebellum convey information back to the motor cortex via the thalamus, which serves as a mediator.

The **hypothalamus** is part of the **limbic system**, which lies above the brain stem and beneath the cortex. The limbic system is involved in hormones, temperature control, and emotion. One part of the limbic system, the hippocampus, is involved in memory formation and long-term memory. Neurons affecting heart rate and respiration are concentrated in the hypothalamus, which directs most of the physiological changes associated with strong emotion. An important function of the hypothalamus is homeostasis, which can be described as keeping bodily functions within sustainable levels. It regulates hunger, thirst, response to pain, levels of pleasure, sexual satisfaction, anger, and aggressive behavior, among other things. "It also regulates the functioning of the parasympathetic and sympathetic nervous systems, which in turn means it regulates things like pulse, blood pressure, breathing, and arousal in response to emotional circumstances."[6] The hypothalamus sends instructions to other parts of the body through the pituitary gland and the autonomic nervous system.

The Biology of Arousal

The parasympathetic and sympathetic nervous systems are part of the autonomic nervous system, which controls many organs and muscles in the body, including muscles in the skin, around blood vessels, in the eye, in the heart, and in the viscera, which include the stomach, intestines, and bladder. The **sympathetic nervous system** produces the fight or flight syndrome, in which the heart beats faster, blood pressure increases, the digestive processes slow down, and the immune system is suppressed. The **parasympathetic nervous system** sends the message that it is time to relax. The heart rate slows down, blood pressure drops, and the digestive and immune systems return to normal. The parasympathetic nervous system permits the body to heal after a period of hyperactivity or stress. The autonomic nervous system also includes the enteric nervous system, which regulates the operation of the viscera, including the gastrointestinal tract, pancreas, and gall bladder.

The amygdala, which are next to the hippocampus, are involved in the "flight or fight" response, a form of arousal. Symptoms include an increased heart rate and "pounding heart," increased muscle tension that may produce tremors, sweaty but cold palms, and in some cases, nausea and diarrhea. It is implicated in post-traumatic stress disorder and panic disorder. It may also be involved in bipolar disorder, though that is still unproved. The fear response and panic disorder are likely to result from both genetic factors and stress, especially stressful events occurring in early childhood.

Biology and Abstract Thought

Among humans, the most elaborated part of the brain is the **cerebrum**, the two hemispheres of the brain that completely cover the brain stem and the midbrain. The convoluted outer layers of the cerebrum are the cerebral cortex, where much of abstract thought takes place, including memory, attention, perceptual awareness, "thinking," language, and consciousness. The outer surface, or **cerebral cortex**, consists of neurons and their unsheathed fibers, whereas the substance below this outer layer consists primarily of sheathed axons that interconnect different regions of the central nervous system.

Vision is concentrated in the occipital lobes located near the rear of the brain. The parietal lobe, located above and in front of the occipital lobe, maps the body's surface area. The parietal, temporal, and occipital lobes process our perception of visual, auditory, and other sensory data involving the body in relation to other objects in the environment. The sensory cortex and motor cortex are located between the parietal lobe and the frontal lobe, which is involved in planning actions and movement, as well as abstract thought. Broca's area and Wernicke's area, which are associated with language, are on the left side of the brain, above the temporal lobe. Broca's area is in front of the motor cortex; Wernicke's area is under and just behind the sensory cortex.

The left hemisphere controls the right side of the body and is important in language and general cognitive functions. The right hemisphere controls the left side of the body and manages nonverbal processes, such as attention, pattern recognition, line orientation, and the detection of complex auditory tones. The two hemispheres of the cerebrum are connected by neurons—the **corpus callosum**—that compare sensory data and coordinate cognitive functions.

SYNAPSES: COMMUNICATION CIRCUITRY OF THE BRAIN

Biological synapses within the human body consist of three kinds: (1) electrical synapses, (2) immunological synapses, and (3) chemical synapses. In all these cases, there is intercellular communication. Communication between neurons—the cells that comprise the brain and other parts of the neurological system—is both chemical and electrical. Communication occurs when the axon of one neuron transmits a signal to the dendrite of another neuron. The axon is the long tentacle of a neuron; the dendrite is the main body of the neuron.

Some of the neurons and almost all of the synaptic connections between them develop after birth, when the individual is interacting with other humans. The growth of the neurons and the synaptic connections among them occur as an individual learns. As we encounter new situations, new synaptic connections develop, producing new synaptic complexity. At the same time, unused patterns of thinking or behavior result in the loss of synaptic connections. This is the electrical and chemical process by which we learn new information and forget information that our brain no longer considers useful. In popular terms, this is called "use it or lose it."

In child development research, this is called "pruning." Synaptic pathways develop very quickly after birth, before the infant has developed the ability to distinguish between types of knowledge it requires. As the infant gains experience and is able to determine which synapses are relevant to its survival, the brain prunes away those synaptic pathways that provide no survival benefit and distract the infant from processing information more relevant to its survival.

The Biochemistry of Synapses

A message is transmitted chemically through the sudden inflow of positively charged sodium ions across the cell membrane followed by the outflow of positively charged potassium ions. This produces a spontaneous change in electrical voltage, which results in an electrical current, or impulse. Within the cerebral cortex, this process happens frequently, whether we are awake or asleep. This is why we have vivid experiences, in the form of dreams, even when we are sleeping.

There is a difference in how the neurons are formed. Some are unmyelinated and others are myelinated, which means that they are either unsheathed or sheathed. If they are **unmyelinated**, they lack the fatty covering over the axon, the long transmitter branch of the neuron. If they are **myelinated**, the axon has sausage-like fatty segments that prevent signals from neurons from interfering with each other. Another function of the myelin sheath is to speed up the conduction of neural impulses, which permits the rapid transmission of information.

Conduction of an impulse occurs differently in myelinated and unmyelinated neurons. A message conveyed by an unmyelinated axon is uncontrolled, since the axon is not protected from incoming messages. Myelinated axons are protected by their fatty covering, which prevents the transmission of incoming messages. Loss of the myelin sheath leads to such disorders as multiple sclerosis, which is caused by erratic nerve signals. As a result, bodily movements are uncoordinated because the axon is subject to competing neural impulses.

It was once thought that neurons were formed before birth or shortly after birth and, therefore, could not be reduplicated. More recent research suggests that even adult brains contain what is called *progenitor* or *stem cells*. That is, they are capable of giving rise to new neurons when conventional neurons are destroyed. The research on this is ongoing, which means we still have not determined the conditions under which a neuron or synaptic connection may be altered or regenerated.

Communication within the human brain is far more complex than any known communication system developed by the human brain. The Internet is primitive compared to the intricate workings of the human brain. This complex communication and information processing system is comprised of about 100 billion nerve cells, or neurons, each of which is connected to other neurons through about 10,000 synapses.[7] This may vary, depending on many factors involving genetics, socialization, and trauma. Though the human brain can sometimes be slower than a human-designed computer, it has qualities that computers have so far been unable to replicate:[8]

- The human brain can process ambiguity and contradiction, which even the most sophisticated computers built to date cannot. The human brain can process such statements as "I might go to a play tonight if I can finish my work in time and if my friend wants to see the same play." An ambiguous statement like this could give a computer a nervous breakdown, but the simplest human brain can compute it easily. Similarly, the human brain can compute the contradictory statement, "He's so smart, he's stupid." To a computer, "smart" and "stupid" are irreconcilable categories; however, to the human brain, both ambiguity and contradiction enhance our ability to communicate.
- The human brain can evaluate its experience and reprogram its responses. In other words, it can learn.
- The human brain can rapidly evaluate environmental cues and produce appropriate behavioral responses to a variety of stimuli. For example, the human brain can correlate the voice tone, body language, facial expression, and verbal expression of an interacting entity (a human) instantaneously and without the need to read a set of instructions. It can do this without conscious awareness.
- According to recent research, the human brain can repair itself. If repair is not possible, the brain can establish new neural pathways that compensate for damaged neurons. Some newer and more sophisticated computers can also perform the repair function, but it is not clear whether this process is identical. At this point, we know more about the repair function of computers than the repair function of the human brain.
- The human brain is conscious of many, if not most, of its own operative functions.

Many operations of the human brain are conscious. We are aware that we are walking through a park, for example. What we may not be aware of is that our emotional responses to what we experience during that walk in the park may be based on interpretations of previous experiences. They are not objective. The sound of surf against the sand may evoke childhood memories of similar experiences with significant others. The rustle of the wind through a cornfield may evoke similar responses, depending on its association with positive or negative experiences.

We may not be fully conscious of these "forgotten" associations. The multiple neural pathways of the unconscious, formed in the process of socialization, and perhaps repressed or integrated into the world view that shapes our responses to external stimuli, also shape our emotional response to our surroundings.

THE SOCIAL CONTEXT OF HUMAN BRAIN DEVELOPMENT

Humans, along with most nonhuman primates and other mammals, are social animals. The offspring of mammals require long periods of care relative to their overall life span. Placental mammals are first nurtured in their mother's uterus, which supplies all the nutrients that the fetus requires to survive and thrive. This environment promotes increased brain development, a characteristic that distinguishes mammals from other animals. After birth, a mammal obtains nourishment from its mother's mammary glands, which produce milk ideally suited for the baby's nutrition. This close contact also promotes a strong social bond in which the baby develops a **cognitive schema**, or world view, within which the infant orders its experience of its surroundings.

During this period of close interaction, the child's brain is rapidly developing. A website maintained by North Dakota State University and the U.S. Department of Agriculture describes the development of a child's brain within the context of social contact: "Brain development allows a child to develop the abilities to crawl, speak, eat, laugh and walk. Healthy development of a child's brain is built on the small moments that parents and caregivers experience as they interact with a child."[9] These interactions are essential to the development of a child's brain and its ability to interact with others.

The website is aimed at instructing parents and other caregivers in the importance of positive interactions with their offspring: "A baby's brain is a work in progress. The outside world shapes its development through experiences that a child's senses—vision, hearing, smell, touch and taste—absorb."[10] Examples provided by the website include (1) the scent of the mother's skin (smell); (2) the father's voice (hearing); (3) seeing a face or brightly colored toy (vision); (4) the feel of a hand gently caressing (touch); (5) drinking milk (taste). "These everyday moments . . . provide essential nourishment."[11]

The opposite may also be true. A study conducted by the Department of Comparative Human Development at the University of Chicago indicates that intergenerational transmission of infant abuse is more likely due to early experience rather than genetic inheritance. The study, coordinated by Dario Maestripieri, was conducted on macaque monkeys, a necessary condition because such intensive observation and alteration of the social contacts of human infants are not legally or ethically possible. Also, the macaques were at a controlled environment at the Yerkes National Primate Research Center of Emory University. This permits researchers to exclude such variables as abuse of infants by older siblings or nonrelated members of the group.

According to the study, most abuse by a mother to her offspring occurs in the first six months of an infant's life, predominantly during the first month. Researchers cross-fostered female infants between abusive and nonabusive mothers, comparing them with a control group who were reared by their biological mothers until members of the control group gave birth. Nine of the sixteen females who were abused in infancy by their biological or foster mothers were abusive to their own offspring. None of the fifteen females reared by nonabusive mothers were abusive to their offspring. Also, none of the offspring who were born to abusive mothers but raised by nonabusive foster mothers developed abusive parenting patterns. Though some personality characteristics, such as impulsivity, may be transmitted genetically, these research results suggest that infant abuse is not among them. This is logical, in evolutionary terms, because infant abuse or child abuse is likely to be selected against. This is because abused offspring are less likely than nurtured offspring to survive long enough to transmit their genetic coding to the next generation.

COMMUNICATION, COGNITION, AND ABSTRACT THOUGHT

The joint North Dakota State University and U.S. Department of Agriculture website notes that the brain grows in sequential fashion from the brain stem to the cerebral cortex. The cerebral cortex is the least developed part of the brain at birth and continues to develop until or beyond adolescence, thus "it is more sensitive to experiences than other parts of the brain."[12] A significant part of this development is the establishment of synapses, the chemical process that controls connections between the neurons. The long duration of human brain development contributes to **plasticity**, the ability of humans to react appropriately to a variety of social situations, as well as to make rapid decisions in a changing environment. Plasticity is an important component of human cognition.

Cognition has been defined as "the process of knowing and, more precisely, the process of being aware, knowing, thinking, learning and judging."[13] Elsewhere, I have defined cognition as the "process of acquiring information about the world, then reordering and interpreting it so that it can be used to operate within that world" (Womack 2001). Cognition is important because the way we think shapes the way we behave in the world. It shapes the way we treat others, the way we treat ourselves, and the way we treat our environment. In the process of cognition, the human animal assesses her or his own feelings and motivations, as well as the feelings and motivations of others. For the most part, this ongoing cognitive process is unconscious.

Most mammals must evaluate the resources and dangers in their environments as a basis for deciding their actions. However, the human brain is especially well-equipped for performance in a complex and challenging environment: society. Even within the primate order, humans have the largest and most complex brain. Social primates have more complex brains than solitary primates because social behavior requires the ability to evaluate the motives and probable behavior of our own kind, as well as that of outsiders.

Humans are especially evolved for communication and evaluation. Compared with other animals, humans have relatively few naturally occurring defense systems. We do not have fangs or claws. Our skin is thin, and we are slow and feeble compared to the other animals on the African veldt where we evolved. But we survived. We could not have survived had it been necessary to go *mano-a-mano* (hand-to-hand) against a lion or other predatory animal. The lion was bigger, stronger, faster, and better-armed than our ancestors. **Hominids** (humans and their ancestors) survived because of their social skills. Humans, of all the animals, are unparalleled communicators. We can communicate at great distances through body language. Up close and personal, we communicate through facial expressions made possible by the reduction of facial hair and a sophisticated system of facial muscles.

Our adaptations for **language** permit us to communicate precisely and definitively. Language is an open system, which means we can generate infinite new meanings by combining a limited number of sounds according to a set of rules. The meanings of sounds used in language are arbitrary, which means they are culturally defined. In other words, we must agree on what a particular sound means. This agreement derives from our socialization into a particular group.

Language has the quality of **displacement**, which means we can communicate about phenomena not immediately accessible or available to the senses. Samuel

Langhorne Clemens, who wrote under the name "Mark Twain" described his crossing over the equator on board a ship early in the twentieth century in a tone of awe: "There it was, stretched out in a silvery line all the way to the horizon." With typical humor, Clemens noted that the concept of the equator is a product of the human mind, made possible through our ability to use language. The term "equator" refers to the equidistant point between the magnetic North Pole and the magnetic South Pole, but it does not exist in the way drawn on maps. There is no visible line drawn around the center of the earth; the line is conceptually drawn by humans around maps and globes that represent the earth.

Adaptations for language in humans include a larynx, which contains the vocal cords, that is lower in the throat than that of other primates. This increases the human ability to make clearly defined sounds. It also increases our propensity for choking since the larynx, which permits air from the lungs to pass over the vocal cords, is close to the opening of the esophagus, which permits food to pass from the throat to the stomach. We must learn to intake air and ingest food as separate actions. Nonhuman primates and very young children, who have not learned to process food and air differently, have larynxes that are higher in the throat.

Humans also have structures in the face that allow us to amplify and precisely define sounds, so that we can distinguish between sounds such as "b" and "p," which differ only in the amount of air that passes between the lips. The spinal column also has larger openings that those of other primates, to allow finer control of breathing so we can produce long sentences, such as "I think that I shall never see a poem lovely as a tree. . . . a tree that may in summer wear a nest of robins in her hair." Joyce Kilmer, the poet who wrote these lines, also makes use of a metaphor, which draws a parallel between a poem and a tree, as well as between a tree and a woman.

Metaphor and Cognition

There is a kind of sublime transition in these metaphors, in which the work of the poet does not pretend to the artistry of the deity (or other power, such as evolution) that produced a tree. The poet also makes a transition between the beauty of a tree and the beauty of a woman. Kilmer's poem "Trees" illustrates an important aspect of human communication and cognition. Our words can draw on imagery to evoke emotions in our listeners (readers). Though Kilmer died fighting in World War I, his poetry lives on.

The linguistic powerhouse for humans is the brain. Whether we perform language or listen to language, the process of communication involves many parts of the brain, some that are specific to language and others that integrate the information that language makes available. What humans lack in physical strength, speed, and biological weaponry compared with other animals, we more than make up for through the power of the brain.

ISSUES IN STUDYING THE HUMAN BRAIN

There are pragmatic and ethical considerations in studying the biology of the human brain. Early explorations of the biology of the brain relied on electrical stimulation of areas of the brain through the use of probes, then observing the behavioral response of the organism. Since it is a violation of experimental ethics to stick foreign objects into a healthy human brain, such research typically used rats, cats, or monkeys as research subjects. Human subjects could only be used in cases where brain damage had already occurred through no fault of the researcher, such as stroke or some other form of trauma to the brain. By using electrical probes on nonhuman subjects, researchers were able stimulate behaviors and emotions, including rage, aggression or fear, measured by assessing the animal's behavior, such as a biting attack.

More recently, Neil McNaughton, of the Department of Psychology at Otago University in New Zealand, has noted that early researchers did not adequately control the relationship between the size of the probe and the size of the brain of the animal being probed, especially in the case of the rat: "stimulation could well be simultaneously activating functionally discrete systems, the anatomical separation of which was not great" (McNaughton 1989:19–20).

As a result, these early researchers described what they called "nonspecificity" in the brain of the rat as opposed to the "specificity" of the "much larger cat brain, where totally different behavioral effects could be obtained with changes in electrode placement of as little as 0.5 mm. The possibility that, in the rat, a relatively large electrode is stimulating a variety of neurally separate structures simultaneously cannot be ruled out" (McNaughton 1989:20).

In recent years, research on the biochemistry of the brain has become much more sophisticated, so that we can measure the electrochemical activity of the brain, rather than rely on behavioral cues. We can also conduct research directly on the human brain through measurements of brain activity that are minimally invasive. One of these is the CT, sometimes called the CAT scan. It consists of using specially designed x-ray equipment to produce multiple images of the brain, then joining them together into cross-sectional views of the brain. Medically, this technique can be used to gain detailed information on head injuries, stroke, brain tumors, and other brain disorders.

Studying Less Complex Brains

Sometimes, however, it is still useful to conduct research on brains that are much less complex than the human brain. Isolating variables is an important aspect of research, and it is difficult to control for all of the possible variables that might account for activity in the human brain. Researchers cannot isolate humans in captivity as they can isolate other research animals, so they cannot control such variables as what the subject had for breakfast (self-reports are notoriously unreliable), whether he or she quarreled with a spouse and is therefore experiencing unusual brain wave activity, or whether the subject heard a disturbing news report on the radio before entering the examination room. Also important is what kind of family the individual grew up in, his or her political beliefs, and feelings of anxiety unrelated to the research environment.

Sea slugs are much more reliable as research subjects, especially if they have been bred especially for the job and therefore have consistent biological and environmental characteristics. Animal activists often accuse researchers of buying stolen pets, but this is a smokescreen. Animals used in research must have a documented genealogy and medical history, which includes their dietary regimen. Depending on the kind of research being conducted, the researchers must also know how much, and what kind of, contact the research animals have had with humans.

Sea slugs have relatively simple brains, and their sexual history is much less complicated than that of humans. Therefore, they make excellent research subjects when studying brain activity. Compared with the approximately 100 billion neurons in the human brain, sea slugs have only about 10,000 large neurons that can be easily identified. "Even so, the animal is capable of learning and its brain cells communicate in ways identical to human neuron-to-neuron" signaling system.[14] The ability of the sea slug (Aplysia) to learn is important because synapses—transmissions of information from one neuron to another—are established during the learning process.

A team of scientists lead by Leonid Moroz of the University of Florida Whitney Laboratory for Marine Bioscience studied gene activity in the sea slug's central nervous system to find out the genetic conductors that facilitate learning and memory.[15] Previous researchers had "identified more than 100 genes similar to those associated with all major human neurological diseases and more than 600 genes controlling brain development."[16] The team led by Moroz focused on the process in which genes switch on and off during a simple defensive maneuver, when the slug withdraws its gills. They studied the transcriptome, "the complete collection of transcribed elements of the genome. In addition to mRNAs, it also represents non-coding RNAs which are used for structural and regulatory purposes."[17] Messenger RNAs (mRNAs) transcribe DNA coding into a form that can produce the proteins that make up a new cell.

The Moroz-led research team found specific genes linked to learning and memory.[18] In an interview with LiveScience, Eric Kandel of Columbia University, a member of the research team, stated, "We've now identified a whole bunch of receptors for serotonin. So we can see what their function is in various cells and which ones participate in the learning process."[19] "The scientists also analyzed 146 human genes implicated in 168 neurological disorders, including Parkinson's and Alzheimer's diseases," as well as genes that control aging.[20]

Serotonin is synthesized from the amino acid tryptophan. "In the central nervous system, serotonin is believed to play an important role in the regulation of body temperature, mood, sleep, vomiting, sexuality, and appetite. Low levels of serotonin have been associated with several disorders, notably clinical depression, migraine, irritable bowel syndrome, tinnitus, fibromyalgia, bipolar disorder, and anxiety disorders.[21] It is still unclear what is involved in producing low levels of serotonin. It is likely that multiple interactive factors are involved, including genetics, early childhood experience, social and physical environment, as well as behavior.

What Is Intelligence?

There are almost as many ways to define **intelligence** as there are specialists who try to define it. Alfred North Whitehead, the British mathematician, logician, and philosopher, writes, "Intelligence is quickness to apprehend as distinct from ability, which is capacity to act wisely on the thing apprehended."[22] A glossary maintained by the American Psychological Association website defines intelligence as the "global capacity to profit from experience and to go beyond given information about the environment."[23] A common component of definitions of intelligence is the emphasis on conceptual flexibility, the ability to respond effectively to conditions in the environment, an ability often described as "problem solving."

Anyone who has observed children, either interacting with others or playing alone, is aware that they display different personalities and talents. Howard Gardner, Hobbs Professor of Cognition and Education at Harvard, has identified what he considers seven types of intelligence: linguistic intelligence, logical-mathematical intelligence, musical intelligence, bodily-kinesthetic intelligence, spatial intelligence, interpersonal intelligence, and intrapersonal intelligence.

Linguistic intelligence involves sensitivity to spoken and written language, the ability to learn languages, and the capacity to use language to accomplish one's goals. This form of intelligence is characteristic of writers, poets, lawyers, and speakers. *Logical-mathematical intelligence* consists of the capacity to analyze problems logically, carry out mathematical operations, and investigate issues scientifically. It involves the ability to detect patterns, reason deductively, and think logically.[24]

Both **deductive reasoning** and **inductive reasoning** are part of the scientific process, but they develop from opposite starting points. Deductive reasoning is based in the process of concluding that something must be true because it is a special case of a general principle that is known to be true. For example, a galaxy consists of a star whose gravitational pull causes planets to revolve around it. The earth and other planets revolve around the sun, therefore we are part of a galaxy. Based on this principle, we can expect that other stars in the universe might also have planets that revolve around them. Inductive reasoning is based on the process of generalizing from specific cases. For example, in the case of clinical trials, if a sample population benefits from treatment by a particular medication or treatment, it could reasonably be expected that the population as a whole might benefit from that medication or treatment.

According to Gardner's model, *musical intelligence* involves skill in the performance, composition, and appreciation of musical patterns. Gardner considers musical intelligence to be structurally parallel to linguistic intelligence. *Bodily-kinesthetic intelligence* involves the ability to use one's body to solve problems, as well as the ability to use mental abilities to coordinate bodily movements. *Spatial intelligence* involves the ability to assess and negotiate within physical space. *Interpersonal intelligence* involves the ability to understand the intentions, motivations, and desires of other people, and thus, to work effectively with them. Gardner considers this form of intelligence to be characteristic of educators, salespeople, religious, and political leaders, as well as counselors. *Intrapersonal intelligence* involves the ability to understand oneself, as well as to appreciate one's feelings, fears, and motivations. Gardner describes this as having an effective working model of ourselves and being able to use this model to regulate our lives.

Clearly, these forms of intelligence are not mutually exclusive. Gardner considers that the unique constellation of intelligences defines the human species. It could also be argued that the unique constellation of intelligences that we acquire through heredity, through socialization, through our interactions with others, and through our experiences could account for the wide variability within the human species.

In his book *What is Intelligence? Beyond the Flynn Effect* (2007), James R. Flynn, an emeritus professor of political science at the University of Otago in New Zealand, writes that I.Q. test scores have been steadily rising in the developed world despite failing schools and stagnant standardized test scores, a phenomenon he calls the "Flynn effect." Flynn attributes the rising I.Q. scores to the Internet and the computer, which teach children to work with shapes and also forces them to solve problems on the spot without being told what to do. However, Flynn adds, children in the developed world today do not have larger vocabularies and are no better at arithmetic. He notes that scores on the PSAT, which measures verbal and mathematical reasoning abilities, have remained stable. The Preliminary SAT provides preparation for the SAT (originally called the Scholastic Aptitude Test), scores of which are important for gaining admission to competitive colleges and universities and for scholarships.

BIOLOGY AND COGNITION

In recent years, scientists have been able to plant electrodes in the human brain that mimic the brain's basic functions. The one patient involved in an exploratory study was able to begin simple sentences and perform simple tasks in spite of extensive brain damage after resuscitation. Is this, however, equivalent to cognition? This experiment also evokes a number of other issues. Will this individual ever be able to live on his own? Could he earn (or re-earn) a college degree? Would he have chosen to be resuscitated in such a manner to such an existence? Cases such as this raise questions about the nature of life, the nature of cognition, and the ethics of medical and scientific technology.

The controversy over the much-publicized Terry Shiavo case illustrates the complexity of these related issues. Shiavo died March 31, 2005, fifteen years after she entered a **persistent vegetative state** due to cardiac arrest at the age of twenty-six. A persistent vegetative state is clinically defined as the complete unawareness, to self and to environment, which occurs in a person who nevertheless experiences consciousness. Over the two years following Shiavo's entry into this state, Shiavo's husband Michael and her parents, Bob and Mary Schindler, tried various therapeutic measures to revive the woman. In one therapeutic attempt, Michael Shiavo took his wife to the University of California, San Francisco,[25] for an experimental procedure involving placement of a thalamic stimulator in her brain. The procedure, which took several months to complete, was unsuccessful.

In May 1998, Michael Shiavo filed a petition to remove a feeding tube that kept his wife legally alive. The Schindlers attempted to get a court order that transferred the right to make therapeutic decisions to them. Thus ensued a long-running dispute that involved religious activists and politicians at the national and local level. The Schindlers insisted that Terry Shiavo could be helped through therapy because she responded to stimuli, including touch. They stated that she smiled, cried, moved, and made childlike attempts to speak. They said she tried to say "mom," "dad" or "yeah" when they asked her a question. They also said that she looked at them and sometimes puckered her lips when they kissed her. The case was taken to the U.S. Supreme Court, which refused to hear it. The feeding tube was removed, and Terry Shiavo died thirteen days later.

An autopsy conducted after Terry Shiavo's death illustrates the biological apparatus underlying the complexity of human cognition and behavior. The autopsy revealed extensive damage to various areas of the brain, including the cerebral cortex, the thalami, the basal ganglia, the hippocampus, and the midbrain. It also found that Terry Shiavo was blind. Since she was blind, it is unlikely that she "looked" at her parents, though she may have responded to other sensual stimuli.

The Terry Shiavo autopsy indicated that her brain was approximately half the size one might expect of a woman her age. The large pyramidal neurons that make up 70 percent of the cerebral cortex were completely lost. The cerebral cortex is the center for processing visual information, information about pressure, pain, touch, and temperature, as well as auditory information. It is also involved in memory, perception, and emotion, the ability to make plans, think creatively, and make decisions. It could accurately be described as the center for cognition. The extensive damage to this area of the brain would have prevented Shiavo from recognizing her parents, remembering anything about her previous experience, or experiencing joy, sadness, love, or anger.

As noted earlier, the thalami are the relay centers of the brain, which receive input from the sensory apparatuses. Jon Thosmartin, who led the Shiavo autopsy, reported irreversible damage to the relay circuits of the thalami, noting that "no amount of therapy or treatment would have regenerated the massive loss of neurons."

Damage to the basal ganglia, which was revealed in the autopsy, could have produced tremors, athetosis (involuntary writhing movements particularly of the arms and hand), and chorea (involuntary constant rapid complex body movements that look well coordinated and purposeful). These involuntary movements could have been interpreted by Shiavo's parents as attempts to communicate with them.

These interpretations could have been reinforced by damage to Shiavo's cerebellum. It is the primary center for regulating motor activity. It was previously thought that motor activity was the only function of the cerebellum. Henrietta C. Leiner pioneered research that has led to speculation that the cerebellum has other important functions as well, which may have been required for the emergence of human language. The cerebellum exists at birth but develops as an individual matures. Henrietta C. Leiner[26] and Alan L. Leiner describe the cerebellum as a computer that interacts closely with the cerebral cortex. The cerebellum may be especially important in streamlining tasks that can be performed automatically, including speech and often repeated actions. They write: "One of the most impressive parts of the human brain, named the cerebellum, has been underestimated for centuries."[27]

Shiavo's movements, as reported by her parents, did not involve cognition, which requires a capacity for abstract thought. However, her parents' interpretation of her movements was a product of cognition shaped by their motivations and culturally defined concepts of what constitutes life. The complex emotions their daughter's condition evoked illustrates the important difference between cognition in humans and the ability of computers to perform complex analytical tasks. Humans care; computers don't.

What Is Life?

A 2006 case in England illustrates an opposite dynamic: The family of a fifty-three-year-old woman in a persistent vegetative state (PVS) wanted her to die with dignity, but a judge ruled she must be treated with Zolpidem, a drug that has caused some patients with the condition to "wake up," before any procedures were undertaken that would result in her death. Zolpidem is a drug that has long been used as a sleeping pill. When it was administered to a young South African named Louis Viljoen, he "woke up." After seven years, he is "awakened" for about two hours by a daily dose of the pill. Repeated doses of the pill within a twenty-four-hour period have no effect.

The cases have raised many issues related to consciousness and volition. Zolpidem does not reverse the brain damage that initially produced the PVS. It apparently acts directly on the thalamus, which regulates the waking and sleep cycle. As noted earlier, the thalamus acts as a switching station that is involved in processing sensory data and coordinating movement. The question arises with respect to the definition of "waking up." Depending on the extent of brain damage, Viljoen could well have been able to respond to environmental stimuli, but he may not have been able to interpret its "meaning," a process that occurs at the level of the cerebrum.

The effects of administering Zolpidem to patients in PVS are variable, and this may be related to the extent and type of brain damage. Marcel Berline, writing in the *Guardian*, notes that patients awakened by Zolpidem are aware of their condition, but adds that none of us can be sure whether they would want to continue life under such limited circumstances.[28] He concluded that none of us will ever know for sure. I would add that the tragedy in these cases is that the patient lacks **volition**. She or he does not have the opportunity to make decisions upon which her/his life depends.

EMOTIONS, HEALTH, AND ILLNESS

About 15 percent of Americans—almost 25 million people—suffer from irritable bowel syndrome (IBS), which is characterized by constipation, bloating, diarrhea, and gas. Most of those suffering with the condition are women. For years, experts in gastrointestinal health debated whether the condition was best treated by medications, dietary changes, or psychotherapy. Some doubted whether irritable bowel syndrome existed at all. They speculated that IBS was "all in a patient's mind." The debate paralleled the Western—especially the American—view that illness is either biological or psychological, rarely both. Patients who exhibited symptoms for which no biological cause could be identified were suspected of being **hypochondriacs**, people who are preoccupied with their physical health and body and fears, or are convinced that they have a serious disease despite medical reassurance.[29]

At the 2006 Digestive Disease Week, a meeting of gastrointestinal specialists in Los Angeles, researchers noted that medications used to treat irritable bowel syndrome were less effective than behavior modification, dietary changes, and cognitive behavior therapy. Patients who were taught relaxation techniques and participated in even short self-help cognitive behavior therapy experienced significant and lasting relief of symptoms. The fact that these patients responded so quickly to treatment indicates that IBS is a **psychosomatic disorder**, rather than a **somatoform disorder**. A psychosomatic disorder is a genuine physical ailment caused in part by psychological factors. Hypochondriasis is a somatoform disorder, which means that it is entirely psychological and has no identifiable organic basis.

Jeffrey M. Lackner, director of the behavioral medicine clinic at the State University of New York at Buffalo School of Medicine, noted that people with IBS tend to have stressful habits, including negative thinking patterns that make them anxious and cause them to exacerbate symptoms. They also have poor coping skills, which predisposes them to react more stressfully to life's ups and downs.

Lackner and co-researchers at SUNY, Buffalo, and SUNY, Albany—Brian M. Quigley and Edward B. Blanchard—note that variance in reports of pain severity by IBS patients is related to negative cognitive patterns such as depression and **catastrophizing**, which refers to taking a pessimistic view of one's life and expectations.[30] One form of catastrophizing characterizes pain as awful, horrible, and unbearable. Catastrophizing has also been linked to fatigue among women receiving treatment for breast cancer, is a predictor of chronic low back pain, and is associated with neural responses to pain among persons with **fibromyalgia**, which refers to pain in the soft fibrous tissues of the body. Catastrophizing is also related to postoperative pain experiences, and may be associated with chronic fatigue syndrome.[31]

Lackner notes that changing these cognitive patterns relieves their symptoms and contributes to the patients' quality of life.[32] This is not equivalent to the popular concept of mind over matter. Though Lackner does not make this point, the added pressure of thinking one can control bodily symptoms by will power alone, in the absence of cognitive and behavioral changes, can increase the physical distress of psychosomatic disorders. Both Lackner and Magnus Simrén, of Sahlgrenska University Hospital in Sweden, note that psychotherapists working with IBS patients should understand the biological implications of the disorder. Simrén states, "It's very important that the therapist does have an interest in bodily symptoms and not just the mind."[33]

The Embodiment of Emotion

A number of anthropologists[34] have written about the embodiment of powerlessness and inability to accomplish one's goals in a particular social context. Powerlessness can be experienced as illness. Just as the person is unable to prevail against overwhelming social forces, the body is experienced as being unable to ward off disease. During two stints of fieldwork in Punata, a rural community in Bolivia, and the city of Cochabamba, Maria Tapias focused on two aspects of emotions and experiences of the body. The Andean town of Punata (population 13,000) is a regional center and has an array of available healing options, ranging from traditional healers to a regional hospital. The social life of the town is organized around a small upper-class elite that is primarily viewed as mestizo, as well as middle- and working-class populations that are primarily Quechua; however, Tapias notes that the class division does not strictly follow ethnic divisions.

Tapias notes that "people are not passive receptors of the dictates of social power. As people interact with others in their social milieu, emotions guide and prepare subjects for social action and enable an expression of agency, even if that agency initially entails not outwardly expressing emotions or taking action at all" (2006:403).

In her initial study, from 1996 to 1998, Tapias focused on the role of emotions in conceptualizing illness. In her follow-up visit in 2003, she focused on breastfeeding women and how they viewed such emotions as rage and sorrow as being potentially harmful to infants. Tapias draws on the view of M. L. Lyon and J. M. Barbalet that emotions are not only embodied, but also mediate between the individual body and the social body. Lyon and Barbalet suggest that emotion is the "experience of embodied sociality" (1994:48). Tapias examines "who holds power to express emotion, what emotions can be expressed and under what circumstances, and how emotions are experienced in the body" (2006:404).

In Punata, emotions are viewed as fluids or substances that have the potential to cause illness. If emotions are not expressed, they cause illness. However, it is not always possible to express emotions, especially if an interaction is public or if one is dealing with a superior social class. Tapias writes: "The damage, however, did not always manifest itself in the bodies of the individuals experiencing the emotions. In pregnant and lactating women, the harm could be passed on to infants" (2006:405).

An infant may become afflicted with *arrebato*, the symptoms of which include stomach aches, incessant crying, severe diarrhea, and vomiting, believed to be transmitted through tainted breast milk of a woman who had undergone social or economic distress. A woman can also transmit *debilidad*, a generalized lack of resistance to illness, if she is distressed or emotionally upset during pregnancy. Tabias writes: "When pregnant, a mother's distress and emotions could reach their children through the placenta. These emotions were seen as the cause of generalized debility among children. Such prenatal exposure rendered these children continuously susceptible to illness throughout their lives" (2006:407).

The behavioral model described by Tabias is complex, involving many levels of interaction, especially involving blame. On one level, it should protect women from abuse if they are lactating or pregnant because any injury inflicted on them is also a cause of potential injury to an infant or fetus. On another level, it suppresses a woman's ability to resist oppression—from her husband or social "superior"—because her inability to control her anger is considered to be inflicted on her infant or fetus as illness.

There is biological evidence to suggest that the emotional condition of the mother can affect the health of an infant or fetus, in view of the fact that emotions are chemical. However, in the Punata case, females are placed in an untenable position because they do not have the social power to resist abuse, and they are likely to be blamed for the health of their offspring. Thus, according to popular culture, it is not social inequities that are to be blamed for the reduced health of lower class infants, but the moral "frailty" of their mothers. This cultural model frees everyone from blame but the women who have invested most in the next generation and have least potential for benefit: mothers.

In a sense, this involves the psychological process of "blaming the victim." Illness, whether emotional or physical, threatens the integrity of the social body. On the personal level, illness threatens our sense that we can resist invasions of disease and disease-causing organisms. Life-threatening or chronic illnesses that do not respond to health-giving treatments threaten not only the individual body of the patient, but the social body of the community. Punata women must not only deal with social inequities in their own lives—in terms of gender and class—they must also deal with blame for undermining the health of their offspring.

4

Metaphor, Labeling Theory, and the Placebo Effect

CASE STUDY
Naming the Loa: Preventive Diagnosis in Haitian Vodou

Scholars have long noted that Haitian vodou is a form of folk psychology that helps practitioners deal with the aftermath of colonial suppression, increasing poverty, and overpopulation. Two of the most cited benefits of vodou rituals involve **catharsis**, in which repressed emotions are expressed in an unthreatening environment, and role playing, in which powerless and impoverished individuals can act out their fantasies of empowerment and abundance. As I have noted elsewhere (Womack 2001), vodou plays another important role, that of defining an individual's psychological profile and allowing him or her to seek aid from the spirit world. **Vodou** is a religion that permits Haitians to integrate three parts of their history, which includes French and Spanish Catholicism, as well as traditional African religions imported to the Western hemisphere by the slave trade. Vodou is based on the idea that spirits play an active role in human life by displacing the human consciousness and acting through the human body. In practice, this idea is related to labeling theory because, through **spirit possession**, an individual can act out different aspects of her or his personality. *Lwa* (possessing spirits) are both ancestral spirits and Haitian representations of African deities. Thus, they link together practitioners' African past with their present experience of Haiti. From a psychological perspective, possessing spirits appear to be idealized and more powerful forms of the *possedé's* personality. The practice of vodou is significant in healing because of the possession career, in which individuals learn to transform the limitations of their circumstances into meaningful relationships with spirit beings that guide them throughout their lives. Naming the *lwa* is similar to medical diagnosis, in that it provides the individual with a model for understanding and coping with the trials and tribulations to which he or she is subjected. Vodou adepts say that Haitians who do not accept the invitation from the spirits to become their *cheval*[1] (horse) become *folie* (crazy), an indication that vodou trance possession provides psychological benefits.

Naming things is an important part of healing and staying healthy. Diagnosis is the process of evaluating symptoms and naming their cause. Naming the loa follows a similar process under the guidance of a different paradigm. The vodou priest bases his or her "diagnosis" on the behavior of a person being possessed. A Western physician bases his or her diagnosis on the "behavior" of clinically defined symptoms. The paradigm that gives rise to the vodou "diagnosis" is spiritual, with perhaps unacknowledged psychological dimensions. The medical paradigm that gives rise to a physician's diagnosis is biological, with perhaps unacknowledged psychological dimensions.

Ultimately, both "diagnoses" and "prescriptions" help relieve symptoms of distress. Labeling provides relief for the patient by defining conditions that explain the patient's experience of symptoms. Diagnosis provides relief for the physician or caretaker by defining parameters within which the patient's condition can be treated. They also provide relief for patients by providing a name for an inexplicable experience.

One problem with labeling and diagnosis is that the powerful metaphors generated by these processes of organizing social relationships can become more significant than the condition being addressed. A medical diagnosis can supplant other definitions of an individual's social status, thus reducing a patient to a medical metaphor and diminishing his or her status as a human being. An individual active in the community can become a "cancer patient" when a diagnosis is tendered. A person who is diagnosed as "terminal" may be treated as though she or he were already dead. The psychiatrist Thomas Szasz (1976) has stated that the power to name has the power to control social interactions.

We use names and labels to define ourselves and others in social space. Prior to the women's movement in the United States, which became specifically defined in the early 1970s, it was the custom in medical practice to indicate differences in gender status through naming. Typically, the patient addressed the physician by his title and last name, whereas the physician would address female patients by their first names.

The United States is a highly stratified society, which likes to consider itself a democracy, a term implying that all of us have equal ability to influence political processes. In fact, we do not have, and the term "democracy" is often used by political leaders to justify imposing their own decisions on the populace as a whole. Thus, naming, labeling, and selective use of terminology has the power to define our experience of who we are, as well as our position in the social group.

If we define ourselves as sick, or are defined as such by others, this definition has both social and conceptual significance. When we see someone in a wheelchair, we adopt attitudes that define that person as "invalidated." It is no coincidence that "invalid" and "invalidated" derive from the same linguistic stem. Our passports may be invalidated, thus canceling our social role as travelers. The definition of ourselves as "invalid" may also cancel important social prerogatives.

WHAT'S IN A NAME?

An Inuit elder explained the importance of having a name to a group of Inuit college students: "Aupilaarjuk is my name and I try to use it to keep me alive. . . . It is my name. It keeps me alive. I think that is how it must be" (Saladin d'Anglure

2001:19). According to Lisa Stevenson, "For Inuit the name has a life of its own that exceeds the body. It enters the human body at birth and leaves again at death."[2] An Inuit infant is named after someone who has recently died and is believed to take on behavioral and personality characteristics of that person. Thus, the personality continues even after the body has ceased to exist. "In passing a name from the dead to the newly born, Inuit understand that the 'life-of-the-name' enters the body of the child"[3] (Stevenson 2006:3). Throughout a person's life, the name does not change except under unusual circumstances. A shaman may give a very sick person a new name in hopes that the person will be "reborn" into the new name and the new life (Boas 1964[1888]; Guemple 1965; Saladin d'Anglure 2001; Weyer 1932).

Names and the Social Order

Names establish one's social position. Among royalty and nobility in Europe, one's personal name has been emphasized, a reflection of the Western focus on personal worth. Thus, we may talk of Alexander the Great, Catherine the Great, Queen Elizabeth, or King Louis XIV. Though these individuals descended from powerful lineages, we emphasize through their names the presumed qualities of these rulers as individuals, rather their lineage membership.

In China, the reverse is true. There have been outstanding emperors and individuals of high status, but the lineage takes precedence. The usual naming custom is (lineage name) (generation name) (personal name). The anthropologist Rubie S. Watson analyzed Chinese naming customs with reference to how they reflect gender roles. She writes, "In Chinese society names classify and individuate, they have transformative powers, and they are an important form of self expression. Some names are private, some are chosen for their public effect" (1993:120[1986]).

Chinese are patrilineal, so names, as well as economic assets, are transmitted through the male line. Watson's ethnographic research is based in the village of Ha Tsuen, in the Hong Kong New Territories. All males in the village share the lineage name Teng "and trace descent to a common ancestor who settled in this region during the 12th century" (Watson 1993:121).

Marriage is based on **exogamy** (out-marrying), which, in this case, means that men marry women from other lineages, who by default, would be women from other villages. Thus, males are embedded in their lineage and remain in their own village, whereas women come from outside the village and do not belong to their husband's kin group. In the case of the Teng, women generally are not employed in wage labor jobs, and therefore, are dependent upon their husband's income. This is true even though Chinese peasant women have traditionally contributed greatly to their husbands' household economy.

Ha Tsuen is in southern China, and therefore, the people are Cantonese speakers. Among Cantonese speakers, a child's soul is not believed to be settled into its body until at least thirty days after its birth. Therefore, both mother and infant are secluded during this time. After the period of seclusion, the child is named by his father or grandfather. The name selected might be based on Chinese philosophical traditions, on some event that took place at or near the child's birth, on birth order, or on some aspirations of the family. The name is also likely to depend on the child's horoscope, as represented in his or her balance of the five elements: fire, water, metal, earth, and wood.

In the United States, names are recorded on the birth certificate and are considered permanent except for women who take their husband's name after marriage. Chinese naming customs are more mutable, depending on circumstances. Though the lineage name is permanent, the first name given to a child, its *ming*, is susceptible to change. For example, in the case of illness, an element deemed to be missing in a patient may be added to his or her name to achieve the necessary balance.

Chinese horoscopes and naming customs emphasize the interdependence of members of the family. Watson notes: "It is particularly important that the five elements of mother and child be properly matched to ensure mutual health. If conditions of conflict arise and nothing is done to resolve this conflict, the child may become ill and even die" (1993:124).

This belief illustrates the ambiguous position of females in Chinese society. On the one hand, a woman is powerless to transmit life to her own lineage. On the other, she is essential for transmission of life through her husband's lineage. She not only has the power to continue her husband's lineage; she also has the power to "kill" her husband's lineage. This "lineage imbalance" is corrected through naming customs. A child's name may be changed to bring its essential qualities more in line with those of its mother. Watson writes: "It is obvious that Chinese personal names *do* things; they not only classify and distinguish but also have an efficacy in their own right" (1993:124).

Naming and Healing: The *Lwa* in Vodou Trance Possession

The lifestyle of most Haitians today is based in poverty and control over small parcels of land. Increased population pressure has resulted in impoverishment of the land through overcultivation, and encroachment on forest lands causes erosion during the rainy season. Alfred Métraux describes how, while watching soil being washed away by a river, a peasant said to him: "*Voila notre vie qui s'en va*" ("That is our life going away") (1958:32).

In a society where prosperity and livelihood are easily washed away, vodou customs involving the naming of the possessing lwa (spirit) provide social and psychological stability and flexibility. In vodou belief, humans have two souls, the '*tit bon ange* and the *gros bon ange*, literally the "little good angel" and the "big good angel." The *gros bon ange* controls the body; the '*tit bon ange* controls the will or consciousness. Possession occurs when a *lwa* (spirit) displaces the '*tit bon ange* and takes control of the *possedé's* body. Because the *gros bon ange* has not been displaced, the *possedé's* body can still move freely, but the individual being possessed is not aware of what the body is doing. This is a very deep state of **trance**, an altered state of consciousness (ASC), in which the individual undergoes profound perceptual and physiological changes.

Not just anyone can undergo this possession state. In vodou belief, the individual must be summoned by the *lwa*. Typically, this involves a possession career. Children of vodou practitioners practice being possessed by mimicking their elders during vodou ceremonies. The first possession usually takes place during puberty and is expected to be *bossal* (wild). *Lwa* have varied personalities, some of which are violent (*pétro*) and others of which are (*rada*), tolerant and forgiving. *Pétro lwa* developed under Spanish rule in Haiti, and *rada lwa* are representations of African gods from the Dahomean religion of West Africa. Typically, *lwa* display both *pétro* and *rada* manifestations, which must be tamed and brought under control of the *possedé*.

The resemblance to psychiatric diagnosis is dramatic. In diagnosis, naming has the power to control symptoms. In vodou, individuals are provided with powerful symbols, identified by name, which possess human characteristics but have the power to impose meaning onto individuals' lives and to mediate extreme social circumstances.

Vodou ceremonies are dedicated to a particular *lwa*, each of which has his or her own emblem, dress, and paraphernalia. Any *lwa* that appears at a vodou ceremony uninvited will be chased away. Thus, order is imposed onto unruly and uninvited "guests," just as order is imposed onto unruly and uninvited economic deprivation.

The personality and imagery of *lwa* reflect syncretism, and the spirits are represented as Catholic images of the saints. Two *lwa* known throughout Haiti are Erzulie and Ogoun. Erzulie is mulatto, and her behavior and tastes are those of a French colonial woman. She must be given beautiful clothing, as well as French champagne and perfume. Her manner is flirtatious and whimsical: If she doesn't like the champagne or perfume she is given, she will pour it out into the dust.

Ogoun is patron of war, fire, and the power of recognized authority. It is said he can protect his petitioners against bullets and other weapons. People possessed by Ogoun may demonstrate their invulnerability to wounds or burns by washing their hands in flaming rum or handling glowing bars of iron. Erzulie and Ogoun may possess either males or females, and the behavior of the *possedé* conforms to the personality of the possessing spirit, rather than to that of the individual being possessed.

The vodou possession career begins in childhood. Children participate in vodou ceremonies from an early age, mimicking the dances adults use to invite the spirits that enable them to enter trance. Children also mimic the behavior of adults in trance. This is not unique to vodou. E. E. Evans-Pritchard writes of the Azande of Africa: "I have seen small children dancing the 'witch-doctors'[4] dance and eating their medicines, in which actions they copy the movements which they have seen their elders make at séances and communal magic meals. Their elders encourage them in a jovial way and the children regard the whole affair as a piece of fun" (1976:90). Through this pattern of interaction, individuals are socialized into the world of spirits, much as people in stratified societies are socialized into the authority of parents.

In vodou, individuals typically become possessed for the first time when they are in their teens, a time when they are preparing to take on the responsibilities of adulthood. Possessions are supposed to take place only during vodou ceremonies, which are presided over by a houngan (male) or mambo (female), people who have had long training in summoning the spirits. Houngans and mambos do not become possessed during vodou ceremonies themselves because an important part of their role is preventing *possedés* from harming themselves.

The first possession may take place outside a vodou ceremonial context and is typically *bossal*, or "wild," because the *possedé* must learn to *marre* (or "tie") the possessing spirit. If an individual experiences his or her first possession outside the ceremonial context, a houngan or mambo will be called to name the possessing *lwa*.

This *lwa* will become the *mâit tête* (master of the head), a guardian spirit. The individual undergoing possession is expected to *marre* his *lwa* by establishing an altar and undergoing a *laver-tête* or "head-washing" ritual to settle the *lwa* in the individual's head. The *laver-tête* is considered a baptism of the *lwa*. As the "horse" strengthens his or her relationship with the *lwa* through repeated possession and offerings to the *mâit-tête*, transition to the possessed state becomes smoother and calmer, and the individual is supposed to acquire increasing control over the *lwa*.

After the onset of possession, individuals maintain a steady and characteristic rate of possession throughout their active adult years. Sometime between the ages of forty-five and sixty, individuals undergo a decline in frequency of possession and soon cease to become possessed at all. This coincides with the release of their social obligations to the next generation.

Elsewhere (Womack 1998, 2001), I have noted that vodou is a form of psychotherapy that provides practitioners with a "possession career" that helps them deal with conditions of economic and social stress. In childhood, individuals are presented with a number of acceptable social personalities. Naming the possessing *lwa* provides the individual with a consistent social personality, as well as with a guardian spirit. Possession occurs between puberty and the end of family responsibilities. In *vodou*, possession is first encouraged and used for its psychotherapeutic value. It is then brought under control and finally extinguished through manipulation of symbols in the ritual of trance possession.

The Power of Medical Labels

Naming or labeling also has the power to change things in medical and psychiatric diagnosis. The power of labeling has been demonstrated by a classic study conducted by David L. Rosenhan (1973). Rosenhan checked himself and others into hospitals located in different states on the East and West coasts of the United States. The pseudopatients included a psychology graduate student, three psychologists, a pediatrician, a psychiatrist, a painter, and a housewife. Three were women, and five were men. The circumstances in the hospitals varied: "Some [hospitals] were old and shabby, some were quite new. Some had good staff-patient ratios, others were quite understaffed. Only one was a strict private hospital. All of the others were supported by state or federal funds or, in one instance, by university funds" (2006:2[1973]).[5]

During intake interviews at the different hospitals, the pseudopatients complained of hearing voices, describing the voices as "often unclear, but as far as he could tell they said 'empty,' 'hollow,' and 'thud.' The voices were unfamiliar and were of the same sex as the pseudopatient."[6] The description of the voices was chosen to suggest that the pseudopatient perceived his or her life as meaningless. All but one of the pseudopatients was admitted with a diagnosis of schizophrenia. Immediately after admission to the psychiatric ward, the pseudopatients began to behave normally, responding to instructions from attendants, to calls for medications, and to dining-hall instructions. In one example, "When asked by staff how he was feeling, he indicated that he was fine, that he no longer experienced symptoms."[7]

The pseudopatients took daily copious notes, an act consistent with their missions as researchers. Though the note-taking was "normal" for researchers, in three cases, the note-taking was viewed by hospital staff as evidence of pathology, specifically as compulsive behavior. Once diagnosed as schizophrenic, the label stuck. Each of the pseudopatients diagnosed as schizophrenic was discharged with a diagnosis of schizophrenia "in remission."[8]

Though staff at the hospitals never recognized the sanity of the pseudopatients, 35 of a total 118 patients on the admissions ward suspected the researchers were sane. One likely explanation voiced by the authentic patients was, "You're not crazy. You're a journalist, or a professor. . . . You're checking up on the hospital."[9] These patients recognized that the pseudopatients experienced a different reality than their own, and they developed their own labels and categories to explain the difference.

Hospital staff, on the other hand, had been socialized into a we-they world view that defined themselves as "experts" and patients as impaired and dependent "others." Though pseudopatients behaved sanely once admitted, behaviors stimulated by the hospital environment were interpreted as characteristic of their "insanity." Their sane and appropriate behavior in the institutional context was regarded as evidence in support of the diagnosis of insanity. Rosenhan notes:

> A psychiatric label has a life and an influence of its own. Once the impression has been formed that the patient is schizophrenic, the expectation is that he will continue to be schizophrenic. . . . Such labels, conferred by mental health professionals, are as influential on the patient as they are on his relatives and friends, and it should not surprise anyone that the diagnosis acts on all of them as a self-fulfilling prophecy. Eventually, the patient himself accepts the diagnosis, with all of its surplus meanings and expectations, and behaves accordingly.[10]

Rosenhan does not reject the idea that deviance exists, nor that mental illness is experienced as anxiety and personal anguish by those afflicted with it. Rather, he asserts that labels can be misapplied and that, once applied, they impose a reality of their own, on both the person who applies the label and on the person to whom the label is applied. As noted above, pseudopatients whose behavior qualified them for release were described as being "in remission." The label of mental illness, once applied, was never removed.

Results of the findings were tested at a research hospital to see whether staff could distinguish between pseudopatients and people with actual psychiatric disorders: "The staff was informed that at some time during the following three months, one or more pseudopatients would attempt to be admitted into the psychiatric hospital."[11] Staff members were asked to rate each patient who presented himself at the hospital or on the ward according to the likelihood that the patient was a pseudopatient. Although no pseudopatients actually presented themselves, forty-one patients were identified, with high confidence, as being pseudopatients. Rosenhan concludes, "However much we may be personally convinced that we can tell the normal from the abnormal, the evidence is simply not compelling."[12]

Humans are social animals. We are able to quickly perceive and analyze, often on an unconscious levels, the way in which we view each other. We interpret signals from others almost as quickly as we apprehend them. An important component of our social lives is the ability to negotiate social space. Labels allow us to attach meanings that facilitate social interactions. Factors that should be considered in evaluating these complex social exchanges is whether they facilitate or impede our ability to attain social and psychological goals.

Labels, Diagnosis, and Healing

Labeling can be healing because it establishes a process of bringing order out of chaos (Larsen 2004). The New Zealand novelist Janet Frame was diagnosed with schizophrenia, but when she won a literary award, her psychiatrists withdrew the diagnosis. She resented losing the label because the diagnosis "had been the answer to all my misgivings about myself" (Angier 2004:12). Stephen J. Kunitz notes, "Naming helps demystify otherwise unknown conditions; it makes possible a community of suffering; and it implies a prognosis and guides treatment. But it can also lead to inappropriate treatment and labeling and neglect of the unique attributes of the individual who is ill. It is thus a double-edged sword" (2006:280).

People who are labeled with a diagnosis of psychiatric disorder do not always experience relief from its symptoms. In many cases, they become labeled as marginal persons (Jenkins and Barrett 2003; Barham and Haywood 1990; Goffman 1961; Barrett 1989; 1996; 1998). If they can establish a community of shared symptoms and goals, they may be able to derive comfort from these shared goals. Psychotherapy can become a shared process of socialization.

A British qualitative interview study found a difference in the way long-term and chronic psychiatric patients explained their illness and the way newly referred patients explained their troubles. All but one of the twenty-two long-term patients held a medical psychiatric model when talking about their problems, while the newly referred patients had a more negotiable model when talking about their problems (Lindow 1986). This is consistent with the long-held psychological view that psychiatric patients are socialized into adopting a psychiatric model. In folk psychological wisdom, Freudian patients have Freudian dreams; Jungian patients have Jungian dreams.

Before consulting a psychiatrist, patients in the British study discussed and negotiated the relevance of a psychiatric perspective with their family and friends. Lindow (1986) describes this as being highly active in the social management of potentially stigmatizing information about themselves. Thoits (1985) describes this process as a dimension in the self-labeling process. Estroff et al. (1991) noted that those who presented a medical/clinical, or a combined medical/clinical and emotional/developmental explanation of their difficulties were most likely to say that they were mentally ill. Through time, participants in the study tended to unlabel themselves as mentally ill. Estroff and colleagues suggested that the hospital context shaped the self-labeling as mentally ill during the first interviews, and that the change in attitude was due to a change in physical and social environment.

Lindow found that self-descriptions changed even within a single interview. When discussing appointments with their doctors, informants described their problems as medical; when talking about attitudes to mental disorder in the workplace they resorted to an insanity stereotype, using such terms as "screwy," "crazy," or "mental" (1986:385).

In Western medicine, psychiatric disorders are often viewed as being permanent, which means they require permanent intervention. Larson (2004) conducted an ethnographic study of an early intervention program in Copenhagen, Denmark, which included young people diagnosed for the first time within the "schizophrenic spectrum," as defined by the World Health Organization. The treatment program linked the newest generation of antipsychotic medicine with a supportive and therapeutic approach based on cognitive therapy. Frank, twenty, was diagnosed with paranoid schizophrenic psychosis. He was convinced that his psychosis was triggered by his extensive use of drugs, including cannabis, cocaine, and hallucinogenic mushrooms. "After a while, the strange sensations and perceptions came to him even when he had not taken the drugs" (Larson 2005:453).

This may be a case in which the patient is more on the mark than the physicians. Synapses within the brain are formed in early childhood. This is the chemical process in which information is transmitted from one neuron to another. Our cognition is shaped by the synaptic patterns established in early childhood. Hallucinogens temporarily disrupt established synaptic patterns. Prolonged use of hallucinogens can establish new synaptic patterns that do not conform to previously established patterns of interacting with the environment.

The Power of Words

There is a pervasive belief cross-culturally that words have the power to heal. An example is provided by R. Jon McGee, who studied Lacandon Maya in Central America: "Some Lacandon men . . . know therapeutic incantations in which the words themselves have the power to heal" (2002:156).The words were considered powerful independently of the social power of the person chanting them: "The beneficial effects of the words could be felt within a few minutes simply by reciting the incantation and then blowing on the patient. Curing incantations were used for headaches, stomachaches, nausea, childbirth, even bleeding" (2002:156). As in other societies, among Maya, the power of words is considered to be dangerous for the healer and for others:

> Few men admit to knowing or using healing incantations. These chants are considered dangerous because if they are not recited properly the person attempting the incantation may be harmed. I was lucky that Chan K¹ in Viejo [McGee's chief informant] knew several healing incantations and did not mind if I listened when he used them. He was not, however, interested in teaching me any incantations because he felt that with my imperfect Maya I might harm myself. Consequently, I never recorded any incantations." (2002:157)

Much evidence has been produced in psychology, sociology, and anthropology to demonstrate that words have the power to change the course of human events. However, we do not, at this point, have the tools to determine whether words are powerful beyond their social and psychological context.

FOLK TAXONOMIES AND EXPLANATIONS OF ILLNESS

Though naming a disorder can bring order out of chaos, thus facilitating the process of healing, labeling can also contribute to a negative prognosis. Cassandra White describes the importance of naming in her study of defining Hansen's disease (leprosy) in Rio de Janeiro, Brazil. White compared the **folk taxonomy** of the disease with diagnoses provided by medical professionals. The anthropologist notes, "The name of a disease and the metaphorical associations with that name can have a significant influence on how people respond to their diagnosis" (2005:317).

Such names as plague, tuberculosis, and AIDS take on associations that lead to social stigma because the diseases are conceptually linked to social behavior that has been deemed inappropriate. In other cases, such as cancer, the name itself evokes terror because it is conceptually associated with death.[13] The Brazilian folk name for the disorder studied by White is *lepra* (leprosy), a term that connotes uncleanness in the public mind. A number of the patients White studied linked *lepra* to conditions considered unclean in Brazilian folk taxonomy, such as dogs and sexual promiscuity, whereas the biomedical diagnosis linked the disorder to a bacillus, *Mycobacterium leprae*, an organism that multiplies very slowly and produces a disease that mainly affects the skin, nerves, and mucous membranes.[14]

According to the U.S. Centers for Disease Control, Hansen's disease is a chronic infectious disease that "usually affects the skin and peripheral nerves[15] but has a wide range of possible clinical manifestations."[16] In 2002, 763,917 new cases were detected worldwide, with ninety-six cases occurring in the United States. According to the World Health Organization, 90 percent of cases of Hansen's disease occurred in Brazil, Madagascar, Mozambique, Tanzania, and Nepal.[17] Worldwide, 1.2 million people are permanently disabled as a result of the disease, but the disease can be treated with an antibiotic regimen.[18]

In Brazil, the etiology described by biomedicine and the folk taxonomy described by patients overlap. The folk taxonomy described by four patients interviewed by White is that *lepra* is spread by the wind (*o vento*). Health care workers explain to patients that Hansen's disease is "transmitted by droplets emitted by a contagious person while breathing, thus, 'through the air'" (White 2005:314). The U.S. Centers for Disease Control notes that, "Although the mode of transmission of Hansen's disease remains uncertain, most investigators think that *M. leprae* is usually spread from person to person in respiratory droplets."[19]

In Brazil, patients who suffer from Hansen's disease and medical people who treat it agree on the etiology that it is transmitted by air; however, explanations and treatments for the disease are linked to class. Patients interviewed by White came mostly from *favelas* (shantytowns) or from low-income working-class neighborhoods. By contrast, health care workers interviewed by White came from the middle class or upper class and were college educated. White writes of middle- and upper-class health care workers who "unaware of what patients' daily lives are like, often assume that patients will be able to follow biomedical directions (such as washing clothes or performing manual labor) that would increase resorption of bone in the hands, and purchasing adequate shoes that protect feet with nerve damage from injury" (2005:313).

An intermediary factor in addressing Hansen's disease in Brazil are **NGOs** (nongovernmental organizations). White notes that workers for NGOs could often provide a communications bridge between patients of the lower classes and health care providers of the middle- and upper-classes because of their own class affiliations and experiences: "many of the NGO volunteers I met came from some of the same working-class neighborhoods as patients and thus were better equipped to communicate with them and help them understand their illness" (2005:313).

White's model of differences in social class, and its implication for communication, is applicable to other treatment contexts. She writes that class distinctions developed in nonmedical contexts extend into the medical contexts, so that lower-class individuals defer to the opinions of individuals in higher social status of their own, and therefore, will not voice their concerns or question the judgments of their "superiors":

> In biomedical settings, this deference usually takes the form of silence and nodding on the part of patients and false acknowledgement of understanding. This communication style results in misunderstanding on the part of both health care workers and patients; health care workers in Brazil, as in the United States, expect some degree of responsibility on the part of patients for their own health. (2005:313)

Differences in expectations between health care workers and their patients can affect the outcome of a diagnosed disorder:

> Health care workers tend to blame patients for problems that result when patients claim to understand something they did not or when patients failed to provide them with important information about their symptoms. This situation can be frustrating for physicians and potentially life threatening for patients. In addition, health care workers' decisions about what information they should reveal to patients about their condition are related to traditional paternalistic attitudes of the upper and middle classes in Brazil toward members of the lower classes. (2005:313)

Traditional Wisdom, Folk Taxonomies, and Medical Paradigms

The paternalism White identifies as being part of the medico-patient interaction is pervasive. An individual who has earned a medical degree may consider herself or himself superior to a patient who has no such certification. In some cases, however, it appears that this difference in understanding may be due to a difference in terminology and world view, rather than a basic misunderstanding of the etiology of a disease.

In a study of nightblindness in a Hausa community in northern Niger, anthropologists Lauren S. Blum et al. compared medical diagnoses with indigenous explanations for the condition. They then analyzed folk treatments within the context of Western models of causation. Explanations for nightblindness involved multiple levels. The medical model attributed nightblindness in young children and pregnant women to vitamin A deficiency. The **indigenous** model attributed nightblindness to lack of "good food." Hausa associated nightblindness in pregnant women with the lack of "good foods" and increased nutritional demands of pregnancy.

Hausa ranking of "good foods" is as follows: liver, red meat, dairy products, and dark green leafy vegetables. For Hausa, liver and red meat are preferred preventatives of nightblindness, as well as the preferred cure. If liver and red meat are not available because the family is too poor to provide them, the leaves of baobab, red sorrel, or bean are recommended by Hausa. Hausa prescriptions for avoidance or treatment of nightblindness are virtually identical to those prescribed by international health organizations, while using different terminology.

According to KidsHealth, an online resource funded by the Nemours Foundation, the nutritional sources identified by indigenous beliefs among the Hausa are precisely those that prevent and are helpful in treating visual disorders. The KidsHealth website states: "Vitamin A prevents eye problems, promotes a healthy immune system, is essential for the growth and development of cells, and keeps skin healthy."[20]

Information provided by the KidsHealth website supports the folk beliefs of Hausa-speakers in a community in northern Niger. The KidsHealth website lists the following foods as good sources of vitamin A: milk, eggs, liver, fortified cereals, darkly colored orange or green vegetables (such as carrots, sweet potatoes, pumpkin, and kale), and orange fruits such as cantaloupe, apricots, peaches, papayas, and mangoes.[21] Most of these fruits and vegetables are outside the Hausa ecological zone, with the exception of pumpkin and mangoes, which are seasonal.

Though medical diagnosis and Hausa folk explanations derive from different paradigms, they identify the same source of the ailment and prescribe essentially the same treatment. The "good foods" identified by Hausa are all good sources of vitamin A. A lack of vitamin A leads to nightblindness, and the treatment preferred by both Hausa and Western medical personnel is based on replenishing the sufferer's access to vitamin A. Whether administered in medication or through foods rich in vitamin A, the outcome is the same: Symptoms of nightblindness are relieved within hours.

Medical Discourse

Language and use of terminology have special significance in conversations about health and disease. Some words, such as "cancer," imply negative outcomes for patients. In discussing a patient's diagnosis and prognosis, this can affect the outcome of the treatment. In his book *Talking with Patients* (1985), Eric J. Cassell notes that doctors who view language as a means of accurately referring to medically defined diseases may not understand what these terms mean to patients. Cassell recommends paying attention to paralinguistic cues, such as intonation and pitch, to assess the patient's underlying beliefs and unconscious assessment of what those terms mean for his or her diagnosis. A number of researchers have noted that the patient's understanding of a physician's use of words can affect whether the patient complies with the physician's recommendations.

To a large degree, a medical diagnosis can produce the same effects that diagnosis of sorcery can produce in traditional societies. As Claude Lévi-Strauss and others have noted, a diagnosis of sorcery can result in social and literal death:

> the community withdraws. Standing aloof from the accursed, it treats him not only as though he were already dead but as though he were a source of danger to the entire group. On every occasion and by every action, the social body suggests death to the unfortunate victim, who no longer hopes to escape what he considers to be his fate. (Lévi-Strauss 1963:167)

Having been deprived of his social support network, the victim of sorcery surrenders to the inevitable: death. He is socially dead for some time before he is physiologically dead. As Lévi-Strauss notes, the death results from physiological causes triggered by the individual's certainty of death:

> the activity of the sympathetic nervous system becomes intensified and disorganized; it may, sometimes within a few hours, lead to a decrease in the volume of blood and concomitant drop in blood pressure, which results in irreparable damage to the circulatory organs. The rejection of food and drink, frequent among patients in the throes of intense anxiety, precipitates this process; dehydration acts as a stimulus to the sympathetic nervous system, and the decrease in blood volume is accentuated by the growing permeability of the capillary vessels. (1963:168)

Lévi-Strauss notes that this process has been observed among victims of bombings, battle shock, and even surgical operations. The victim dies, even though an autopsy does not reveal physical trauma sufficient to cause death. Lévi-Strauss' colleague Michel Foucault notes that discourse constitutes the social order. Discourse becomes translated into practice (behavior and social interaction) (1972:49[1969]).

In Foucault's view, the words of the doctor become authoritative. The patient must either comply with the doctor's instructions or become "noncompliant," a term that suggests that the patient is responsible for the negative course of his or her own disorder. The power relationship in medical discourse favors the physician or other medical practitioner: "You did not follow my instructions; therefore you died (or your condition got worse)." This is akin to "blaming the victim." However, the more widespread implication is that the medical practitioner has knowledge that is not usually available to the patient. Thus, the medical practitioner has the real power of specialized knowledge, as well as the social power of access to medical discourse. The "noncompliant" patient challenges the social power of specialized medical knowledge.

Medical Discourse and the Negotiation of Social Space

The practice of medicine is negotiated in social space. Richard Frankel (1983) notes that the physician uses touch and conversation to draw the patient's attention away from physical manipulations of his or her body. The doctor-patient relationship involves a physical intimacy rivaled only by sex. Conversation, used as a distraction, can be beneficial to the patient, in that the patient can accept intrusions that could otherwise be viewed as aggressive. We tend to think of verbal exchanges between doctor and patient as being entirely informative, but they can also defuse the volatility of such close physical proximity.

Jay Katz (1984) notes that physicians use a complex organization of silence and speech in face-to-face interaction with patients. He adds that we assume the doctor-patient interaction involves only medical intervention, typically in the form of machines and medications. In fact, the doctor-patient interaction involves negotiation of social and physical space. In her analysis of informed consent, Kathryn Taylor (1988) notes that physicians feel stress in telling patients bad news. As a result, they may not fully inform the patient of what their condition implies. In order to minimize their own personal involvement, physicians may develop a routine that obscures complete disclosure of the patient's condition.

Frankel (1984) notes that the form of medical discourse favors the physician in terms of power. Candace West (1984) observes that doctors are more likely to interrupt patients than vice versa, especially if the patients are female or minorities. On the other hand, female patients are more likely than male patients to interrupt physicians.

On some levels, the asymmetry between doctor and patient may work to the patient's benefit, if it reinforces the patient's confidence in the physician. On other levels, the asymmetry may be detrimental to the patient, if the patient feels too intimidated to ask questions that could affect the course of treatment. It may be difficult for a physician or other medical personnel to determine which approach is likely to yield the best results. That is one of many reasons why the doctor-patient relationship can be mandated by law or other forms of rules imposed from outside. It is also why physicians and other medical personnel should be trained in communication skills.

Perhaps the most important of these communication skills is paying attention to the patient's reaction to the information provided by the physician or medical caretaker. Patients react in different ways, depending on their cultural background and particular circumstances. Medical personnel are trained in the biological manifestations of particular diseases, and increasingly, they are trained in formulas for informing patients of the particular ramifications of their disorders. A more subtle issue, and one that may never be addressed, is how to tailor a diagnosis to the psychological needs of a particular patient. This may be an area in which shamans (traditional healers) are better trained.[22]

The Placebo Effect

Physicians have long known that any diagnosis or course of treatment will produce a positive effect as long as it does not discourage the patient from participating in the treatment. The question is not whether placebos are effective but why they are effective.

The most common explanation is based in psychology: Placebos are effective because people believe in them. Irving Kirsch and Guy Saperstein evaluated the placebo effect in nineteen clinical trials conducted on 2,318 patients with a primary diagnosis of depression. These patients had been randomly assigned to either antidepressant medication or a placebo. The researchers concluded that 75 percent of the benefit from the active drug resulted from the patient's expectation of improvement, rather than adjustments in brain chemistry from the drug itself. Kirsch and Saperstein extended their analysis of the placebo effect further by suggesting that the 25 percent of patients whose symptoms were relieved by the drug may have been persuaded by its side effects:

> This study suggests that antidepressants might function as active placebos, in which the side effects amplify the placebo effect by convincing patients that they are receiving a potent drug. So if a patient takes a pill that causes side effects, he or she feels better because they believe they have been given an actual antidepressant and that the pill must be working.[23]

Much of the effectiveness of placebos may be due to the social context of healing. As a number of scholars have noted, illness is experienced as chaotic, disorderly, and out of control. It feels as if our bodies are rising up against us. Naming the disorder can confer real benefits by explaining the source of our discomfort. In an article in the *Psychiatric Times*, the psychiatrist Walter A. Brown notes, "Most physicians make at least some use of the placebo effect to enhance treatments, whether they realize it or not." He adds:

It is instructive to note a feature of virtually every antidepressant efficacy trial: In outpatients with moderately severe depression whose symptoms are assessed using the Hamilton Rating Scale, most of the improvement occurs during the first 2 weeks of treatment, and during this time, no differences in outcome between active drug and placebo are evident. After about 2 weeks, the placebo response reaches a plateau. Response to medication may continue to increase for a time, but during the period when most of the improvement occurs, placebo and medication produce similar responses.[24]

Brown suggests that many psychological factors are important components of the healing context: "In my opinion, the term placebo is misleading. In fact, patients who receive 'placebo' treatment get much more than a sugar pill, whether they are enrolled in a placebo-controlled clinical trial or are the recipients of ordinary medical care."[25] Brown enumerates important elements of what he calls the "treatment situation": recognized healer, healing symbols, evaluation, healing rituals, diagnosis, prognosis, and plausible treatment. He adds, "People benefit from getting an explanation for their distress. It brings the problem down to size and makes their suffering seem more manageable. Suggesting honest, appropriate, and positive expectations about a patient's illness can be worthwhile."[26] Brown concludes:

What we call the placebo response is probably a complex interaction of expectation, conditioning, endorphin effects, and distress relief. Our role as psychiatrists is to be aware of the conditions in which the placebo response may be likely to play a strong role in recovery. We have an important part to play in inspiring confidence, evaluating the patient and providing a diagnosis, and enhancing the treatment response. Many of these facets of the placebo response are components of "bedside manner." We do not need to have a full understanding of how the placebo response works in order to harness some of its benefits in practice.[27]

The issue of what constitutes health and healing is complex. Does a relief of symptoms constitute healing? Certainly, optimism and a sense that one is getting better can promote both psychological and biological healing.

II

MAINTAINING HEALTH AND HEALING THE WHOLE PERSON

There is wisdom in this beyond the rules of physic. A man's own observation, what he finds good of and what he finds hurt of, is the best physic to preserve health.

—Francis Bacon, *Essays, Of Regimen of Health*

The tepee is much better to live in: always clean, warm in winter, cool in summer, easy to move. . . . Indians and animals know better how to live than white man; nobody can be in good health if he does not have all the time fresh air, sunshine, and good water.

—Flying Hawk, *Statement in old age*

In the United States, health and healing are typically viewed in biomedical terms, so that the life cycle and lifestyles are often considered only in terms of biology, narrowly defined. This **ethnocentric** view disregards the intricate interrelationship of biology, psychology, and social interaction. Thus, modes of maintaining health and promoting healing are framed in terms of regimens imposed on the body. In Part II of *The Anthropology of Health and Healing*, we take a cross-cultural view of the human life cycle and lifestyles to evaluate factors that appear to contribute to health and longevity, as well as those that appear to cause illness.

Chapters 5, 6 and 7, "The Human Life Cycle," situate health implications within each stage of the life cycle, from birth to death. Chapter 5, "Coming of Age" examines childbirth and childrearing practices. Chapter 6, "The Reproductive Years," explores expectations attending adolescence, sexuality, and parenthood. Chapter 7, "Aging and Endings" follows the trajectory of the human life cycle from grandparenthood to old age. Chapter 8, "Lifestyle and Health," explores ways in which we can promote our own health and avoid illness, based on data from cross-cultural comparisons of lifestyles and their health implications. This chapter also considers the importance of play and pleasurable activities in sustaining health.

5

The Human Life Cycle

Coming of Age

CASE STUDY
Horticultural Models for the Human Life Cycle

Hindus and Hopis link their view of the stages of human life to the life cycle of plants, which are central to their survival. Hindus of South Asia are agriculturalists; Hopis of the U.S. Southwest are horticulturalists. The difference between the two is that Hindus produce a surplus to be sold at market, whereas Hopis produce crops for their own use. According to Hindu cosmology, the entire universe, including humans, undergoes a continual tripartite cycle of birth and childhood, maturity and fruition, followed by decay and death. Death precedes a period of dormancy, after which the cycle begins again. The creator god Brahma presides over the first stage, when plants emerge from the ground and humans emerge from the womb. The sustainer god Vishnu presides over the second stage of life, when plants become productive and humans become householders, who provide for their families and produce the next generation. In the final stage of life, after the harvest and after the productive stage of human life is over, the plants and the human body begin to decline in health, vigor, and strength. Both the fields and humans must be cleared away so the new crop can be planted and the new cycle of life can begin. Śiva, the destroyer, is the god who accomplishes this task, but he serves a dual purpose: He both sweeps away decay and plants the seed that will later emerge through the ground. Just as the seed seems dead but contains life, the spark of life in humans will return in a new incarnation. For Hopis, on the other side of the planet, water is the symbol of life. In their arid region, crops grow only if there is water; humans live only if there is breath, which is moist. Corn, the mainstay of Hopi life, is female because females, like the stalks of corn, produce new life. Hopis are matrilineal, tracing their group membership through the female line. Thus, females convey the life of the lineage. Just as women bear children when they are adults, the stalks of corn bear ears of corn, their children. The digging stick men use to plant the corn is male, thus the digging stick prepares the way for the new life. When humans take their last breath, the moist breath becomes a cloud that travels to the land of the ancestors. When Hopis need water for their crops, the breath of their ancestors returns as rain.

Humans enter life through birth and leave it through death. Both reorder the experience of the individual and the alignment of social relationships within a group. Both events are universally addressed through rites of passage. **Rites of passage**, analyzed by Arnold van Gennep in his book *Les Rites de Passage* (1908), are rituals that accompany a "passage from one situation to another or from one cosmic or social world to another" (1960:10[1908]). According to Van Gennep, rites of passage involve three processes: (1) *rites of separation* sever the individual from his or her previous social status; (2) *transition rites* address the time when an individual has lost his or her previous social status, but has not yet acquired a new status; and (3) *rites of incorporation* settle the individual into his or her new social status.

Van Gennep describes these three phases as preliminal, liminal, and postliminal rites. The word "liminal" refers to a marginal state in which the social persona of an individual has been stripped away to be newly defined. In the preliminal phase, the individual is about to lose the social persona he or she and his or her social group have built up over the years. The initiate will enter a new territory, in which his or her social identity is not clearly defined, and is therefore, "dangerous" both to the individual and to the group as a whole. Thus, a rite of passage conducts an individual and a group through the "dangerous" transition from one social status to another.

Rites of passage include baptisms and naming ceremonies, in which social identity is conferred onto a new member of a group, as well as coming-of-age ceremonies, in which an individual acquires a form of social identity that leaves the unencumbered state of childhood behind and initiates the beginning of adult identity. Marriage marks the onset of socially responsible fertility. Typically, a man and woman exchange vows of responsibility to each other and to the children they will eventually produce, as well as to the society as a whole. End-of-life ceremonies, such as funerals, mark the cessation of social responsibilities for an individual and the group.

The fecundity of women, and the dramatic way in which their bodies "embody" the life cycle, provide a powerful metaphor for the circularity of life, as well as the demands the life cycle makes upon us. Van Gennep adds, "Such changes of condition do not occur without disturbing the life of society and the individual, and it is the function of rites of passage to reduce their harmful effects" (1960:13[1908]).

The human life cycle is biological, psychological, and cultural. We acquire life through conception and birth, and we acquire the skills we need to sustain our lives through physical growth and the process of socialization. We try to transmit our skills to the next generation, but human life is complex, and many life skills are acquired only through experience and experimentation. At some point, different depending on genetics and circumstances, we lose control over our bodies and over our lives. Eventually, we die.

In this and following chapters we examine consistencies and variability in how human groups define and organize the human life cycle. Our object is to analyze how phases of the life cycle are defined cross-culturally, as well as how attitudes and practices associated with these phases factor into definitions of health and the practice of healing.

Though life cycle transitions are universally considered dangerous because of the alteration in social relationships they engender, there is a dramatic difference in how these disruptions are viewed cross-culturally. Folk beliefs in societies that are not organized around Western medicine view them as disruptive situations that can be controlled through ritual. In Western medicine, they are often viewed as disorders that can be treated through medications.

CONCEPTS REGARDING CONCEPTION

Trobriand Islanders, studied by Bronislaw Malinowski early in the twentieth century, considered that the human essence, the soul, journeyed after death between the islands where humans live, to Tuma, the island of the dead, then back again as a new human in the form of an embryo. It is not surprising that Trobrianders see the process of death and rebirth as a journey from one island to another, since their daily lives involve journeys between islands. The Trobriand Islands, now known as the Kiriwina Islands, are a cluster of islands off the northeasternmost part of what is now Papua, New Guinea.

In describing the journey of the human spirit, Malinowski asserts, with his usual flair, "the new life, in Trobriand tradition, begins with death" (1929:170). After death, the human spirit or *baloma* "moves to Tuma, the Island of the Dead, where he leads a pleasant existence analogous to the terrestrial life—only much happier" (1929:170). On the island of Tuma, the human spirit undergoes a continual process of rejuvenation. If the spirit's hair grays and its skin becomes wrinkled, the spirit sloughs them off and returns to a youthful appearance. Eventually, however, the process of rejuvenation palls: "when a spirit becomes tired of constant rejuvenation, when he has led a long existence 'underneath' as the natives call it, he may want to return to earth again; and then he leaps back in age and becomes a small preborn infant" (1929:171).

Baloma float in the sea until they are rescued by a spirit, who will guide them to their human mothers. Malinowski's account of this process was provided by one of his consultants, Tomwaya Lakwabulo:

> A child floats on a drift log. A spirit sees it is good-looking. She takes it. She is the spirit of the mother or of the father of the pregnant woman. . . . Then she puts it on the head, in the hair, of the pregnant woman, who suffers headache, vomits, and has an ache in the belly. Then the child comes down into the belly, and she is really pregnant. She says: "Already it (the child) has found me; already they (the spirits) have brought me the child." (1929:173)

Malinowski notes, "These rejuvenated spirits, these little pre-incarnated babies or spirit-children, are the only source from which humanity draws its new supplies of life" (1929:171). Trobrianders are matrilineal, and a spirit-child can only be reborn from the womb of a woman who belongs to the same matrilineal clan and subclan as the spirit-child. Thus, the child's essence is inherited from its mother.

When Malinowski tried to explain to Trobrianders that sperm causes conception, they replied that this might be true for other people but not for them. Trobrianders connected sex with conception, but they did not consider sex sufficient cause for producing a child. They assured Malinowski that a virgin cannot conceive because there is no open passage through which the spirit-child can enter. Malinowski sought to impose the Western biological model onto Trobrianders, but they resisted such conversion in favor of a social and conceptual model of conception.

Malinowski's data led him to believe that Trobrianders did not understand the biological basis for conception. Other anthropologists generalized this view to Pacific Islanders as a whole, many of whom have similar explanations for conception. The idea that Pacific Islanders did not understand the biological basis of conception prevailed among anthropologists until the 1950s, when a young anthropologist named Jane G. Goodale traveled to Australia to conduct her fieldwork among Tiwi women of Melville Island, off the northern coast of Australia. One of her primary goals in conducting this research was to examine the question of whether Pacific Islanders understand the biological basis of conception.

Biological and Social Paternity

Early in her fieldwork, Goodale approached a group of men and women and asked them, "Who makes babies and how do they get inside the mother?" Their reaction was entirely unexpected to her, but entirely reasonable to Tiwi. Goodale writes:

> The men and women stopped their talk and looked at me questioningly. When I said nothing, they looked at each other and began to giggle, then broke into uncontrolled laughter. They paused only to repeat my question to each other and to those who, hearing the uproar, came to investigate. Each time my question was repeated, the laughter resumed with renewed convulsions. Finally, one woman dried her streaming eyes and caught her breath enough to answer my repeated question: "Boy make him," she said and looked so contemptuous at my innocence that I feared for my future ability to get any useful information from these people. (1994:136[1971])

Tiwi sophistication in the matter of biological and social paternity became clear later in Goodale's fieldwork after she had learned much more about relationships within the group. She writes, "Without a doubt, the Tiwi today know that sexual intercourse between a man and woman is likely to result in pregnancy, that husbands and lovers both can *make* babies" (1994:137[1971]).

Goodale describes the case of a man who returned to the group after having worked in Darwin, capital of Australia's Northern Territory, for more than a year. He was returning to see his wife and newborn son. When Goodale asked the woman "who was the father of her child, she replied with the name of her husband, but when I asked her who *made* the baby, she gave me the name of another man" (1994:137[1971]). Other women shared this view of the relationship: "I asked the other women how they knew the name of the man who *made* the baby, and they said, 'That is easy. The baby looks like B., its mother's lover,' and indeed the infant was the image of its biological father" (1994:137[1971]).

The relative ease with which Tiwi women move between relationships with husbands and lovers is largely due to two factors: their matrilineal inheritance pattern and their **subsistence practices**, in which women contribute a great deal to the economy. Because Tiwi are matrilineal, a child belongs to its mother's kin group. The child's social father is important in the life of the child because he contributes to the social identity of a child born to his wife.

Tiwi believe that the pregnancy of a man's wife is announced to him in a dream. Like Trobrianders, Tiwi consider the child to be the reincarnation of an ancestral spirit, and further, Tiwi assign to the husband the role of identifying that ancestor and giving the name to the child. These customs—dreaming the baby, identifying the ancestor, and naming the child—establish a social bond between the child and its mother's husband, whether or not he is the man who "made" the baby.

On the surface, Tiwi attitudes toward conception and kinship appear very different from those of people in the United States; however, there are some striking similarities. The American legal system distinguishes between biological and social paternity by defining a child's father as the man married to its mother at the time of its birth. Further, a man can acquire paternity rights and responsibilities by adopting a child. Men who donate sperm for purposes of insemination cannot claim paternity even though the child produced by his sperm carries his genetic heritage.

Anthropologists have noted that, cross-culturally, paternity is culturally defined. A common phrase is, "You always know who your mother is, but you don't necessarily know who your father is." This is based on the idea that pregnancy is a visible sign of impending motherhood, whereas the father's biological contribution to parenthood is not so apparent. Under certain circumstances, however, social parenthood is extended to women. A woman can become a mother by adopting a child. In the United States, a woman who becomes a surrogate gives birth, but does not become a mother. The mother is the woman for whom the surrogate carries and gives birth to the child.

The Biology of Feeding the Baby

People of the rural community of Zumbagua, in Ecuador, emphasize social parenthood over the biological parenthood of procreation. A woman does not become a mother simply by giving birth. Similarly, a man does not become a father simply by having had sex with a child's mother. In Zumbagua, men and women become parents through another biological act, feeding the child. Mary Weismantel writes: "In the parish, any act involving food performed in the presence of others expresses important social facts" (2001:141). Weismantel adds:

> Andean beliefs and practices about illness, death, and healing reveal an underlying conception of the human body as a material object built up over time through various substances and acts: ingesting food and drink, sharing emotional states with individuals or spirits, being physically close to people or objects. Bonds between people are created in the same way—gradually.[1] The two processes are interrelated: the bodies of individuals are linked through shared substances to the bodies of family members.[2] (2001:141)

Weismantel concludes, "Those who eat together in the same household share the same flesh in a quite literal sense: they are made of the same stuff" (2001:142). In this conceptual world, it is not the sexual union of female and male, nor the union of sperm and egg, that defines parenthood. Rather, it is the sharing of food and social intercourse that defines the relationship between parent and child. This view ensures that all children have the opportunity to obtain parental caretakers, even if the woman and man whose sexual union gave birth to them do not want them. A child's parents are the people who demonstrate social responsibility for the child by feeding it and otherwise investing in its well-being.

Sperm Donors: Genetic and Social Parenthood

One of my colleagues in graduate school at UCLA supplemented his income by donating sperm. It was a matter of great interest to the rest of us to wonder what it might be like to encounter a half-dozen Harolds on a bus some day. At that time, it was assumed that our physical appearance was determined by biology but our attitudes and behavior were determined by socialization. Since that time, children conceived by sperm donation have reached maturity, and our understanding of the relationship between biology and behavior has become much more complicated.

Children conceived through sperm donation, and increasingly egg donation, have become an important resource for investigating the relationship between biology and culture, a debate originated by the anthropologist Franz Boas early in the twentieth century. One issue involved in the quest for biological ancestry has to do with genetically transmitted disorders. Michelle J. noted that her daughter Cheyenne exhibited behaviors that had not previously been observed in her family. The child was extremely sensitive to sound and walked on her toes. After checking out this tendency on the Internet, Michelle J. connected with six other children who displayed similar behavioral patterns. Two had autism and two others displayed symptoms of a sensory disorder related to autism. The donor whose sperm conceived the children is protected by anonymity, as is necessary for legal reasons. No one would donate sperm for a few hundred dollars if they were later to be sued for medical costs.

In another case, a sperm donor decided to end his anonymity. Jeffrey Harrison was responding to an article in *The New York Times* in which two of the children bearing his contribution to their genetic code were seeking to get in touch with him. As of this writing, the children and their genetic father shared two things in common, his distinctive forehead and his love for dogs. The distinctive forehead is easily understood because it is biologically determined. The love for dogs is more difficult to explain.

Another case of donation of **gametes** (sperm and eggs) had a less optimistic outcome. A gay male couple who conceived a child through anonymous donation of an egg, fertilized through their sperm, discovered the child had Tay-Sachs disease, a neurological disorder that typically limits a child's life span to approximately five years. The egg donor was not aware that she carried genetic coding for the Tay-Sachs **allele**, a variation in genetic coding. The allele for Tay-Sachs is **recessive**, which means it will only express itself if the other biological parent also carries the Tay-Sachs allele. In this case, one of the male biological parents carried the Tay-Sachs allele, so that the resultant child was **homozygous** for Tay-Sachs, which means that she did not have a "normal" allele that would have cloaked the expression of the Tay-Sachs allele.

Early in 2008, largely, as a result of this example and others, representatives from the Society for Assisted Reproductive Technology (SART), which represents the fertility industry, announced that they intended to establish a registry to record the histories of sperm and egg donors, as well as surrogate mothers, in an attempt to prevent matches that inadvertently pair sperm and egg donors who carry recessive alleles for debilitating diseases. As of this writing, the SART website does not mention the establishment of a registry.

"Natural" and "Social" Conception

Even when conception occurs "naturally," as the result of sexual union between a woman and a man, it is still bound about with social conventions. Humans, as well as other animals that reproduce sexually, have a strong sex drive. This is selected for, since sexual reproduction produces diversity in the gene pool. Diversity in the gene pool is important because it increases the likelihood that some members of a species will survive even if there are dramatic changes in the environment.

A singular characteristic among mammals is that sexual reproduction in some species creates an ongoing bond between the parents and between parents and offspring. Female placental mammals nurture their offspring through their gestation period, thus providing them with all they need to survive during this period of body and brain development. After birth, female mammals nurture their offspring through mammary glands, a defining characteristic of mammals.

The gestation period and the development of a close mother-child bond after birth promotes brain development, so that learning plays an important part in the survival of mammals. Unlike fish and snakes, which swim or slither away from their offspring, mammals must stay around to ensure the survival of their offspring. The offspring of fish and reptiles are encased in eggs that provide the nutrients they need, and they emerge from their egg cases when they have reached a stage of development that allows them to survive on their own. Mammalian babies are entirely dependent on their mothers, and in some cases, their fathers as well.

This relationship of dependency becomes more important among our closest relatives, the nonhuman primates. Among a number of primate species—including chimpanzees, gorillas, and some species of baboons, among others—immature offspring must rely on the protection of both their mothers and fathers.

Since the identity of the mother is biologically obvious, the identity of fathers must be defined by other means. This results in a number of reproductive strategies, including pair bonding, that ensure the protection of both parents. Among humans, pair bonding is called marriage. A man married to a child's mother, or otherwise pair-bonded with her, is expected to assume responsibility for her dependent offspring. As a result, both human and nonhuman males may seek evidence that the offspring of a woman is also their biological offspring.

Because of the need to care for important economic resources and preparing sexually mature offspring to care for their own dependent offspring, romantic love or strong sexual attraction are typically not considered sufficient for socially approved conception. Marriage not only assigns paternity, it also establishes economic and other social bonds that promote the likelihood that the human infant will survive. Producing and socializing a child require a great economic investment. Cross-culturally, humans seek means to ensure that the investment will result in a successful reproductive effort. In most societies marriages are arranged, establishing a bond that lasts long enough to ensure that a child will be provided with social and economic resources that increase the likelihood that the child is likely to survive into adulthood.

PREGNANCY: WHO OWNS THE EMBRYO?

Traditionally, in the United States and elsewhere, the unborn child was the property of the family. Today in the United States, the fetus has become state property. In the guise of protecting the fetus, the state has stripped families of their right to make decisions about their own fertility. A woman's womb is now state property, out of reach of herself, her husband, and the family as a whole. There is logic here: Because an aborted fetus will never be able to pay taxes, the state has a vested interest in the woman's womb; however, in the United States, the state does not have to underwrite the investment of producing a child—that expense is borne by the family. The fetus is a future taxpayer or soldier.

Overproduction of babies reduces the cost of labor and increases the consumer market, as well as the tax base. These are rational concerns on the part of government. How can one run a large corporation, which in fact all governments are, without a strong economic base? However, since this is a book on medical anthropology, rather than on the economics of government, we must focus on the costs of unbridled fertility on families and individuals. This cost falls largely on the poor and uneducated. Affluent families have the leisure and economic base to underwrite the cost of birth control. They can also afford the cost of large families if they choose. Usually, they do not produce large families because they can afford the cost of restricting fertility and because excessive fertility reduces the economic base of its members. This reproductive strategy increases the investment in individual family members, who may add to the overall well-being of the family.

Abortion as a Collective Family Decision

In most societies cross-culturally, a fetus is the property of the family, however the family is defined. The anthropologist Tine M. Gammeltoft examined abortion decisions in postwar Vietnam in Hanoi, specifically with respect to the abortion of deformed fetuses. This discourse has been largely shaped by new reproductive technologies, including ultrasound, which allows prenatal diagnoses of fetal abnormalities. In a report for *American Anthropologist*, Gammeltoft describes two cases with different outcomes.

In the case of Tuyét, the fetus she was carrying was diagnosed as having water on the brain. She was advised by physicians to end the pregnancy. Tuyét and her husband Huy returned to their village and advised his father of the situation. As head of the patrilineage, Huy's father would play an important role in deciding whether or not to abort. Although he had ultimate authority, Huy's father decided to include all those who would be affected by the decision of whether to keep the fetus. Gammeltoft describes the complexity of the father's decision, as described by the paternal household head:

When the children [Tuyét and Huy] came home after the scanning in Hanoi, they discussed it with us. First of all we had to find out what the children themselves thought. Second, after hearing their opinion, I asked for the opinion of my elders on both sides—that is, the children's grandparents on both sides. Even though I am Huy's father, I cannot decide about this on my own. This has to be a collective decision. In case problems or regrets arise later, it is important that no one can say it is anybody's fault. Our elders said: "We are simple people, we cannot imagine what this fetus is like. So first of all, we have to trust the experts. If the experts have given their opinion, we should believe them." Both sides of our family then made the decision together to [long pause] . . . give it up. In short, this is the story. (2007:154)

It is clear from Gammeltoft's account that all members of both sides of the family experienced great sadness at "giving up" the fetus. After the abortion, Tuyét lay in her hospital bed, with her husband and mother sitting by her bedside. Tuyét paled as she heard the cry of an infant in the delivery room next door. The child had lived for a few minutes because **feticide** is illegal in Vietnam. A woman in the next bed said to Tuyét's mother, "Grandmother. The child cried. Now it is your turn to cry for the child" (2007:153). Gammeltoft writes:

Toyét's mother had left, then came back with the body of the newborn in her arms, tightly wrapped in blankets. Later she told me: "My arms trembled so much that I could hardly hold it. But I did as she said. I cried for it for several hours. Here in Vietnam you must cry when someone in your family dies, to show your love for that person. This child cried. This means it was a human being." (2007:153)

The outcome was different for Xuân, who learned after two 3-D (three-dimensional) scans that the fetus she was carrying lacked a left hand. A 3-D ultrasound scan can monitor the development of the fetus with greater accuracy than with the traditional 2-D ultrasound technique.

In Xuan's case, doctors recommended against abortion, since the fetus was otherwise normal and its weight indicated that terminating the pregnancy could result in a premature birth rather than an abortion. In this case, as well, the decision rested with the family as a whole. They decided that the woman should keep the pregnancy, even though she would have preferred an abortion. Their reasoning was that her health was not strong and they felt that she could not cope with the physical and emotional trauma of a late-term abortion. They also considered that she had only one living child, even though she had been pregnant five times. Among other considerations they offered was that a missing hand was a minor defect and that the scans had demonstrated that the two most important organs (to them), the heart and the brain, were normal.

Xuân lamented to the anthropologist, "My family forced me to keep it. The entire kin-group forced me to keep it" (2007:159). Two months later, Xuân gave birth to a healthy boy with both hands, though the fingers on his left hand were rudimentary. Gammeltoft concludes:

In contrast to citizens of societies that emphasize personal autonomy and individualism, women in northern Vietnam live in a social world that enables them to turn prenatal diagnosis into an issue of social belonging rather than individual moral pioneering and to frame the issues at stake in terms of social connectedness rather than personal moral conviction. Living in a society that provides them with powerful cultural means for seeing themselves as tied to others through mutual obligations and commitments, women are enabled to share with others the burdens of excruciating existential decisions. (2007:161)

The two cases presented here illustrate alternative strategies associated with social embeddedness. A woman facing abortion of an abnormal fetus does not have to absorb the cost of making that decision alone. She does not need to feel guilt, because the choice of abortion has been taken from her. On the other hand, a woman who wishes to abort a fetus can blame family members for forcing her to bear a child she does not want.

CHILDBIRTH

When an infant is born, it is thrust from the dark, cozy warmth of the uterus into a bright, noisy world. This new world is beset by air currents and other environmental stimuli that the newborn has never before experienced. While in the womb, the infant floats in a warm, watery environment that restricts its movements, but keeps it secure. The religious scholar Lex Hixon writes, "the infant's landscape, before and after birth, is simply mother. For nine months, her heartbeat is our rhythm, our primal music" (1994:3). Hixon links this primal experience to the prevalence of goddess imagery throughout the world.

The infant's entrance into its social world has been described by some as traumatic. Its limbs flop helplessly. For the first time, the infant must gain air and nutrients by its own efforts, through breathing and sucking. It must learn to focus its eyes and control its movements.

The invasion of what some have called the "little stranger" alters the social universe into which it enters. Childless women and men become mothers and fathers. Parents of the mothers and fathers become grandmothers and grandfathers. Siblings of the parents become aunts and uncles. All these newly created social positions imply some degree of responsibility for the little invader. The shift in social status for all concerned can be both welcome and burdensome. It requires a redefinition of one's place in the social group.

All societies provide rites of passage aimed at readjusting the social relationships involved. Among Hopis of the U.S. Southwest, birth mothers and their new infants traditionally remained secluded for one month after parturition. The woman's usual chores would be assumed by other women in the matrilineage, the maternal line. The birth mother was attended by members of her matrilineage, and was instructed in care of her infant by older female relatives. After one month, the infant would be introduced to the outside world by its maternal grandmother, who would show the child the world it would now inhabit. The grandmother would place a little ground corn in the infant's mouth and say, "This is what you will eat while you live among us." The ritual act of introducing the child to his physical and social world eases the transition for all concerned. The lost physical security of the womb is replaced by the social security of the matrilineage.

Biological and Social Birth

During her pregnancy, a woman's body becomes social property. She is the object of advice from all who know her, and even from people who do not know her. Her bulging belly identifies her as someone who will significantly alter the social landscape. At birth, the biological bond between mother and infant is irrevocably severed. From that point, both infant and mother must negotiate a complex social territory in which outsiders stake competing claims.

Brigitte Jordan and Robbie Davis-Floyd investigate the contested territory of the mother and newborn in their comparison of birth in four cultures: Central American Maya, the United States, Sweden, and Holland. Jordan and Davis-Floyd discuss the ways in which different cultures make the biologically complex process of producing a human infant socially and culturally coherent. Since biological processes are intricately linked to social and cultural processes, cultural concepts relating to childbirth can shape the birth process for mother, infant, and others.

All mammals arrive in the social universe through birth. Among humans, the process is especially complicated because the bony structure of the infant's head and the bony structure of the mother's pelvis are nearly equivalent. Thus, a comparatively long and difficult childbirth is the heritage of Homo sapiens species. The cranial case, within which the cerebral cortex is located, is large. Relative to the gigantic Homo sapiens brain, the female pelvis is small. There is a selective relationship here. At birth, the human cranium is collapsible. The skull emerges in fragments in order to pass through the birth canal. Recent studies have indicated that the infant's brain bleeds a little in the transition through the birth canal. This apparently does not result in permanent damage, but it does illustrate that birth is traumatic for the infant as well as for the mother.

In some cases, the birth transition requires a caesarian section because the bony structure of the infant's head cannot pass through the bony structure of the mother's pelvis. Were childbirth inevitably fatal or socially unproductive, it would have been selected against millennia ago and the human species would have been an evolutionary dead end. Thus, it remains to explain how sociocultural processes contribute to the production of the next generation, without which the human species could not continue.

Based on the Jordan and Davis-Floyd analysis, the experience and outcome of childbirth are linked to the social context in which they occur. Variables in all cultures include the birth setting, the view of who should be present when childbirth occurs, what kinds of prenatal care a woman receives in preparation for childbirth, and postpartum care. Jordan and Davis-Floyd note that pregnancy and childbirth among Yucatec Maya are embedded in the social life of the family. A birth typically takes place in the woman's home, either in the compound where she lives or in her mother's home, if it is a first birth. The birth is most likely to take place in the main house of the compound, usually consisting of a single room. The room may be divided by a blanket, or the main house itself may be devoted to the birth. The woman is surrounded by the sights, sounds, and smells of the familiar activities taking place around her.

Jordan's study of Yucatec Maya birthing processes is based on **participant-observation** with an experienced midwife, Doña Juana, who was respected both in the community and by the head of the local hospital. Doña Juana is the daughter of a midwife, though she did not herself take up midwifery until after her mother's death. According to the midwife's account, she received formal medical training from her mentor, Dr. Sanchez, who provided her with both instruction and equipment. Doña Juana also attended a course for midwives offered by a Mexican government agency.

Though Doña Juana emphasizes her formal medical training, her practice draws heavily on both traditional midwifery indigenous to the region and on her familiarity with the customs and social relationships of the people among whom she works. Indeed, it seems likely, based on Jordan's description of her fieldwork, that a key component of Doña Juana's midwifery practice is her ability to negotiate the delicate social relationships within which childbirth occurs. Doña Juana's midwifery combines technical knowledge of childbirth with sensitivity to social relationships, as well as attention to concerns of the mother and family. She also exhibits qualities that inspire confidence.

Doña Juana's prenatal care consists of several visits, the object of the first of which is to calculate the probable date of birth, expected to occur nine calendar months from the day following completion of the woman's last menstrual period. Jordan and Davis-Floyd note that this is equivalent to Nagele's Rule, a calculation of birthdate used by biomedical practitioners. As is typical of traditional midwives, Doña Juana is familiar with the family, having attended other births. During her prenatal visits, she gains further information about family relations and attitudes, such as who would be a likely "helper" during the birth and what kind of person the birthing mother is:

> Doña Juana forms an estimate of how well the woman will be able to withstand pain, whether she is apt to complain for trivial reasons, how important considerations of modesty are to her, whether she is reassured by traditional practices (such as the reciting of prayers, or the burning of rosemary under the bed to ward off evil spirits) and so on. (1993:25)

At the same time, the pregnant woman becomes acquainted with Doña Juana. There is a formal quality in these visits, consisting of three stages: greetings, massage, and leave taking. Though the order is formal, the interactions during each phase are relaxed and leisurely. It is a social occasion involving members of the family other than the pregnant woman.

During prenatal visits the midwife gives the pregnant woman a massage (*sobada*). During the massage, Doña Juana attempts to find out the position of the fetus and determines whether it needs to be "turned," or manipulated into a more favorable birthing position. The midwife discusses with the pregnant woman how she has been feeling and reassures her as to the condition of the baby. Though the procedure and communication center on the woman's condition and experiences, other topics unrelated to the pregnancy are discussed with whoever happens to be present. This may include the women of the household, related men, and children. During the formal leave taking, Doña Juana negotiates with the senior woman of the household as to the timing of the next visit.

When the pregnant woman's contractions begin, Doña Juana is summoned to the woman's household, typically by the woman's husband. The midwife takes with her an equipment case when she goes to the house to assess the situation. The equipment case includes a clear plastic sheet to place under the expectant mother; a heavy clear plastic apron that Doña Juana will don during the later stages of the birth; a gown, cap, and face mask; a metal box with a syringe and two needles; and two stainless steel bowls, for washing her hands and for sterilizing the scissors used to cut the umbilical cord. Her equipment case also includes a rubber squeeze bulb for extracting mucus from the newborn's nose and mouth, eye drops, a glass jar of cotton balls, a metal soap box, a small hand brush, and a closed glass jar containing alcohol in which the waxed thread for tying off the umbilical cord is soaking.

Doña Juana begins her visit by a "friendly exchange of greetings with the family," (1993:31) followed by inquiries about the frequency and strength of the contractions. She then has the mother lie down for a massage, during which she feels for the position of the baby's head "to see if it is engaged or still moving" (1993:31). As the woman's labor progresses, she and the family go about their familiar routines, gossiping, doing chores, and sharing a dinner that may include the birthing woman.

The birthing woman may herself tend a child or perform other household tasks. As the contractions become stronger and more frequent, conversations and interest center on the birthing woman. The husband is expected to be present. If he is not, any calamities experienced during the birth will be attributed to his absence. The woman's mother is also expected to be present for the birth. Women who have not given birth are not permitted to be present. As the moment of birth nears, the husband or other helper takes his place behind the woman's hammock, and she is instructed to brace herself for the final push by wrapping her arms around his neck.

Men can only be present for the birth of their own children, but a long and difficult birth may attract the presence of other women, including mothers-in-law, godmothers, sisters, sisters-in-law, close friends, and neighbors:

> This group of helpers substantially contributes to a successful birth. Jointly and by turns, they give the woman mental and physical support. They encourage her, urge her on, and sometimes scold her, always letting her know that she is not alone, that the business of getting this baby born will be done. It will take time and work and pain, to be sure, but 'we have done all this before and this baby will arrive, soon now.' (1993:33)

If the birthing mother's strength appears to be flagging, the onlookers engage in "birth talk," encouraging her by chanting *"Ence, ence, mama"* (Maya for "make it come") *"jala, jala, jala"* (haul, haul, haul), or *"ko'osh, ko'osh"* (come on, let's go). The rhythmic stream of words is paced to the birth contractions. Jordan and Davis-Floyd suggest that the shared experience of birth, including the women observers' stories of their own childbirth experiences are not intended to frighten the birthing woman, but to assure her that her birth experiences are normal. Furthermore, the husband's witnessing of his wife's pain increases his willingness to engage in birth spacing.

Pregnancy and Childbirth as a Medical Condition

In the United States, early in the twenty-first century, biomedicine began to preside over conception, pregnancy, and childbirth, as well as over the process of aging. Botox, the injection of the organism causing botulism to reduce wrinkling, breast

enhancement for women, penile enhancement for men, and various cosmetic surgical procedures offered the promise of eternal youth. Medical interventions such as
in vitro fertilization, on-demand caesarian sections, and induced births offered the
promise of disengaged, pain-free, and biomedically controlled reproduction.

Within months of her marriage, a woman of my acquaintance began researching
in vitro fertilization. Since she was years away from menopause, I wondered why
she might prefer artificial insemination over the old-fashioned kind. This was
before I grasped the full implications of the baby-production business in the
United States.

Though biomedicine is often portrayed as a monolithic institution, it includes
many subcultures with respect to childbirth techniques. Jordan and Davis-Floyd
compare the intimacy and communality of the Mayan birthing context to the biomedical context of birthing in the United States, Holland, and Sweden. They note
that, for some decades, Sweden and Holland have had some of the lowest birth-
related mortality figures in the world, whereas the United States lags significantly
behind.

Jordan and Davis-Floyd observe that both Sweden and Holland provide abortion
on demand, so that all babies are wanted babies. Though all three countries take a
biomedical approach to birthing, birthing practices differ according to cultural attitudes toward childbirth and the biomedical practices followed. The authors describe
the varying cultural attitudes toward childbirth in the four cultures studied as follows: Yucatan Maya view childbirth as a stressful but normal part of family life; people and physicians in the United States view childbirth as a medical procedure
under the control of the attending physician or practitioner; in Holland, childbirth
is viewed as a natural process; in Sweden, childbirth is viewed as an intensely personal, fulfilling achievement.

All births in the Yucatan, except the most troubled births, take place at home; in the
United States, 99 percent of all births take place in hospitals; in Sweden, all births take
place in hospitals under the management of highly trained midwives; in Holland, 55
percent of births take place at home, with a midwife being the typical attendant
whether at home or in the hospital.

Jordan and Davis-Floyd state that the U.S. view of childbirth as being a medical
event is consistent with attitudes toward physiological processes in this country. Such
issues as nutrition, sexual adjustment, sleeping patterns, mood swings, obesity, learning difficulties, alcoholism, drug use, violence, dying, and other forms of "deviance"
are viewed as suitable objects for medical intervention. Physicians or other medical
personal diagnose the "condition" and control the course of treatment. Being defined
as deviant strips the individual of his or her autonomy. Similarly, defining a pregnant
woman as a "patient" strips her of both agency and responsibility.

In terms of pain management, Jordan and Davis-Floyd write that, in all societies,
pain is recognized as being a part of the birthing process. Given the narrow fit
between the bony skull of the infant and the female pelvis, pain is for the most part
a natural accompaniment of childbirth. The degree of pain involved in childbirth is
variable, involving the relationship between the size of the baby and the size of the
mother's pelvic opening, whether it is a first birth, and the conditions under which
childbirth occurs. Jordan and Davis-Floyd state that the experience of pain is observ-
ably more visible in obstetric wards in the United States than in Holland, Sweden,

or Yucatan. They attribute the highly observable exhibit of pain during birth in the United States to the need of birth mothers and medical personnel to negotiate competing definitions of the degree of pain involved.

Medical attendants in the United States withhold pain medication as long as possible out of concern for its effects on the course of labor. The decision to administer pain medication is made by medical personnel. In order to obtain pain relief, a birthing mother in the United States must anticipate and demonstrate her need for pain medication. Jordan and Davis-Floyd argue that the need to demonstrate a high degree of pain provides a feedback mechanism that increases the subjective experience of pain. The ability to exhibit symptoms of pain can serve to equalize the balance of power in the birthing process. The birthing mother's ability to demonstrate pain counterbalances the power of the birthing attendant to give or withhold pain medication.

In contrast, the decision of whether to give or withhold pain medication in the Swedish birthing process is made by the mother. Analgesics and anesthetics are commonly given for pain relief, but Swedish women are informed about the kinds of medications available, "the conditions under which they are not advisable, and the known and possible side effects on the baby" (1993:53). Thus, the locus of control remains with the mother. She is able to evaluate her own experience of pain against the well-being of the child she is producing.

Jordan and Davis-Floyd note similarities between the Yucatec views of birthing and those in Holland, in that both view childbirth as a normal process. Both hold the view that "the woman's body knows best and that, given enough time, nature will take its course" (1993:53). Therefore, birthing women in Holland typically do not seek pain medication because they consider pain a part of the natural and inevitable process of producing a new human life.

The Political Context of Childbirth

In biomedicine, childbirth is viewed as a medical condition, requiring the assistance of medically trained doctors and nurses. Traditionally, in most societies, childbirth was conducted under the care of midwives, who typically had no formal training, but who had experience in birthing procedures. The transition from midwifery to medically assisted childbirth was reversed in war-torn Iraq early in the twenty-first century. The U.S. invasion of Iraq in 2003 overthrew the prevailing social institutions, so that chaos erupted among the many factions kept under control by Saddam Hussein's dictatorship. Insurgents began targeting hospitals as places where people were required to seek medical aid.

As it became too dangerous to seek help at hospitals, women and their families turned to midwives and birth assistants. In one case reported in the *Los Angeles Times*,[3] a woman gave birth shortly after she had watched her father and uncle die in a bombing attack. Thus, she was in a state of shock. In such a situation, it is difficult to determine whether birth attendants were appropriately credentialed, either by medical personnel or by local cultural standards. In more stable situations, midwives can gain a reputation of having presided over a number of successful birth outcomes. Under such unstable conditions, the situation is more likely to be under the control of anyone who is willing to take responsibility.

The female infant delivered under the circumstances reported in the *Los Angeles Times* did not breathe on its own; however, the midwife had been trained in birthing by her mother, so she was prepared for this emergency. She breathed into the baby's mouth "to give her life."[4] She then pricked the baby's ear, and the baby began to cry. With the cry came an intake of breath, signifying life. At the time of this writing, Iraq no longer licensed or trained midwives or birth attendants, hoping to "steer women to government clinics."[5] However, in war-torn Iraq, delivering at a clinic or hospital was fraught with danger, even greater than that of giving birth in the absence of bio-medical care.

In all societies, giving birth is a life crisis, one often hidden from view in societies such as the United States, which downplays biological dramas. Biomedicine, especially, hides birth and death behind curtains and antiseptic conditions. For the patient, however, the processes of birth, death, and illness are far from clean and simple.

Maternal Mortality and Infant Well-Being

Late in 2007, reporting in *Lancet*, a medical journal, the United Nations and related agencies noted that the United States ranked forty-first among 171 nations in rates of maternal survival, well behind all western European countries, including poorer countries, such as Macedonia and Bosnia. One in 4,800 U.S. women dies from complications of pregnancy and childbirth, the same as Belarus and slightly better than Serbia. The major direct causes of U.S. pregnancy-related deaths are blood clots, complications of preexisting medical conditions, eclampsia, and pre-eclampsia.

Pre-eclampsia and eclampsia are forms of high blood pressure occurring during pregnancy. These conditions are accompanied by protein in the urine and edema (swelling).[6] Eclampsia is accompanied by seizures. Women are considered high-risk for pre-eclampsia and eclampsia if the following conditions are present: (1) it is a first pregnancy; (2) there is a family history of pre-eclampsia or eclampsia; (3) the woman is carrying more than one baby; (4) the woman is a teenager; (5) if she is over 40; (6) there is a pre-existing condition such as high blood pressure, kidney disease or diabetes; (7) the woman smokes; (8) she is obese; or (9) she suffers from malnutrition; or (10) if she is carrying an infant with "non-immune hydrops."[7] "Non-immune hydrops" is a condition in which a fetus has fluid in one or more body cavities, plus has edema at birth.[8]

In 2007, the most favorable international statistics for low maternal mortality were registered for Ireland, with one in 47,600 women dying during or just after childbirth. Bosnia had the second-lowest rate, one in 29,000. Among the ten top-ranked European and other industrialized nations (which does not include the United States), fewer than one in 16,400 women die of pregnancy and childbirth complications.[9] The report linked the high survival rates to guaranteed good-quality health and family planning services that minimize the lifetime risk of death from pregnancy and child-birth.

The report from the United Nations and related agencies noted that in the ten lowest-ranked countries, the lifetime risk of dying in pregnancy or childbirth is one in 15. The four lowest-ranking countries are Chad with one in 11 women dying in pregnancy or childbirth, Afghanistan and Sierra Leone with one in eight, and Niger with one in seven. The United Nations report was based on figures from the World Health Organization, the World Bank, the United Nations Population Fund (UNFPA), the United Nations Children's Fund (UNICEF), and The World Bank.

Based on statistics compiled by the United Nations, UNICEF notes that close to 600,000 women, more than one woman every minute, die from complications related to pregnancy and childbirth. This has important implications for the health and well-being of children who survive their mother's death: "these complications contribute to more than three million infant deaths within their first week of life and another three million stillbirths."[10] A joint statement by UNICEF and the World Bank attributes high rates of mother and infant mortality to the low social status of women in developing countries: "Low social status limits women's access to economic resources and basic education, impeding their ability to make informed decisions on childbearing, health and nutrition. Poor nutrition before and during pregnancy contributes to poor health, obstetric problems, and poor pregnancy outcomes for both women and their new-borns."[11]

The report recommends addressing these life-threatening health conditions by ensuring that women are empowered to make reproductive health choices, that they have access to maternal health services including midwifery, and that they have access to family planning information and services: "As many as half of all pregnancies are unplanned and unwanted. Prevention of unwanted pregnancies is one of the key strategies for reducing maternal mortality. Thus, in addition to midwifery and referral services, there is also a need to provide client-centered family planning services with safe and effective contraceptive methods and counselling."[12]

INFANCY

Among the Swazi, the anthropologist Hilda Kuper writes, "Until the third month of life a Swazi baby is described as a 'thing.' It has no name, cannot be handled by the men, and, if it dies, it may not be publicly mourned" (1963:59). Cross-culturally, an infant does not have a social identity until it is named. Traditionally, in Roman Catholic custom, an infant who died before it was baptized could not be buried in hallowed ground, defined as a Catholic graveyard. It had to be buried outside the fence, and its soul was believed to be consigned to limbo. Limbo is an intermediate state in which the infant's soul could not enter heaven because it had not been baptized, and therefore, had no Catholic identity conferred upon it.

It is common cross-culturally to distinguish between the biological entry of a child into the group and its social entry, when it acquires a name and social identity. Kuper links the withholding of social identity among Swazi until the third month of a baby's life to a high rate of infant mortality. She suggests that Swazi are reluctant to invest social identity in the child until it has demonstrated its ability to survive. In the third month, the infant is symbolically introduced to the world of nature and culture. It enters into the category of persons, and is given a name, which may be sung to it in its first lullaby.

The infant remains a "baby" until it has "teeth to chew" and "legs to run," at which time it is weaned and treated as a full and interactive member of society. Kuper writes, "Obedience and politeness are inculcated from the beginning of awareness" (1963:50). A child who behaves in appropriate ways is addressed as "Chief," or encouraged with such phrases as "Now you are really a man [or woman]." When the mother returns to work in the fields or goes to gather firewood, the newly emancipated child is socialized by peers. But with emancipation comes responsibility:

> Discipline becomes more strict and punishment more physical as the child grows older, but the over-all impression is that Swazi children are reared with unself-conscious indulgence, relatively free from constant adult supervision. They also learn unconsciously through riddles and verbal memory games, said to "sharpen the intelligence," and there are songs and dances to "make a person grow into a person." (1963:51)

Parental Investment and Early Childhood Socialization

In societies where resources are scarce, there may be little investment in an infant until he or she demonstrates the ability to survive. In her article "Lifeboat Ethics: Mother Love and Child Death in Brazil," Nancy Scheper-Hughes notes that women in a favela (urban slum) do not invest in their offspring until the child demonstrates a "will to live." This results in a high infant mortality rate, but also conserves limited food resources.

By way of contrast, people in the United States invest heavily in their offspring, almost from the point of conception. Typically, from the point a pregnancy becomes apparent—usually after the first missed menstruation—a woman's pregnancy becomes a medical condition, and the fetus becomes a patient. Its viability and physical condition are closely monitored through ultrasound and other measures. Once born, the infant is almost as much the property of its pediatrician as of its parents. Nothing is left to chance.

In a classic analysis published in 1946, the anthropologist Ruth Benedict compared the rigid structure of an American infant's life with that of a Japanese infant. She remarked that this early socialization was in marked contrast to the demeanor expected of an adult in these two societies:

> Japanese babies are not brought up in the fashion that a thoughtful Westerner might suppose. American parents, training their children for a life so much less circumspect and stoical than life in Japan, nevertheless begin immediately to prove to the baby that his own little wishes are not supreme in this world. We put him immediately on a feeding schedule and a sleeping schedule, and no matter how he fusses before bottle time or bed time, he has to wait. A little later his mother strikes his hand to make him take his finger out of his mouth or away from other parts of his body. His mother is frequently out of sight and when she goes out he has to stay behind. He has to be weaned before he prefers other foods, or if he is bottle fed, he has to give up his bottle. There are certain foods that are good for him and he must eat them. He is punished when he does not do what is right. (1989:253)

By way of contrast, Benedict writes, Japanese children are not subjected to such rigid discipline so soon after birth: "The arc of life in Japan is plotted in opposite fashion to the United States. [The Japanese life cycle] is a great shallow U-curve with maximum freedom and indulgence allowed to babies and to the old" (1989:253–254).

The freedom and indulgence a Japanese child infant enjoys is short-lived: "Restrictions are slowly increased after babyhood till having one's own way reaches a low just before and after marriage. This low line continues many years during the prime of life, but the arc gradually ascends again until after the age of sixty men and women are almost as unhampered by shame as little children are" (1989:254).

Benedict describes the gradual process of socializing the Japanese child largely in terms of shaming, but it has multiple layers of subtlety. I was privileged to witness a contemporary example of Japanese socialization in a near-empty train in Tokyo in the 1990s. The car was nearly empty because it was in the middle of the day and most people were at work. A man in a business suit, a young woman with her child, and I boarded the train at the same time and sat within easy observation of each other. The woman and her child, a boy who appeared to be about four years old, sat across from the well-dressed businessman. As we boarded the train, the child was in the midst of a tantrum. He was flailing his arms, kicking his legs, and crying.

The mother held the boy's hands tightly and spoke softly as she compelled him to interact with her. The businessman opposite her signaled his approval of her socialization style by nodding and smiling at her as she gradually brought the boy under her control. Within what seemed like minutes, the child seemed to forget whatever had caused his displeasure and began to interact calmly with his mother. Her attention appeared to be totally absorbed by her interaction with the child, but she and the businessman frequently exchanged glances, as he signaled approval, and she, through her expression, signaled her acknowledgement of his approval. It was a microcosm of interaction involving the child, his mother, and the businessman, a representative of the society as a whole. Together—the mother and the businessman—imposed culturally appropriate behavior on the child without using physical or vocal censure.

I mentally contrasted this interaction with scenes of tantrums I had observed in the United States, of children kicking and screaming on the floors of supermarkets, of toy stores, of department stores. The American mothers glared at their children, spoke harshly to them, and in some cases, carried the child bodily out of the store, as onlookers glared at both mother and child. Ruth Benedict contrasts the arc of life in Japan with its opposite trajectory in the United States:

> Firm disciplines are directed toward the infant [in the United States] and these are gradually relaxed as the child grows in strength until a man runs his own life when he gets a self-supporting job and when he sets up a household of his own. The prime of life is with us the high point of freedom and initiative. Restrictions begin to appear as men lose their grip or their energy or become dependent. (1989:254)

Benedict notes that both the American and Japanese approaches to socialization are aimed at ensuring an individual's full participation in society at the prime of life. Both societies apply restrictions, but the restrictions are imposed at different points of the life cycle. Americans are restricted early in their life cycle to prepare them for the rigors of adult life; Japanese are socialized gradually into the connections they must make with the social group as preparation for the obligations they will assume as adults.

Ruth Benedict's friend, Margaret Mead, did much to liberalize American child rearing patterns, based on her field research in Samoa. During the time of her fieldwork, a Samoan child was breast-fed until it was two or three years old. During that time it would sleep with its mother. After that, it would be cared for by an older child in the village, who may have been only a few years older than the newly weaned child.

> From birth until the age of four or five a child's education is exceedingly simple. They must be housebroken, a matter made more difficult by a habitual indifference to the activities of very small children. They must learn to sit or crawl within the house and never to stand upright unless it is absolutely necessary; never to address an adult in a standing position; to stay out of the sun; not to tangle the strands of the weaver; not to scatter the cut-up cocoanut which is spread out to dry; to keep their scant loin cloths at least nominally fastened to their persons; to treat fire and knives with proper precaution; not to touch the kava bowl,[13] or the Kava cup; and if their father is a chief, not to crawl on his bed-place when he is by. (1968:31–32[1928])

Margaret Mead's observations of Samoan childrearing practices were more admiring than critical, and she incorporated the relaxed childrearing of Samoans into her own rearing of her daughter, Mary Catherine Bateson. At the time, American mothers maintained a strict schedule of feeding and sleeping. Mead introduced the concept of "demand feeding" into American culture. This is the idea that an infant should be fed whenever she or he appears to be hungry. Bateson's pediatrician was Dr. Benjamin Spock, author of *Baby and Child Care*, at this writing in its seventh edition. Mead's ideas about relaxed feeding and sleeping schedules found their way into that influential book. Bateson writes:

> Spock was blessedly relaxed about letting my mother do as she wanted, abandoning the fixed schedules that were regarded as essential to health, but he seems to have been only partly aware of the innovation taking place in front of his eyes, for he wrote later that the first experiment in "self-demand feeding" took place in 1942, an example of the limited willingness of physicians to learn from their patients. (1984:23)

Bateson notes that her mother's anthropological research in a number of the world's cultures contributed to her own pattern of mothering:

> I have wondered sometimes about her assurance, since she was doing things that were widely believed to be wrong or unhealthy for infants, calmly planning how to bully doctors and vamp nurses into allowing all sorts of irregularities at a time when most women find themselves easily bullied by those who represent medical authority. When Vanni [Bateson's daughter] was born, I was enriched by my mother's confidence, becoming able in my turn to reject the kinds of advice that undermine breast-feeding and invade the intimacy of mother and child. (1984:25–26)

Modern Western medicine is reacting, in part, to the disease-ridden cities of the European Middle Ages, when people kept pails in their bedrooms for convenience in excretory functions and disposed of such "night soil" by throwing it out the window into the streets. Also, one method of postnatal population control was "sleeping over," in which a woman smothered her newborn and explained it as inadvertently rolling over onto the child while sleeping. In fact, it was a form of postnatal birth control. Margaret Mead's cross-cultural experience, especially in more temperate climates, led her to understand that Western childbirth and infant care behaviors developed in cold, crowded, and germ-ridden European cities were maladaptive to contemporary societies, in which antiseptics and antibiotics are part of the everyday accoutrements of childbirth and childhood. Bateson notes that Mead's "revolutionary" ideas about child care—based on essential components of human evolutionary survival—helped her to feel comfortable with her own child.

> It was splendid, for instance, to have Margaret robustly declare that it was rubbish that I should never nurse Vanni in bed for fear of dozing off and suffocating her, as all the nurses insisted. All around the world mothers and infants sleep side by side and the danger of suffocation arises mainly when mothers are drunk or sick, not under normal circumstances—it is the American habit of leaving an infant alone in a crib in a separate room that is at odds with the normal range of human behavior. (1984:26)

Cosleeping and Infant Health

Much research has been conducted on the biological benefits of cosleeping for human infants. Cosleeping refers to the common cross-cultural practice in which infants sleep with their mothers, or in come cases, with both parents. Relindis D. Yovsi and Heidi Keller (2007) describe cosleeping as offering an evolutionary advantage because human infants are born neurologically immature. Because of their neurological immaturity, infants need care even when they are asleep. (See also McKenna 2000; McKenna et al, 1997; and Small 1998). A classic study by Roger Burton and John Whiting (1961) determined that of 100 societies surveyed cross-culturally, only middle-class families in the United States put their children to sleep in rooms separate from their parents.

Yovsi and Keller link parent-infant sleeping patterns to economic activities among the Nso, one of the largest ethnic groups in the western grasslands of Cameroon in Africa. The anthropologists compare agricultural Nso with "an elite cohort [that] has emerged as a result of urbanization and education" (2007:69). The "wage-earning group consists of professionals such as nurses, teachers, civil servants, tailors, carpenters, and traders" (2007:69).

Yovsi and Keller write that the traditional agricultural way of life among Nso is organized around the "family," which may include friends and neighbors, as well as individuals related by descent or marriage: "All family members are expected to support each other, and an individual predicament is considered a family one" (2007:69). They add: "The farming families depend solely on their farm products for their livelihood. Farming is a joint venture among men and women, as well as children" (2007:70).

Families depend on the common agricultural source for their livelihood, and life centers on compounds that may include several households, as well as a "big house," a sitting room used mostly for senior male visitors and family members. Also in the compound is a kitchen building: "The kitchen building is a room in which cooking, eating, and conversations among women take place. It is also used for storing farm products and firewood. The kitchen is also an area where parents sit together with their children in the evening to learn about the children's day and teach them through moral stories" (2007:70).

Sleeping arrangements reflect communality organized around the mother and children: "The mother and father sleep in the same room in the big house, but in separate beds. The mother sleeps with all her children, who lie according to their birth order, with the youngest one nearest to her" (2007:70). The sleeping arrangements reflect the overall family household arrangements. Both males and females are involved in farming, but the wife/mother makes the greater investment in providing food for the family. Males join each other in such community work as digging, maintenance of roads, or constructing bridges. Maintaining ties with neighbors outside the family through rituals and other communal activities is part of the role of the father.

Urban wage-earning families among the Nso reflect a different pattern of economics and sleeping arrangements. At least one parent earns wages from his or her professional activities. The parlor where the family eats, sits, and receives visitors also contains urban goods such as sofas, a television, radio, and refrigerator. Thus the central area retains its role as a gathering place. Child care, on the other hand, becomes professionalized: "Wage-earning families are able to send their children to school and ensure the health of their members because they can pay for hospital services" (2007:72).

Urban wage-earning families can also pay for child nurses and household staff: "The nurses or helpers are the ones who mainly care for the children, and they generally spend more time with them than the parents do. If the mother is a housewife, she generally invests more time in household management than in childcare, which is still left with the baby's nurse" (2007:72).

The family still spends time together watching television, playing games, or helping children with their homework; however, sleeping arrangements reflect the affluence of the wage-earning family: "Children go to bed independently of their parents. Apart from the youngest child who sleeps in the conjugal bed, other children usually sleep with other siblings or with the baby nurse in other rooms" (2007:72). If the child who sleeps with the parents awakens, he or she will be cared for by the baby nurse. Yovsi and Keller conclude that cosleeping is not the product of poverty or necessity, but of cultural conventions that reinforce relationships of parents to their children:

> Nso parents cosleep with their children not because of insufficient space but, instead, because it facilitates nocturnal nursing and care. Parents also share the bed with their children to prevent them from crying. Infant nocturnal crying is an ominous event in Nso land because of the belief that the night is a malicious phase and can be dangerous for a crying baby because evil spirits might *tah kitu ke waàn* (want the child). (2007:78)

Yovsi and Keller suggest that cosleeping practices among Nso combine Western and traditional parenting practices that produce a new form of integration of the self: "The Nso wage-earning families portray a culture in the process of change, particularly within the family, related to socioeconomic development. This change has implications for the development of a self that integrates both autonomy and relatedness" (2007:80).

Infanticide

In societies where effective birth control is not an option, infanticide is a common practice. Netsilik lived on the northeast coast of Canada above the Arctic Circle. They were foragers, subsisting primarily on seal and caribou. The terrain was harsh, and the danger of starvation was always imminent. The birth rate was high, a factor that threatened a group's survival in such a fragile ecosystem. Boys were needed for hunting, the primary means of survival. Girls reduced the chances of a group's survival by producing children.

Twenty children were born to one family described by Asen Balikci. Ten were boys, and ten were girls. All the boys were allowed to live, but only one of the girls was allowed to survive. She survived because her father was celebrating a particularly good fishing catch. Balikci writes: "The decision to kill a child could be made by the mother, the father, the grandfather, or the widowed grandmother" (1970:149). This case illustrates the strong relationship between infanticide and the availability of resources.

Infanticide was not practiced if a child had already acquired a name. Netsilik believed that a person's name referred to a dead person who wished to reincarnate and who had chosen their new infant bodies at the time of a child's birth. A woman undergoing a difficult childbirth could enlist the aid of ancestors who might be attempting to reincarnate by calling out their names. The name she called at the time of the infant's birth would become the name of the infant, in the belief that the spirit of that ancestor had entered the child's body. Out of respect to the ancestor, the child would be allowed to survive. A child acquired a social identity when it acquired a name.

CHILDHOOD

In his book *Gleanings in the Buddha-Fields*, Lafcadio Hearn describes his impressions of the life and culture of Japanese during the nineteenth and early twentieth centuries. Hearn, son of an Anglo-Irish surgeon major in the British Army stationed on the Greek Island of Lefkas, and a Greek mother, took up residence in Japan in 1890 and stayed there until his death in 1904. Previously a journalist, Hearn supported himself in Japan as a teacher. While reflecting on Japanese psychology and philosophy, Hearn chanced to overhear a girl instructing her brother in calligraphy:

> The cooing voice of a little girl dissolves my reverie. She is trying to teach a child brother how to make the Chinese character for Man, —I mean Man with a big M. First she draws in the dust a stroke sloping downwards from right to left . . . then she draws another curving downwards from left to right . . . joining the two so as to form the perfect *ji*, or character, *hito*, meaning a person of either sex, or mankind. . . . Then she tries to impress the ideal of this shape on the baby memory by help of a practical illustration, —probably learned at school. She breaks a slip of wood in two pieces, and manages to balance the pieces against each other at about the same angle as that made by the two strokes of the character. "Now see," she says: "each stands only by help of the other. One by itself cannot stand. Therefore the *ji* is like mankind. Without help one person cannot live in this

world; but by getting help and giving help everybody can live. If nobody helped anybody, all people would fall down and die."[14]

Hearn observes that "the pretty moral fancy is much more important than the scientific fact. It is also one charming example of that old-fashioned method of teaching which invested every form and every incident with ethical significance."[15]

By way of contrast, the anthropologist David M. Hayano's stay among the Awa of Papua New Guinea during his fieldwork reflects a different set of circumstances and a different type of childhood experience. Hayano's need to conduct research as an anthropologist permitted him to casually observe children interacting among themselves. Hayano writes: "The slew of children always around the house meant a never-ending supply of informal informants. Often I would question them on the use of various plants and their names. Even the tiniest four- or five-year-olds could describe precisely where numerous species of domestic and wild foods could be found" (1990:77).

Since Awa are horticulturalists, it is not remarkable that even small children would understand the importance of learning about plants. Hayano describes another episode that demonstrates the "adult" knowledge of children. Hayano and his wife walked to a little-traversed area near the village, where they talked of future plans and gathered some botanical specimens. On their return to the village, Hayano and his wife were met by children who were clearly upset:

> The moment I stepped over the hamlet fence, the children, who of course knew where we had been, began yelling and pointing. Kuintawe, a bright, attractive, fourteen-year-old girl, rushed toward me and motioned to me to get rid of the plants. I had forgotten that Wopimpa was thought to be one of the most dangerous parts of the village. The people believed it to be the dangerous abode of ghosts and malevolent spirits. . . . One could get seriously ill by falling down on the trail or spending too much time in its cool shade. Collecting plants from Wopimpa to bring home was simply out of the question. (1990:110)

An epidemic of influenza began to ravage New Guinea shortly afterward, leading Hayano to fear that he would be held responsible for the deaths. Even more, he felt helpless that his stock of medical supplies would not be effective against influenza, which is caused by a virus and does not respond to antibiotics. Soon after, a woman gave birth to a stillborn child and did not expel the afterbirth. Hayano's wife was sent for. Though she administered a vial of penicillin, the woman's case was hopeless. Hayano writes:

> The children foresaw Kaera's end and would openly talk about it before the adults. That night an unusually strong breeze blew from the south, disturbing the pitter-patter of rain. The children looked at me and said it was Kaera's ghost. It had separated from Kaera's mortal body, leaving the filth and excrement [that had surrounded her after the unsuccessful birth] and darkness to wander about in a better place. (1990:116)

The sophistication of Awa children's awareness of death stands in marked contrast to the American practice of concealing such facts as birth and death from children. It is likely that American children are aware of the altered circumstances surrounding a life crisis event, but typically do not have the consequences of such an event explained to them.

Formal Childhood Education

Anthropologist Deborah Golden conducted an ethnographic study of how "notions of social order . . . are conveyed to young children in early childhood education" (2006:367).

Her study focused on a kindergarten located in a small town in northern Israel catering to a working-class immigrant population, which during the 1950s was primarily from South Africa and Muslim countries.

The populations shifted beginning in 1989, when immigrants from the former Soviet Union were drawn to the town because of affordable housing. The result was a diverse population. Golden's description of the kindergarten suggests that administration of the kindergarten was organized around a predictable routine, a stable staff, the spatial layout of the kindergarten, and guidelines provided by the State of Israel Ministry of Education Culture and Sport. In actual practice, Golden notes, prescribed daily routines were often interrupted and were seldom carried out with uniformity:

> This somewhat ragged texture of daily life did not mean that the children were unaware of the outer limits of social behavior deemed acceptable. At the one end of the spectrum, there was very little overt physical aggression or violence among the children and any evidence of it was severely curtailed by the teacher. At the other end of the spectrum, too little social engagement—namely, children who wandered around on their own, chose to eat their snack facing away from the other children, or otherwise made it obvious that they were [disengaged from the group] were called to order.

On the other hand, teachers' response to behaviors of children appeared to be unpredictable. It would be more accurate to say that they were not determined by institutionalized principles:

> There appeared to be no clear criteria in the selection of children for various tasks. Moreover, praises and punishments were erratic and inconsistent. Thus, for example, the same behavior on the part of a child, such as hugging the teacher . . . or calling out her name to call her attention during a whole group activity, was sometimes approved (with varying degrees of enthusiasm), sometimes met with disapproval (with varying degrees of severity), or sometimes called up no response at all. (2006:377)

Golden contrasts what she calls the "personalized mode" of attaining acquiescence in Israeli kindergartens to what may be regarded as the more institutional form of the American mode of requiring obedience. American kindergarten teachers persuade children by appealing to the reasonableness of the request, the benefit of compliance to the individual child, threat of consequences in the event of disobedience, citing the child's responsibility to the group, or the need to accede to the teacher's superior rank. In contrast, appeals of Israeli kindergarten teachers were framed in "personal, even intimate, terms" (2006:379). Golden suggests that the relationship of Israeli kindergarteners is modeled on a mother's relationship to her child. One teacher described her role as providing a "warm loving home" and kindergarten as a place where children can "give and receive [love]" (2006:379).

The Evolution of Childhood

Expectations for the body of a modern child in the United States differ greatly from the requirements for movement that facilitated the biological evolution of the human species. As of 100,000 years ago, anatomically modern humans did not have chairs. Our bodies were adapted for mobility. As a forager, this bipedal animal, Homo sapiens, survived by moving from place to place. Humans didn't become sedentary animals until about 10,000 years ago, when many human groups settled down into intensive agriculture. Even then, farmers performed hard physical work. In addition, rulers who wanted to keep their thrones had always to be battle ready.

As I note in my book *Sport as Symbol: Images of the Athlete in Art, Literature and Song* (2003), most sports developed as training for battle. Polo, for example, developed on the Asian steppes as training for raids. It began as an exercise in which players on horseback would battle each other for possession of a headless goat or calf. This prepared them for riding swiftly into a village, grabbing a calf or goat, and racing off before the more sedentary villagers could arm themselves. Foot racing among American Indians trained swift messengers to aid in coordinating battles. Hyperactivity would have been selected for among these populations. But their hyperactivity was controlled and purposeful. It served a social purpose. Hyperactivity in contemporary American classrooms disrupts the desired social order, which is sedentary conformity..

Children are, by definition, "uncivilized." They have not yet internalized the rules of behavior that the rest of us have been persuaded to take for granted. The whole point of parenting and schooling is to turn these little savages into commendable members of society. Usually social interaction with more powerful elders, such as parents and teachers, is adequate for the transition. For some, the brutality of socialization is not enough to coerce conformity. Conformity is a double-edged sword, as illustrated by Mark Twain's opus *Pudd'nhead Wilson*. Pudd'nhead Wilson was a genius who lived among ordinary people in a small town. Since his fellows were not geniuses, they did not understand him. They concluded that he was stupid and, consequently, gave him the nickname "Pudd'nhead Wilson."

People in the United States like to view childhood as equivalent to Adam and Eve in the Garden of Eden. We prefer to regard children as happy innocents. In fact, for most of us, childhood is a difficult time in which we have to learn how to "fit in." We must learn how to form alliances, as well as how to deal with bullies and belittlers. In raising our own children, we try to create an idealized world where bullies and belittlers do not exist. We try to construct an "Eden" that does not adequately prepare our children for adult life.

Childhood as Behavioral Disorder

One area in which contemporary forms of socialization prepare us for adult life is in the area of conformity. The factory system of education, as practiced in industrialized countries, requires conformity. Just as factories turn out identical parts, educational institutions attempt to turn out students who can fit into a particular mold. We prepare them to become good workers who do not question conformity. This occurs at both the management and worker levels.

Genius, by definition, is abnormal, in the sense that genius departs from the norm. Where, on the assembly line or in the corporate office, would genius fit in? Though the owners and managers of the factory or corporate office may consider themselves above the norm, they must also adhere to the manufacturing model. In education, this is evident in the composition of standardized test scores.

In the United States, children who cannot adapt to sitting for long in a chair or heeding the dictates of others are diagnosed as having Attention Deficit Hyperactive Disorder (ADHD). This "disorder" may have served the child well had he or she been a forager in search of new means of survival. In an industrial society, ADHD is a handicap. The manufacturing model of education validates long hours of effort concentrated on production of a result considered adequate by others, but it does not facilitate creative effort. This is not to suggest that ADHD does not impair performance. It is inappropriate for situations that require sustained focus on tasks that do not interest us.

Much of my philosophy regarding early childhood education derives from my own childhood spent on a farm. Variability in personalities was encouraged as long as it did not disrupt the smooth functioning of the corporate unit, the family. Two of my male cousins spent most of their time in the forest. They learned the skill of forestry which, in its traditional form, does not involve the wholesale slaughter of trees. It involves the harvesting of mature trees to provide oak and cedar wood for luxury housing. As students in the factory system of education, they were misfits. As adults engaged in a prosperous business that required ingenuity and technical skill, they fit in perfectly.

Still, creativity typically challenges the prevailing social order. Its association with danger is not unique to industrial societies. In all human groups, creativity flies in the face of norms. Generally, however, geniuses and creative people are tolerated because they contribute to the well-being of other members of the group. Where creativity is stigmatized, as among working classes in industrialized societies, it is likely to be defined as disruptive or "abnormal."

Hyperactivity and the inability to focus are genuine "disorders" in the sense that they do not conform to the social order. In these cases, failure to conform to the norm does not appear to contribute to the overall well-being of the group or to the well-being of the child. Children with ADHD do not appear to engage in activities that provide them with satisfaction and self-esteem. I had an opportunity to observe hyperactivity in a child in a play group. This child seemed unable to form bonds of empathy with others in the play group. Had the play group not been under the control of the mothers, this child would probably have been excluded from the group. Because this was a social occasion, I could not ask the mother whether the child was taking medications for his "condition." Therefore, I could not assess what role this might have played in the child's behavior; however, it was clear the mother did not consider her child's behavior to be "normal."

Beginning in 1990, when ADD became part of the medical terminology and the American's public psyche, the recommended treatment for ADHD or ADD was prescribing stimulants containing either methylphenidate or amphetamine. The biochemistry of adults and children with respect to stimulants and sedatives is almost exactly opposite. Children calm down under the influence of stimulants and become hyperactive under the influence of sedatives. In the first decade when attention deficit disorder was defined as a medical condition, almost 2 million American children were diagnosed as having ADD.[16] Diagnoses continue to rise.

Who Owns the Child?

At the time of this writing, there is a conflicting trend in the United States concerning who owns the right to control early childhood socialization. On the one hand, educators are playing an increasingly important role in determining family priorities. On the other hand, in legal decisions about child welfare, parental rights often take precedence over the welfare of the child. Children may be placed under control of parents or other caregivers who have demonstrated their inability to provide a safe and positive environment for children.

Early in 2007, *The New York Times* reported on the case of a six-year-old girl who drastically cut back on eating after educators at her school sent home a note in her report card stating that the girl had a body mass index (BMI) in the 80th percentile. The normal body mass index is between the 5th and 85th percentile. Thus, the girl's body mass index was within the normal range. As the article reports, however, a note from educators is typically interpreted by children as chastisement for misbehavior. In this case, the first-grader thought she was being chastised for overeating. She immediately undertook an extreme dieting regime similar to one followed by anorexics.

In spite of the mother's attempts to get the child to eat normally, she continued to subsist on a diet insufficient to support a growing child. The educators in this instance exceeded both their authority and expertise. Children develop at different rates. The child's pediatrician, in close consultation with the parents, is the one best able to evaluate his or her overall health, much of which is influenced by activity levels rather than by body mass index. In this case, the educational institution inadvertently inflicted on a child of normal weight a dietary regimen that may impair her health for the rest of her life.

Another case reported in *The New York Times* involved a four-year-old girl who died from an overdose of psychiatric drugs she had been taking since she was two years old. At that time, she was diagnosed with attention deficit disorder and bipolar disorder. As the American Academy of Child and Adolescent Psychiatry suggests, behavior the girl exhibited may have been within the normal range for a child of that age. The child was taking Seroquel, an antipsychotic drug; Depakote, a powerful mood medication; and Clonidine, a blood pressure drug. The parents were charged with deliberately poisoning their daughter by giving her overdoses of prescription drugs to sedate her.

During the same period, a California Juvenile Court commissioner halted the adoption process in the case of a two-year-old girl who was born with severe heart defects, a cleft lip and palate, and mild cerebral palsy, to consider whether the child should be returned to the custody of her father, a registered sex offender. The father had previously pleaded guilty to raping a developmentally disabled woman incapable of giving consent and to having unlawful sex with her 16-year-old sister. A counsel for Los Angeles County offered the opinion that "Generally speaking, parents have a fundamental right to parent their kids. That would include child molesters." This opinion ignores the right of the child to be socialized by a parent or parents who would place the safety and psychological needs of the child above their own sexual impulses.

In Los Angeles County, advocates for the homeless objected to a plan to find homes for children of skid row. Skid row in Los Angeles has long been known for its rat-infested homeless camps, drug bazaars, and prostitution. The effort to remove children from skid row was opposed even though the effort was supported by offers to help secure welfare benefits, mental health services, and housing for the family as a whole. These examples illustrate the important issue of whose rights take precedence: Authorities who make decisions for which they are not qualified, parents whose lifestyle choices endanger the lives and well-being of their children, or the rights of children who live in dangerous circumstances through no choice of their own.

6

The Human Life Cycle

The Reproductive Years

CASE STUDY
Acquiring a Bra

"We didn't have school because of the snow today. I miss Kelly. I don't know why, because I've seen him all week except for today. P.S. Please help me to be more mature and help me fill out my bra." This is an entry in a diary by an American teenaged girl who as an adult read it to a highly entertained audience on Cringe Night at Freddy's in New York City. This event is held at a neighborhood bar, initiated by Sarah Brown, who had moved to the city from Tulsa, Oklahoma. Cringe Night attracted overflow crowds and spilled over to a blog site. The popular event spread to other cities in the United States and Canada, and gave rise to a stage show called "Mortified Live." Reading publicly the most embarrassing secrets of one's adolescent angst appears to have a therapeutic effect for those who choose to do so. Laughing at, and hearing others laugh at, one's most carefully guarded secrets is cathartic. It is comparable to the public confessions at an Alcoholics Anonymous meeting. It permits the individual to acknowledge his or her errors and accept forgiveness from the audience. The term "cathartic" was used by a thirty-year-old news anchor who described his teenaged self as a "pudgy kid with bad skin who didn't talk to anybody in junior high."[1] He compares the catharsis of looking back as an adult to the years "when they're laughing at you and you're not laughing at all." The shared experience of confessing our flaws to an appreciative audience provides a way of revisiting them, moving beyond them, and acknowledging that painful and humiliating episodes are a part of human social development. In the process of growth we learn how not to repeat the experiences that make us feel bad about ourselves. Hearing the appreciative laughter from the audience provides a form of ablution, in which the "sins" of the past are released from the private prison of the unconscious and moved to the stage of public acceptance.

Airing one's adolescent angst before an appreciative audience is apparently unique to the United States. However, the transition from childlike dependency to the assumption of adult responsibility is complex in all societies, and all societies provide mechanisms to ease this difficult transition.

Anthropologists have noted that the human life cycle is especially shaped to promote the acquisition of social and cultural knowledge, while facilitating the ability to transmit that knowledge to offspring. Humans cannot survive without sophisticated social skills. This is true of all primates, but it is especially marked in humans. Childhood in the human species is a drawn-out process in which the individual acquires the social and cultural skills to survive in human groups. The "delayed puberty," which defers the onset of reproductive capacity, permits intensive socialization by parents, peers, and public groups designed for this purpose. In most egalitarian societies, much of this socialization takes place within the peer group, where status relationships become established and individuals are coerced into conformity to the group. In stratified societies, schools and other entities participate in the process of socialization.

Puberty begins with the onset of sexual maturity, which occurs rapidly. Anthropologists have suggested that the rapid onset of puberty is selected for as an adjunct to the long period of childhood. The long period of childhood promotes plasticity, the ability to rapidly assess a situation and behave appropriately. After the intense period of learning during childhood, individuals rapidly mature sexually to ensure that they survive past the long period required for their own offspring to mature and reproduce. In general, sexual maturity occurs more rapidly than psychological maturity.

Among domesticated animals, humans take longest by far to acquire sexual maturity, from ten to sixteen years for females. Males typically do not reach full maturity until their early twenties. Chimpanzees, once considered our closest primate relatives, mature at about the same age as humans: thirteen to fourteen years for females and fifteen to sixteen years for males. Recent research has suggested that bonobos are closer to humans than chimpanzees, though research in this area continues. In addition to resembling most closely our maturation rates, our closest primate relatives are most similar to humans in their degree of social complexity. This supports the theory that the slow maturation rate of humans is due to the need to prepare them for their complex social roles.

The relevant categories in considering maturation rates for mammals are body size, life span, complexity of the brain, and social complexity. Primates exhibit a number of characteristics that distinguish them from other mammals. A chief distinction is increased cranial capacity (brain size), with a focus on the cerebral cortex, the area that facilitates abstract thought. **Abstract thought** is the ability to conceptualize phenomena that are not available to the senses. Humans excel in the area of abstract thought.

The pace of the rapid biological change during puberty varies by individual. Childhood friends can suddenly become strangers, as one continues to be fascinated by dolls, while the other becomes fascinated by "boys." Neither can understand the other because their differing chemistries are sending conflicting messages. One girl is receiving a message that says, "Let's play at being mommy." The other, at a similar age, is receiving a message that says, "I need to *be* a mommy." A similar disparity of messages takes place among males. This is why those participating in

Cringe Night, either as one who reads his or her teenaged diaries or as a member of the audience, find catharsis. The teenaged disparity is equalized by the common experience of having to undertake a confusing, and often humiliating, experience in which contradictions that arise during puberty are resolved.

One website[2] aims to reassure those undergoing puberty that their seemingly inexplicable experiences are "normal": "Puberty is the period of time when children begin to mature biologically, psychologically, socially and cognitively. Girls start to grow into women and boys into men." The biological changes at puberty are produced by hormones that stimulate sexual differentiation. Consequences of this rapid biological differentiation are experienced socially and psychologically; however, the manner in which they are experienced differs cross-culturally.

Coming of Age: The Samoan Example

In her book *Coming of Age in Samoa*, Margaret Mead compares the lives of Samoan adolescent girls with adolescent girls in the United States. She notes that, in the United States, adolescence is considered to be "a period of mental and emotional distress for the growing girl" (1961:144–145[1928]). Mead suggests that the image of a turbulent adolescence does not hold true for Samoan girls. She attributes this to a difference in the Samoan lifestyle: "The Samoan background which makes growing up so easy, so simple a matter, is the general casualness of the whole society. For Samoa is a place where no one plays for very high stakes, no one pays very heavy prices, no one suffers for his convictions or fights to the death for special ends" (1961:146[1928]).

Since conflict is a part of all groups, it is almost certain that Mead overestimates the general harmony. It is possible that Samoans do not express their discontents because it is not considered culturally appropriate. That Mead recognizes this is evident in a later statement: "we may say that Samoa is kind to those who have learned the lesson of not caring, and hard upon those few individuals who have failed to learn it" (1961:146–147[1928]).

Margaret Mead notes that adolescence is especially difficult in the United States because this society lacks the social and cultural mechanisms characteristic of other societies. In *Coming of Age in Samoa*, Mead identifies several aspects of Samoan childrearing practices that ease the transition from childhood to adulthood. Among these are a limited choice of careers and adult lifestyles. Though people in the United States cherish the concept of freedom, lifestyle choices can complicate the transition from childhood dependency to adult responsibility. At the same time individuals are coping with the biological changes that occur at puberty, they must choose careers, of which they have little knowledge, but which will determine the trajectory of their subsequent lives.

In both cases, that of Samoan and U.S. teenagers, the career choices that teenagers make are imposed by socioeconomic class.[3] However, there are differences. A Samoan youth must strive to uphold the status of his lineage, whereas in many U.S. subcultures, a young person is encouraged to exceed the status and wealth of his or her forebears. In both cases, the youth must live up to the social expectations of elders.

U.S. teenagers must also make seemingly unrelated choices that affect their ability to implement their careers and lifestyles. For example, a teenager's choice not to use a condom may make him a parent. It may also expose him or his partner to infectious diseases, some of which are incurable. As a result, career or educational aspirations may be limited. The urgency of the moment may supersede the aspirations of a lifetime. In all societies, fertility is dangerous. It is bound with rules, rituals, and restrictions. Mead asserts that, in Samoa, there is general agreement about appropriate moral choices, whereas U.S. teenagers are faced with conflicting moral views, in their own families and in the society as a whole.

Mead also notes that adolescents in U.S. society must break free of parental restrictions at the same time they are undergoing hormonal changes and facing life-altering career choices. Whereas U.S. children are economically dependent on their parents, Samoan children traditionally made an economic contribution to the household. Even small children could bring sticks to fuel a cooking fire. Older children could tend younger children. Therefore, children were not dependent on their parents. They could leave their natal home and be welcomed by a family in need of the services the child could provide.

Adoption was not unusual among traditional Samoans. A family with more children than needed could provide children for a family with fewer children than needed. This differs greatly from adoption patterns in the United States, where children are treated as property. In the United States, adoption may transfer a child from one state to another or even from one nation to another. In traditional Samoan society, an adopted child would simply begin sleeping in another household close by and provide labor for that household. The child would also continue to interact with the same cadre of playmates and with the same society of adults.

Mead suggests that, during the time of her study, a Samoan child could be part of a social milieu including as many as half a dozen adult females and males, all exercising parental roles of nurturing and discipline. As a result, she noted, Samoan children "do not distinguish their parents as sharply as our children do" (1968:153[1928]). In the process, Mead writes, "The Samoan baby learns that the world is composed of a hierarchy of male and female adults, all of whom can be depended upon and must be deferred to" (1968:153[1928]).

Parental Control and Emotional Disorders

In contrast to the Samoan case, U.S. children are economically and socially dependent upon their parents, a dependency that can allow parents to impose restrictions upon their children. This is illustrated by a story in *The New York Times* about the difficulties teenagers in the United States face when they have been diagnosed as mentally ill by their parents and by health care providers. The story dealt with issues confronted by these teenagers when they left home to attend college. In one case, a young woman confronted a mother who intended to visit her daughter every few weeks to monitor her daughter's "bipolar disorder." The daughter responded by saying "I am so totally aware of the control you have over me right now. In a few months the power dynamic is going to be different."[4]

Where is mental illness located in this case? The mother writes the checks, and therefore, controls the diagnosis. The seventeen-year-old assumes that college will free her of her mother's domination. But will it ultimately free her? The mother will also pay her daughter's tuition, and therefore, maintain a high degree of control over her. The diagnosis of bipolar disorder guarantees that the daughter could be under her mother's control for the rest of the mother's life.

In another case in the same report, C., a young man also diagnosed with bipolar disorder surrenders control over his life to his parents, who had directed every aspect of his mental health care. He says, "If it was up to me, I would just have it so you could make those decisions for me up until I was like, 22. I mean, you've raised me well up to now. You know me better than anyone."[5]

A part of the dependency in these two cases involved control over medications. J., the young woman, rejected medication for her "condition" when she was fourteen because the side effects of the medications left her feeling "out of whack and emotionally inauthentic."[6] Her parents respected her choice, and as she prepares to leave home for college, she states: "I don't feel vulnerable about this transition because this is very much my decision. This is a very autonomous move, very much me structuring my own life. I feel like I am putting myself in a situation with really clear intentions."[7]

Mead suggests that Samoan youths do not feel the same need to resist parental control because the authority of elders, though strong and important, is more diffuse. Parents do not "own" children, and children assume a great deal of responsibility at an early age. Samoan teenagers are still subject to a great deal of social pressure, but much of this pressure comes from the peer group among which they have been socialized. Whereas teenagers in the United States are socialized from the top down—by parents, teachers, and other authority figures—Samoan teenagers have traditionally derived much of their socialization from their peers. Teenagers in the United States are also socialized by their peers, but this socialization often centers on defying authority figures.

The Psychology of Puberty

A report on the online site LiveScience.com states that "Teenagers do crazy things. They take drugs, have unprotected sex, ride with drunken drivers, and pretend to be asleep when it's time to do the dishes."[8] What the website doesn't say is that biologically mature humans often do the same things. Both adults and teenagers are motivated by peer group pressure and the need to define one's social identity.

Adults assume that teens do not take risks into account when making decisions. A study by Valerie Reyna and Frank Farley indicates that [U.S.] teens take about 170 milliseconds longer than adults in weighing the pros and cons of engaging in high-risk behavior and teens often overestimate the odds of a bad outcome. Teenagers are more likely to engage in risky behavior because of their desire for acceptance among peers. Studies of Western European and American teens suggest that their brain wave patterns differ from those of adults, but whether this difference is due to biological development or experience is difficult to measure. A study authored by Sarah-Jane Blakemore of the University College London Institute of Cognitive Neuroscience indicated that the area of the brain associated with "higher-level thinking," empathy, and guilt is "underused" by teenagers. In the study, teens and adults were asked how they would react to certain situations, and researchers measured their brain waves as they responded.[9] Though their responses were similar, their brain activity differed. "The medial prefrontal cortex was much more active in the adults than in the teens; however, the teenagers had much more activity in the superior temporal sulcus, the brain area involved in predicting future actions based on previous ones."[10] The medial prefrontal cortex is involved in decision-making.

This research supports the findings by a Cornell/Temple research team, that teens do consider the possible outcome of their actions. Teens take even longer to consider these possibilities than adults, but their decisions are based on considerations that differ from those of adults. Blackmore notes, "We think that a teenager's judgment of what they would do in a given situation is driven by the simple question: 'What would I do?' Adults, on the other hand, ask: 'What would I do, given how I would feel and given how the people around me would feel as a result of my actions?'" Teenagers consider the consequences of an action for themselves, whereas adults consider the social consequences of their actions. Blakemore adds:

> Thinking strategies change with age. As you get older you use more or less the same brain network to make decisions about your actions as you did when you were a teenager, but the crucial difference is that the distribution of that brain activity shifts from the back of the brain (when you are a teenager) to the front (when you are an adult).[11]

The back of the brain processes sensory data, whereas the front of the brain is involved in decision making.

Blakemore notes that children start taking into account other people's feelings when they are about the age of five, but the ability to factor in this equation increases with age, perhaps both as the result of experience and of shifting brain-wave patterns: "Whatever the reasons, it is clear that teenagers are dealing with, not only massive hormonal shifts, but also substantial neural changes. These changes do not happen gradually and steadily between the ages of 0-18. They come on in great spurts and puberty is one of the most dramatic developmental stages."[12]

In another study, subjects between the ages of nine and twenty were tested on their ability to multitask. They were "given multiple pieces of information, then asked to re-order the information to formulate an accurate response to a question. In another of several tests, they were asked to find hidden items using a high degree of strategic thinking."[13] The study determined that "the ability to remember multiple bits of information developed through age 13 to 15 . . . but strategic self-organized thinking, the type that demands a high level of multi-tasking skill, continues to develop until ages 16 to 17."[14] Monica Luciana, lead researcher of the study, concludes, "Our findings . . . indicate that the frontal lobe is continuing to develop until late adolescence in a manner that depends upon the complexity of the task that is being demanded."[15]

The Acquisition and Socialization of Fertility

Biological and psychological changes taking place at puberty occur within a particular social context, and our survival requires us to adopt a degree of conformity to that context. Though humans are unique in their DNA coding,[16] they must sacrifice some of that individuality to survive and function within a particular social group. This does not imply that conformity requires uniformity. Robert B. Edgerton notes that "behavior can often vary greatly without violating any rule or calling forth any punitive action. All societies provide for acceptable variation in many areas of behavior" (1978:466).

A degree of variability confers benefits on both the group and the individual. The group benefits by continual introduction of new ideas. This allows the group to survive in the event of change, such as the introduction of new technology. Both the group and the individual benefit from variability through the process of negotiation, which permits innovation and the continual adjustment of social relationships.

Puberty requires a major adjustment of social relationships. Children acquire fertility, which involves the power to introduce new members into the social group. Customs such as puberty rituals and marriage allow elders to control the introduction of these intrusive new members into the group. It would be a mistake to assume that the need for control by elders is entirely personal and psychological. Though these rituals confer power on older members of the group, they also ensure that new members of the group are provided for.

As noted earlier, parenthood is not automatically conferred biologically among the Zumbagua of Ecuador. A woman does not socially become a mother until she has demonstrated her ability to feed her child. Similarly, a man does not become a father through his sexual relationship with the child's mother, but by demonstrating his ability to feed the child (Weismantel 1998). Thus, the child's need to be fed is guaranteed by the group as a whole, rather than by the inclination of particular individuals. If the biological parents do not demonstrate their ability to feed the child, the child can be claimed by a member of the group who does demonstrate that ability.

As noted in chapter 2, females are cross-culturally identified with nature, whereas masculinity is viewed as being socially constructed. Carol P. MacCormack notes that females, as well as males, must undergo puberty rites that tame their biological potential: "the very point of the [female] rite of passage is to teach girls to bring the biological events of their lives under careful control" (1993:181; see also Richards 1956).

The puberty rite of passage for girls among the Sande society, a women's religious society in Sierra Leone, includes a period of seclusion, after which their sexual behavior is carefully controlled. The sexual behavior of human females is culturally distinguished from the uncontrolled sexuality of animals and involves instruction in practical techniques for the bearing and rearing of children. These instructions include Sande knowledge about hygiene, nutrition, medicine, and other practical matters.

This initiation ceremony takes place after the first stage of the female life, which lasts from birth until the onset of menstruation. The second stage, which involves initiation and instruction, lasts until the girl marries. The third stage involves marriage, reproduction, and cohabitation with a man. The final stage occurs after her physical death, when she becomes an ancestor.

The Sande ritual that prepares a girl to become a wife and mother begins with the excision of the clitoris and part of the labia minora. Sande women state that this stage of the puberty ritual permits women to be prolific bearers of children. They also explain that the ritual makes women clean by excising the clitoris, which is biologically the female manifestation of the penis. Excising the residual penis permits a girl to become fully a woman, without any vestige of the male sex organ. The male equivalent of this operation is cutting away of the foreskin, which for the Sande is symbolically equivalent to the labia. The labia enclose male sexuality, and therefore must be cut away. The point of initiation ceremonies is not biological or medical fact, but the imposition of cultural and social models onto biological reality.

Menstrual Seclusion

Among Athapaskans, which includes a number of hunting societies who occupied the forested regions from central and south Alaska to the Hudson Bay, the onset of a girl's menses was prepared for by the entire community because it indicated that she was ready for marriage:

> At the beginning of her first menstrual period a girl would leave the camp for a special hut where she remained in complete seclusion for a given period—among the Slave, for ten days, but among the upper Tanana for a month. Food and water were brought by other women, liquids being sucked through a special bone tube. . . . After the period of seclusion, the girl might venture out occasionally, but always with her face covered. She had to make a special effort to avoid men, and, if the band was forced to travel at this time, she had to break her own trail or travel in her own boat. (Vanstone 1974:80)

James W. Vanstone's account of menstrual practices describes what male anthropologists of his generation considered "seclusion." The menstruating girl was clearly not secluded from other women, since they brought her food; however, she was secluded from men. "Seclusion" of females—or more precisely, segregating them from males—is a means of protecting a group's resources by controlling fertility. These practices also ensure that the child born from a sexual union has a recognized social identity that entitles it to group protection and resources.

Controlling Fertility

Westerners have often criticized female seclusion rituals as examples of male dominance over females or as "superstition," the belief that spirits control human lives. In fact, these rituals have developed during 100,000 years of human evolution in which females controlled female fertility rituals. Female seclusion rituals are aimed at containing the power of female fertility within the resources required to sustain it. Fertility is a double-edged sword. It is essential for continuing the existence of a population, whether that is reckoned at the level of a family, of a village, or of a nation. At the same time, excessive fertility stretches the ability of a population to provide resources.

This was recognized in the scientific literature as early as 1798, with publication of Thomas Malthus' *An Essay on the Principle of Population*. In it, Mathus noted that, in nature, plants and animals produce far more offspring than can survive.[17] Malthus was from a prosperous family that was well able to provide for his existence and education, but based on his observations of poverty in eighteenth century England, he concluded that humans, like other animals and plants, could reproduce at rates greater than the environment could support. Malthus' *Essay* became an important part of Charles Darwin's concept of natural selection, in which he noted that members of a species compete with each other for access to environmental resources. Those members of a species best able to compete for resources are most likely to survive and pass on their traits to their offspring.

On the other hand, a species that reproduces beyond the capacity of its environment to support it can become extinct. Before this happens, however, other selective factors come into play. Among humans, these include disease, war, and starvation. As of 1900, the earth's human population stood at 1.9 billion people. Between 1900 and 2000, the population more than tripled, to about 6.7 billion. That century saw the rise of wars and regional conflicts, the development of new diseases, and widespread famine, especially in Africa, where the human species originated. The social and biological crises now afflicting the African continent had all been predicted by population demographers and the World Health Organization.

Though fertility and reproduction are often viewed as being beyond human control—as a gift from God or as a revisiting of the ancestors—reproduction in human groups serves, or subverts, human goals. Reproduction is power. It continues lineages, assures control over wealth, and provides armies that assert control over new territories. Reproduction is risky because it strains resources, but absence of reproduction can be fatal to the survival of a group. The two most common means of controlling fertility are seclusion of females and marriage.

Controlling Fertility: Separation of the Sexes

On the Butaritari atoll, in the southwestern Pacific, the freedom and play of a girl's childhood ends with her first menstruation: "At the first sign of bleeding, the girl is taken into the care of her mother and mother's sisters and confined to the house for three days" (Brewis 1996:27). Menarche marks the transition from girl to woman, and during her seclusion, the girl is instructed in her new responsibilities as a woman. She is fed little during this time of instruction, as a means of teaching her that she must put the needs of her husband and children before her own. Her mothers and aunts teach her how to take care of herself during menstruation and they say incantations to make her beautiful and hard-working. "Effort is made to enhance her beauty: Her skin is rubbed with oil, her hair combed, and her stomach bound tightly to make it flat. On the third day, the woman emerges from the hut to an evening feast in her honor" (Brewis 1996:27).

From this time on, the woman will be watched to ensure that she will be a virgin when she marries. On the evening of her wedding day, her family gathers outside the home of her new in-laws, who join her family in a boisterous celebration outside the house. The bride and groom are left alone to consummate the marriage. Prior to this time they have never been alone together. When the marriage is consummated, the woman must bleed to prove that she is a virgin. This custom is similar to Mediterranean traditions, in which the marriage is consummated while the families celebrate. The purpose of these rituals is to ensure the social identity of children who might be produced by conjugal sexual acts.

The virginity of the bride is important in societies where effective forms of birth control are not available and where inheritance is traced through the male line. The people of Butaritari atoll were traditionally organized under a king, a position inherited through the male line. Similarly, social position is traditionally inherited through the male line in most Middle Eastern groups.

Cross-culturally, the rules of female seclusion before marriage are imposed and controlled by women. During puberty, hormones that drive the urge to procreate are both intense and erratic. Where birth-control measures are inadequate, the only effective form of birth control is abstinence. The only effective way to control abstinence is to spatially separate teenaged boys and girls, preventing their interaction. Since females bear the brunt of reproduction, their seclusion protects them from both their own reproductive urges and from the seduction by males who are not willing to incur the costs of providing for the resulting child.

Historically, in England and the United States, seclusion was effected by establishing different educational models for boys and girls. In England, boys from privileged families were educated in public schools at great expense; girls were educated by private tutors at home.

Controlling Fertility: Marriage

Anthropologists note that marriage does not provide access to sex. Marriage limits access to sex by prescribing socially accepted sexual relationships. An important role of marriage in all societies is providing a stable environment within which children can be raised. This is a necessity because of the long period of dependency characteristic of humans. In human groups, some benefit by fertility, others lose economically and socially through excessive fertility. Still others benefit by exerting control over the reproductive capacity of others. Marriage gives males access to female fertility.

Some form of premarital seclusion for women is a recurring theme in marriage customs cross-culturally. In the United States, the bride is secluded on the morning of her wedding before she is escorted down the middle aisle by her father. It is considered unlucky for anyone outside her immediate family to see either the bride or her dress before she begins that journey down the aisle. In times past, the bride would be heavily veiled as she made that life-altering journey. Her veil and dress would reach to her feet, and the neck of her dress would reach all the way to her chin. Her sleeves would cover her arms and end in a point just above her fingers, allowing her to carry her bouquet and allowing the groom to slip a wedding ring onto her finger. Contemporary wedding gowns in the United States are much more revealing, but the symbolism of veiling continues.

Among Athapaskans a girl was considered ready for marriage shortly after emerging from the seclusion related to her first menstruation. Vanstone writes:

> The selection of a daughter's husband rested in large measure with her family, particularly her mother and other female relatives. It was natural that the girl's parents would look with favor on an older and wealthy suitor. In any event, arranged marriages were the rule and those based on individual choice, while they did occur, were often believed to be less successful. (1974:81)

Because of the changing world economy, the reproductive role of women in some parts of the world has undergone revision. Rachel R. Chapman notes, "For many

African women, bearing children who survive continues to be a sign of female and maternal lineage health, female competence, and female social status. The cultural emphasis placed on female reproductive capacity is reflected in the gender socialization process that, from a young age, prepares girls for their role in reproduction" (2004:230–231). According to Chapman, the term *"nova vida"* represents opportunities for a new life based on the acquisition of commodities as well as the predicament of those who cannot afford these new luxuries. Chapman suggests that the transition exerts new pressure on the reproductive capacity of women:

> A key feature of the *nova vida* is the commoditization of reproduction (which is signaled by the explosion of sex-work in urban and rural settings) and the shift to cash instead of gifts, cattle, tools, and labor for seduction fees, bride wealth payments, and the offerings of respect paid for birth assistance at a time when access to money is more important to survival than it has ever been. As a result, women experience multiple levels of vulnerability—biological, social, and economic—and their bodies bear the brunt of the commoditization of reproduction when sex, marriage, birthing, and births have cash value to parties with competing interests. (2004:232–233)

The reproductive power of women has always played an important role in African gender relations, as is the case in all other societies. According to Chapman, however, a shift from an exchange economy to a cash economy brought about by international forces has divested women of traditional familial support systems, which may include co-wives, to a system in which men establish relationships with women in dispersed regions, so that women cannot form support networks with their co-wives or other family members. As a result, women who cannot produce surviving children may be divorced or abandoned for a more fertile partner. This promotes an increasingly competitive reproductive environment in which women provide children that increase the status of males and reduces the ability of females to control their own fertility.

BECOMING A PARENT

Any woman who has ever been pregnant, or any man who has ever lived with a pregnant woman, would never deny that pregnancy is an essentially biological process. In addition, it entails many changes in attitude, self-definition, and social relationships. For the most part, males are helpless observers to this powerful demonstration of female fecundity. The renegotiation of social space is managed in different societies by different means.

Pregnancy emphasizes the female power of fecundity over male social power. At the same time, a pregnant woman becomes social property. For example, in the United States, strangers feel they have the right to stroke the pregnant woman's stomach, prescribe for her appropriate foods, and tell her how to raise her still enwombed child.

In most societies, including the United States, pregnant women may have special privileges or gain the right to make demands on others. In an analysis of food cravings of pregnant women in Laggala, a village in Sri Lanka, Gananath Obeyesekere proposes that pregnancy cravings are "a culturally constituted structure, built on [a] psychobiological base" (1974:204[1963]) The Sinhalese word for food craving in pregnant women is *dola-duka*, a term that includes *arrack* (a strong alcoholic drink distilled from fermented fruits, grains, sugar cane, or the sap of coconuts or other palm trees), cigars, or cloth.

Obeyesekere notes that, ordinarily, males in the family, especially the father-husband, are associated with authority, whereas wives are expected to be subservient and submissive: "Women are considered physically and mentally weak (though actual facts belie these prejudices). . . . The ideal wife according to a village moralist is one who does not question her husband, but merely obeys him" (197:205[1963]). As Obeyesekere implies, this "ideal" state is seldom found in actual practice.

Obeyesekere writes, "The social situation fosters antagonism between the sexes. . . . The most obvious manifestation of intersex antagonism is overt hostility, in the form of physical violence on the part of the male, and vituperation on the part of the female" (1974:210[1963]). Men beat their wives, sometimes to the point of serious injury, and the wives may respond with curses and obscenities. A favorite swear word of women is *pittambaya*, the Sinhalese word for "penis." In its vituperative form, *pittambaya* is used much as the English word "f—k!" Accommodation of these conflicting viewpoints takes place over the course of a marriage. Beating is mostly aimed at young wives, rather than wives who have passed the age of menopause.

Obeyesekere attributes the intersex hostility he describes to socialization and marriage patterns. Young children, both boys and girls, are raised with great love and attention until girls are about six or seven, when they begin to help with domestic chores. Girls still have a high degree of freedom until menarche, the onset of menstruation, when they begin to be viewed as unclean. They are expected to marry soon after, and marriages are arranged. There are some instances of **uxorilocal residence** after marriage (residence with or near the wife's family), but most residence after marriage in Sri Lanka is **virilocal**, which means that a woman will most likely move to her husband's village. Even if she marries within her own village, her family will consider her well-being to be the province of her husband.

Laggala households typically consist of a nuclear family, consisting of the procreative and reproductive family, which excludes family members outside the procreative unit. Therefore, a woman will have to perform all domestic duties herself, plus assist her husband in fieldwork, until her daughters are old enough to help.

Like menstruation, childbirth among Sinhalese is viewed as unclean. Further, until children are of an age to help with chores, they increase a woman's workload. Owing to their life circumstances, women do not want to have children. But, due to the absence of effective birth control, women can expect to bear children throughout their fertile years. One woman told the female component of the anthropological team: "Oh, lady, if there is some medicine that could rid me of this [fetus], I shall take it immediately" (1974:211[1963]). Some women expressed an interest in being sterilized, even after it was explained to them that they would be infertile for life.

Sharing the Reproductive Burden: Food Cravings

Obeyesekere states that foods and objects chosen by pregnant women of the village are a means of dealing with the psychological problems caused by the sociocultural context of the village. Among these psychological problems are (1) the problem of adjustment, (2) ambivalence toward children, and (3) female envy of males. "Dola-duka is an institutionalized nonidiosyncratic defense provided by the culture itself for coping with these problems" (Obeyesekere 1974:211[1963]).

With menarche, which marks the beginning of a woman's fertility, her life changes from that of a loved and carefree child to the overworked and undervalued role of wife and mother: "Dola-duka . . . gives the woman an opportunity to escape from her adult roles into the emotionally gratifying phase of childhood" (Obeysekere 1974:211[1963]).

A woman's pregnancy and dola-duka invert the superordinate-subordinate husband-wife relationship. The Sinhalese are patrilineal, so a man's status and continuation of his lineage rest on his wife's ability to produce a son. There is some evidence that the strong public assertion of male power may mask an unstated, and perhaps suppressed, awareness that male status is based on female productivity (see Lederman 1993).

During the first trimester of her pregnancy, a Sinhalese village woman is expected to be weak, which finds expression both culturally and physically. Her body becomes "cold." She develops perverse tastes, which must be satisfied by her husband. She is aided in many of her domestic duties—cooking, pounding rice, drawing water, gathering firewood, looking after her children—by her female kin; however, the husband may take on many of these duties, even cooking on occasion. Ordinarily, a woman must serve and obey her husband. During her first trimester of pregnancy, her husband must serve and obey her: "He has to yield unto her 'perverse' demands, often walking long miles and incurring great expenditures and inconvenience in order to bring her the required foods" (Obeysekere 1974:214[1963]).

Dola-duka does not precisely conform to the phenomenon of "morning sickness" experienced by American women, but both require a man to meet his wife's needs. Nausea and vomiting characteristic of American women during the first trimester typically occur during the early hours of the day. Dola-duka can occur at any time of the day. Further, nausea is rare among the Sinhalese village women studied by Obeyesekere. Dola-duka most commonly manifests as spitting. Outside the context of dola-duka, spitting expresses disgust.

During dola-duka, a Sinhalese woman does almost no work. She lies around most of the day and her demeanor changes: "She is petulant, easily irritated, 'behaves like a child,' as one informant put it" (1974:214 [1963]). This informant's description of dola-duka conforms to Obeysekere's view that dola-duka permits a return to childhood.

Types of food and objects rejected and craved by pregnant women reflect the reversal of roles. Typically, rejected dishes are those cheaper and easier for a man to acquire and those that require greater effort on the part of women. For example, rice requires hard work to produce and prepare, and much of this work is performed by women. Pregnant women in their first trimester find rice and the smell of rice cooking repugnant. *Kurakkan roti* is a tortilla made from millet, as important in the Sinhalese diet as rice. Kurakkan prepared as a porridge is preferred by some pregnant women, "since this is a rarer and tastier dish [than rice]" (Obeyesekere 1974:215[1963]). Some women reject everyday curries prepared with coconut milk in favor of the more expensive curries made with coconut oil.

Cold water is scorned. Obeyesekere writes: "Water is strongly associated with the social role of women—one of their major tasks is to bring water from the river in pots for domestic purposes. Bathing, too, is a part of the daily workaday activity. These activities are symbolically rejected" (1974:216[1963]). Because of dola-duka, the husband must boil water, or brew tea, for the "sick" woman to drink.

Foods "craved" by pregnant Sinhalese woman reflect social differentiation. Obeyesekere identifies nine food categories craved by pregnant Sinhalese women: (1) Sweets are associated with childhood. They are used to placate unhappy children. Or, in the case of dola-duka, they are used to placate unhappy pregnant women. (2) Sour foods are associated with childhood, but these cravings may also be based in biology. Sour foods favored by pregnant Laggala women are tamarind, citrus fruits, and pickles. Women who crave them say they stimulate the palate. Pregnant American women also crave pickles, so there may be a biological connection, perhaps because pregnancy may dull the palate. (3) Festival foods are associated with fun and relaxation. Obeyesekere notes that festivals and other celebrations are the only times Sinhalese women are able to set aside their daily tasks, to shop and indulge in leisure. (4) Expensive and rare foods force the husband to spend both money and time in acquiring them. Typical foods in this category are ginger beer, canned fish, dried fish from the Maldive Islands off the coast of southern India, grapes, and meat of the the sambhur deer. Sambhur deer are indigenous to Sri Lanka and southern India. Their numbers are threatened by poaching, expansion of human settlement, and leopards, as well as by the scarcity of water. (5) Pineapple has strong symbolic significance in Sinhalese culture. It is considered bad for the fetus, and "is eaten by women in all Sinhalese villages who wish to [bring about] a miscarriage" (Obeyesekere 1974:218[1963]). The husband is required to supply pineapple if his pregnant wife demands it, even though the fetus may be destroyed. (6) Similarly, honey is associated with menstruation, which is referred to as *pani berana kale* (honey dripping period). During dola-duka, a woman who asks her husband for honey is saying "I want my menstrual flow back" (Obeyesekere 1974:219[1963]). Thus, in the Laggala cultural symbolic idiom, Obeyesekere suggests, this is equivalent to saying, "I want to abort the fetus." Yet the husband must accede to her wishes, even if these wishes endanger his future child. (7) Male foods include *kiroti* (milk pancake), the traditional foods eaten by males during the *adukku* ritual, where ancestral gods are worshipped. Women cannot participate in these rituals because of female ritual impurity. All pregnant women in Laggala craved *kiroti*. In addition, village women craved cigars, cigarettes, and arrack, an alcoholic beverage ordinarily consumed by males. In Sri Lanka, it is fermented from the milky coconut sap produced by palm trees before they bloom. Under ordinary circumstances, "male foods" are taboo to women, so Obeyesekere suggests, the desire to "consume" male food indicates the desire to assume male social roles. (8) Penis symbols are foods that, Obeyesekere holds, are related in villagers' minds with the male sex organ. *Dandulena* or lumpy squirrel (a large squirrel found in Sri Lankan jungles) is linguistically associated with the penis. The term may refer to either the squirrel or the penis. The term may also refer to foods that are associated with males. In Obeyesekere's analysis, the craving for penis symbols is equivalent to eating the penis. (9) Idiosyncratic foods are those unique to a particular case. As Obeyesekere notes, these are hard to interpret because one must know the personal psychological history of the craving person. In one instance, a woman craved green cloth. In another, a woman craved mangoes and *kurumba* (drinking coconut), items that were only available, at great expense, from her natal village. She demanded that they be brought by her mother and brother. In this case, Obeyesekere contends that the woman was seeking to reestablish sentimental ties to the people from whom she had been separated. She may also have been expressing her repressed anger at being separated from her kin, among whom she had felt supported and respected.

Obeyesekere interprets the dola-duka complex as women's desire to have a penis, which represents male social power. However, the prevalence of penis symbolism—especially the use of the Sinhalese word for penis as a pejorative—may indicate the opposite: the desire to cast off the penis on multiple levels, as male social control, as a penetrating object, and as a weapon that inflicts upon women increased social responsibilities. The symbolism could well be that of overthrowing male authority.

Sharing the Reproductive Burden: Couvade

Obeyesekere's description of pregnancy cravings in a Sinhalese village illustrates the negotiation of relationships that ensues when males and females have disproportionate access to public power. Dola-duka moves female social power from the private to the public realm. This is reflected to some degree in U.S. customs when a woman sends her husband out at midnight to acquire ice cream and pickles, the American equivalent of unusual and socially demarcating foods, at considerable cost to a husband's comfort. Pregnancy beliefs and customs express contesting between female and male realms. Since the pregnant female has absolute biological power over the fetus, males must contest for power and access to the fetus and resulting offspring through social means.

Couvade is the term for parenting behavior in which a man shares his wife's experiences, "including her birth pains, postpartum seclusion, food restrictions and sex taboos" (Counihan 1999:69). Anthropologists have explained couvade as a means in which the father can share with some degree of equality the wife's more immediate experience of pregnancy and giving birth. Couvade may also have a biological basis produced by the profound psychological process of becoming a father: "Couvade has been seen as an expression of somatized anxiety, pseudo-sibling rivalry, identification with the fetus, ambivalence about fatherhood, a statement of paternity, or parturition envy. It is likely that the dynamics of couvade may vary between individuals and may be multidetermined" (Klein 1991:57).

Bronislaw Malinowski notes that, among Trobriand Islanders of the western Pacific, a man "takes over the symptoms of post-natal illness and disability while the wife goes about the ordinary business of life" (1985:215[1927]):

> If it is of high biological value for the human family to consist of both father and mother; if traditional customs and rules are there to establish a social situation of close moral proximity between father and child; if all such customs aim at drawing the man's attention to his offspring, then the *couvade* which makes man simulate the birth-pangs and the illness of maternity is of great value and provides the necessary stimulus and expression for paternal tendencies. (1985:215–216[1927])

Pregnancy and motherhood are two realms in which feminine personal and biological power threaten to overthrow the public social power of males, at least temporarily. Couvade may permit a man to stake a social claim to parenthood that equals or rivals the biological claim of the mother.

Children require a committed social environment for their biological and social development. Throughout human evolution, this social environment has been provided by families. Couvade engages the male parent in the social and biological development of the child, a process that is often explained by anthropologists as a social phenomenon in which the father can share some degree of equality with the wife's more biologically immediate experience of gestating and giving birth.

SHARING THE BURDEN: THE BIOLOGY
AND SOCIOLOGY OF PATERNITY

Though pregnancy and childbirth are often viewed as "female disorders" in the United States, males involved in the transition from husband to father experience emotional and physical symptoms related to the lifestyle transition. According to the Mayo Clinic, a man's life situation shapes whether becoming a father contributes to his health and well-being or whether it can lead to health problems: "Every father's experience is different. If you're happily married and gainfully employed, you may be more likely to reap the health benefits of fatherhood. If you're divorced and lose custody of your children, you may be at special risk of developing serious physical and mental illnesses."[18] Specifically, the Mayo Clinic notes:

> During your partner's pregnancy, you also may develop some physical signs and symptoms. Compared with men who aren't expecting children, you may be more likely to catch colds, become irritable, gain weight and have trouble sleeping. It's even possible that you could develop pregnancy-like signs and symptoms such as nausea, vomiting, fatigue and decreased sex drive. But this phenomenon, known as couvade, hasn't been well studied and appears to be uncommon.[19]

The Mayo Clinic analysis notes: "Several studies suggest that expectant fathers experience hormonal changes that mimic those of their partners. These include decreased levels of the male hormone testosterone and the stress hormone cortisol, and an increased level of the female hormone estradiol."[20]

These hormonal changes may be selected for in humans and other mammalian species because they increase the probability that their dependent offspring will survive by reducing the male parent's aggressive levels and enhancing his nurturing tendencies: "Although the significance of these hormonal changes is unclear, it's possible that they're nature's way of priming you to become a nurturing father. Similar changes occur in males of other species who actively participate in raising their young."[21]

Mammalian offspring require a high degree of parental investment because they remain dependent on their parents for almost one-third of their lives. The degree of parental investment increases dramatically for primates by requiring the acquisition of survival skills through learning. The need for learning survival skills reaches its pinnacle in the human species. The anthropologist Clifford Geertz (1973) called humans "the incomplete animal" because humans must learn virtually all of what they need to survive: how to acquire food, how to keep themselves clean and free from disease, how to recognize danger and organize a defense, and how to interact with that most subtle of organisms, fellow members of the human species.

Mothers, as well as fathers, must learn how to parent. We were not provided with an instinct for parenting. We must learn that skill, and our own parents and children are our best teachers. The Mayo Clinic suggests that this learning process may ultimately improve our own lives and health:

> When your partner gives birth and becomes absorbed in caring for your newborn, you may feel excluded or even irrelevant. But over time, fatherhood inspires many men to make lifestyle changes that improve their physical health. The possibility of premature death becomes less abstract when you have children. You want to be around for them as long as possible, and you want to be a good role model.[22]

Nadya Pancsofar, the lead author of a study conducted at the Frank Porter Child Development Institute at the University of North Carolina, suggests that, in families with two working parents, fathers may have more impact on a child's language development than mothers. The study was based on researchers who recruited 92 families from 11 child care centers before their children were a year old. Variables in the study included family income, level of education and child care arrangements. Subjects in the study were well-educated middle-class families with married parents living in the home.

Children in the study were observed over a period of two years, involving videotapes at home in free-play sessions with both parents, in which all their speech was recorded. Researchers measured the total number of utterances of the parents, the number of different words they used, the complexity of their sentences and other aspects of their speech. In analyses of the children at the age of three, the predictors of high scores on the test were the mother's level of education, the quality of child care, and the number of different words used by the father.[23]

Trouble in the Nuclear Family Paradise

The number of parenting magazines aimed at middle-class families in the United States may provide a clue that there is trouble in the paradisiacal view of parenting. A study conducted by Robin Simon at Florida State University indicated that parents have significantly higher levels of depression than other people. Simon's study was published in the February 2006 issue of the *Journal of Health and Social Behavior*, a publication of the American Sociological Association.[24] The study was based on a population of 13,000 adults. In all cases, no parent reported less depression than nonparents, regardless of the parenting style practiced. The highest rates of depression occurred among parents of grown children and those who do not have custody of their minor children. Simon suggests that one basis of the problem is that parents in the United States don't get as much help in parenting as they once did, or as is still the case in most other countries.

The extended family, which has been the tradition in agricultural families such as in the United States prior to World War II, provided many hands for helping with cultivating crops, tending farm animals, and caring for children. Thus, the burden of parenting did not rest on the parents alone. The nuclear family, which is associated with industrialization and has become idealized in the United States, does not provide all the labor necessary to cover economic necessities and socialize dependent children.

Affluent families can cover this lack by hiring skilled labor, including cooks, housekeepers, gardeners, and child care specialists. Less affluent families are left to cope on their own. In both cases, the child's well-being is in the hands of nonfamily members (as in the case of affluent families) or of overworked and overstressed near kin. The idealized urban nuclear family—consisting of a working father, stay-at-home mother, and dependent children—may not be the ideal context within which to raise children. Certainly, it is not the norm, even in the United States.

GRANDPARENTHOOD

As a child growing up on a farm in southeast Missouri, I had vastly different experiences with my grandparents. My paternal grandfather died the year before I was born, and my maternal grandfather was an imp who did not display much more maturity than my cousins. My maternal grandmother was an eternal child who recounted many stories of her childhood that would have been shocking to my paternal grandmother. I heard these stories as an interested onlooker. My paternal grandmother was a wise woman who offered counsel to her sons but displayed little interest in her grandchildren.

My maternal grandmother and I had many adventures that my mother and father would never have permitted. One afternoon, my maternal grandmother decided that we should gather and cook mussels from a local stream on their farm. We gathered about fifty "mussels" and put them in a large pot of water. After several hours, my grandmother and I were both surprised that the mussel shells failed to open. When my uncle, then in his twenties, came home from work, we apprised him of the failed attempt. His bemused reply was, "That's good, because they are poison."

My mother offered a different episode involving this grandmother, who once collected wild turtles and made them into soup. After returning from his fields, my maternal grandfather took one look at the "turtle soup," packed their children (including my mother) into his car, and drove them into town for lunch at a restaurant. Though I didn't notice it at the time, I had an unusually instructive and colorful childhood, thanks mostly to my maternal grandparents..

In writing this part of *The Anthropology of Health and Healing*, it struck me as remarkable that so little of the anthropological literature, which values holism, deals with the relationship between grandparents and grandchildren. What literature is available in popular media deals mostly with grandparent-grandchild relationships characteristic of the nuclear family. Since the nuclear family is an anomaly associated with mobile societies, such as those of foragers and industrialists, it seems a great loss that grandparent-grandchild relationships among extended families characteristic of horticultural and agricultural societies are so little represented in the literature.

In foraging through my ethnographies, collected over a thirty-year career as an anthropologist, I found only one account of what might come close to a grandmother-grandchild relationship.[25] In her book *Tiwi Wives: A Study of the Women of Melville Island, North Australia,* Jane G. Goodale describes the relationship of the senior wife to the children of junior wives:

> She can direct the other mothers in her domestic group in what she considers to be the proper management of their children's upbringing. These are her given rights as a *taramaguti* (senior wife). Whether or not she exercises these rights depends on her own personality. Some women demand the respect and obedience due to them. Others receive it without demand and exercise their power "behind the scenes." And still others are content to relegate their power to another co-wife or at least make no attempt to exercise these rights. (1994:228[1971])

Goodale adds, "While a *taramaguti's* powers appear to be restricted to her co-wives, in actuality they may extend much farther because of her control over their children: she is their 'supreme' mother" (1994:229[1971]).

In the United States, the September 12, 2007, comic "Family Circus" shows four young children with smiles on their faces and hearts drawn above their heads sitting on a woman's lap. The caption reads, "Most adults pursue happiness. Most children create it." Significantly, the woman is the children's grandmother. Most of the comics in the series depict an unsmiling woman dealing with a problem caused by one or all of the children. She is the children's mother.

The contrast between indulgent grandparents and overburdened parents is a common theme in American popular culture. This is due in large part to the emergence of the nuclear family in the industrialized United States between the first and second World Wars. It was common for the grandparent generation to stay on the farm while their children moved to the city to take wage-labor jobs. This migration gave rise to the model of the contemporary urban family in which grandparents do not live with, or even near to, their grandchildren. According to that model, the role of the grandparent was to wait patiently until the children and grandchildren came to visit.

Since that era, that image of the grandparent has become obsolete. Grandparents may themselves live in cities and remain active in wage labor jobs. As a result of the shift from farming to wage labor jobs, grandparents may live in cities far away from their grandchildren. Industrialization and a wage labor economy require mobility in the work force. Wage earners take the jobs they are qualified for, and which provide economic benefits, regardless of whether they are close to, or far from, their extended families.

As a result of immigration, parenting and grandparenting customs from other countries have been introduced into the United States. Grandparents, parents, and grandchildren may retain the customs of their own countries, including the traditional attitudes toward economic and social interdependency. Grandparents may expect to be actively involved in rearing their grandchildren, and parents may welcome their assistance or resent their "interference."

Research on Grandparenting in American Families

In 1995, the U.S. National Institutes of Health solicited applications to obtain funding for studying the role of grandparents in U.S. culture. The desired research focused on five topics: (1) As a center of interest for grandparents in an aging society; this aspect focused on **demographic analyses** of grandparenting and economic research. Demographic analysis refers to the statistical dimensions of human populations, such as age and income; (2) the role of grandparents in the family unit, which includes family relationships, caregiving, and family change; (3) grandparents in the network of aging, including social, community, and legal affiliations such as churches, aging support, and advocacy groups, as well as neighborhood organizations and school-affiliated groups; (4) grandparents as aging individuals, including roles, expectations, and identity of grandparents; (5) special populations and grandparents in special circumstances, such as minority families, custodial grandparents, great-grandparents, and impoverished familes.[26]

Research objectives cited by the Institutes of Health are as follows:

> Grandparents have always been acknowledged as influential in family life and grandparenthood has been a marker of aging within society. However, only within the last half century has increasing longevity meant that most older people live long enough to become grandparents, that these elders continue as robust and active in family life and society, and that grandparenthood is now a status and role affecting middle-aged adults through the oldest.[27]

The NIH bulletin notes that "it is known that grandparents provide care for other family members, particularly grandchildren, either on a part-time day care basis or as a custodial caregiver."[28] The bulletin added that, in 1990, 4.2 million children lived with grandparents and in one-third of these cases, the child's parents were absent.[29]

To track these issues, in 2008, the *Journal of Grandparenting Research* was established online for professionals and researchers. It publishes abstracts of research on grandparenting. A number of the abstracts deal with stress felt by grandparents if they were the primary caregivers. Other research indicated that grandmothers continued to be active in the lives of grandchildren whereas grandfathers did not.

A study by Philip Cohen at the University of Utah linked human longevity to grandmothers. Cohen studied modern groups that subsist on wild foods. He discerned that grandmothers continue to gather large quantities of food and that they often gave the surplus to their grandchildren. Cohen notes, "This would have helped humans to compete against species with self-sufficient young and could also explain why humans live so long. The researchers also suggest that the late maturity and small size at weaning that have evolved in humans were driven by grandmothers."[30]

A Limited Survey

In 2008 I undertook a limited survey of multicultural students in my introductory cultural anthropology classes in the polyglot region of Los Angeles. I promised the students anonymity and extra credit for their descriptions of their relationships with grandparents. This study was too limited to produce a statistical analysis or even a comprehensive analysis of grandparenting in Los Angeles; however, it did produce some expected and unexpected results.

Reports by Latino groups showed that students experienced strong intergenerational relationships with both maternal and paternal grandparents. These relationships were reinforced by participation in ritual occasions, such as Day of the Dead, Cinco de Mayo, and family events, including birthdays, weddings, and funerals. Several students who were predominantly Anglo or of mixed parentage stated that they had never known their grandparents.

Asian students, whether immigrants or Asian-American, described their relationship with paternal grandparents as formal and restrictive. This surprised me, since most Asian groups figure kinship through patrilineal lines. The Asian students in my classes described close emotional ties with their maternal grandmothers. This came as a surprise to me until I considered that the formal relationships established by patrilineal inheritance of status and property would necessarily be formal, whereas matrilineal grandparental relationships would not carry the responsibility of transmission of property and status.

7

The Human Life Cycle

Growing Old and Growing Good

CASE STUDY
Views of Happiness in L.A.'s Chinatown

Wong Yee, ninety-two, catches the bus every morning at 7:30 and journeys to the nearby Chinatown district in Los Angeles. He has coffee and sweet bread at a Mexican bakery and then sits down to play Chinese chess or mah-jongg at the Hop Sing clubhouse. He bets on the game, but not too much. Steve Lopez, a columnist for the *Los Angeles Times*, asked Jimmy Wong, a cousin of the venerable chess and mah-jongg player, if there was a "chess king." The younger Wong replied, "There's no such thing as the best. We do this for happiness. That's the reward." The elder Wong emigrated from China in 1931 at the age of seventeen. His first job in the United States was delivering newspapers in San Francisco. After that, he worked as a kitchen boy in a Chinese restaurant in Fresno, in central California. He then moved to Los Angeles. During World War II, Wong was ferried to Catalina Island, where he helped build ships for the Pacific fleet. After the war, Wong worked for a Trader Vic's restaurant until he retired. He has been hanging out at the Central Plaza in Chinatown for more than fifty years. Wong interrupted his interview with the *Los Angeles Times* columnist to check his cell phone. Lopez asked whom Wong Yee had called on the cell phone. "His girlfriend," the columnist was told.[1] Culturally, Chinese differ from Americans in their views on growing old. For Chinese, growing old is a mark of merit. Traditionally, Chinese invested in their work and health when they were young. They took care of their families with the expectation that their families would take care of them when they grew old. Thus, old age is viewed as a time when people reap what they have sown. By way of contrast, Americans view old age with dread. When she was about forty, a Hollywood actress known for her beauty was asked by a reporter, "How does it feel to get old?" She replied, "It beats the alternative."

Not all societies consider forty to be old. This is an artifact of the Hollywood youth culture, which ascribes beauty only to smooth skin and a skillful application of makeup. A number of photographers and artists have recorded the beauty of aging, which implies the accumulation of experience. Linda L. Richards, an art reviewer, describes Annie Leibovitz's powerful portrait of her mother, Marilyn Leibovitz: "Perfect in unforgiving black and white, the light on the subject's face is sharp and diffused at once, while her hair is illuminated by a halo of light. Marilyn is meeting the camera full on and it is impossible not to see the strength in this woman's face. A lifetime of love and hard work fairly emanate from her."[2]

The dynamic beauty of real life contrasts with the static beauty of media figures, who are burnished by experts trained in erasing the flaws that life imposes on the human body. The image that emerges from media figures is that of ancient Greek statues of gods, which aim to portray perfection, in contrast with Roman sculptors, who recorded the imperfect features of living humans. Leibovitz's photography does both.

Cheryl L. Reed, an art reviewer for the *Chicago Sun-Times*, prefers Leibovitz's portrayal of real life over her homage to celebrities. In writing of Leibovitz's book *A Photographer's Life: 1990–2005*, Reed contrasts her "photos of glitzy actors and musicians" with the "real-life black-and-white photographs" of Leibovitz's own family and friends. Reed states that the celebrities "become static eye candy amidst a compelling personal photo narrative. With her family, Leibovitz has captured emotion and drama between generations and couples."[3] The reviewer adds, "If ever a case was to be made that photographs of beautiful people become monotonous after a while, this is it."

Vincent van Gogh considered the Roulin family in Arles to be remarkable art subjects, not because of their beauty, but because of the way they represented the human condition. He painted a number of portraits of the postman, Joseph Roulin, in his blue uniform with gold buttons. In a letter to Emile Barnard, van Gogh wrote, "I want to do figures, figures and more figures. I cannot resist that series of bipeds from the baby to Socrates, and from the woman with black hair and white skin to the woman with yellow hair and a sunburned brick-red face" (Pickvance 1984:90).

The Gift of Growing Old

Not everyone has the good fortune to grow old. I take the term "good fortune" from a Chinese philosophy that views growing old as a mark of good fortune. Dying before reaching an advanced age does not permit fulfillment of one's karma. On the wall next to my bed is a Chinese scroll decorated with 100 characters that represent 100 ways of saying "longevity."[4] I don't know of any culture other than the Chinese that places such linguistic emphasis on celebrating the gift of living a good, long life.

The difference between the Chinese and American views of old age is due, not just to the cultures, but to the cultures shaped by the economy. The Chinese have not come far from their agricultural roots, whereas Americans have forgotten that they ever had agricultural roots. The extended family of agriculturalists consists of at least three generations and is linked to a **unilineal kinship system**, in which descent is traced through either the male or female line, but not through both.

In an agricultural society, the knowledge and experience of elders is essential for the prosperity of the entire family. Young, vigorous adults provide strength for the daily chores, for planting, harvesting, cooking, and cleaning. Children contribute their share through running errands and tending younger offspring. Each member of the family has much to contribute. Thus, prosperity depends on making a long-term investment in one's family because family members are the source of one's health, happiness, and prosperity.

In contrast to the extended family characteristic of agricultural societies the nuclear family centers on a single reproductive unit, a parent or parents and children. Members of the nuclear family are economically dependent on each other, but they cannot count on economic support from outside the reproductive unit. The nuclear family is characteristic of industrialized societies and other groups in which mobility is more important than stability. The nuclear type of family organization is based on short-term investment in one's children, who are socialized into fending for themselves after their parents have provided them with a home and education during their early years.

In the nuclear family system, parents expect to provide for themselves when they grow old. When they are no longer able to care for themselves, their health and well-being often depend on professional caretakers, rather than on their families. Elders who have invested in their children's futures instead of their own are viewed as lacking in foresight. They are "unwise" in their financial planning. The extended family is still characteristic of rural communities in industrialized societies. Having grown up on a farm in the American Midwest, in a loosely knit extended family, I was appalled when I arrived in Los Angeles and realized I had no safety net.

In all societies, regardless of family organization, we try to transmit our skills and resources to the next generation; however, human life is complex, and many life skills are acquired only through experience and experimentation. At some point, depending on genetics and circumstances, we lose control over our bodies and over our lives. Eventually, we die. I have made the tasteless joke that the death rate from cancer in my family is 60 percent, but the overall death rate is 100 percent. We all die eventually. If we are fortunate, we will grow old before that happens.

In Chapter 5 we examined consistencies and variability in how human groups define and organize the human life cycle with respect to conception and birth, infancy and childhood. In Chapter 6 we described the reproductive stage of the human life cycle. In this chapter we follow the trajectory of the human life cycle into grandparenthood, old age, and finally, into death and mortuary rites.

Our objective is to examine how phases of the life cycle are defined cross-culturally and how attitudes and practices associated with these phases factor into definitions of health, as well as into patterns of diagnosis and healing. Though life cycle transitions are universally considered dangerous because of the alteration in social relationships they engender, there is a dramatic difference in how these disruptions are viewed cross-culturally. Folk beliefs in societies that are not organized around Western medicine view them as disruptive situations that can be controlled through ritual. In Western medicine, they are typically viewed as disorders that can be treated through medications.

ATTITUDES TOWARD AGING

Though aging is often viewed as a disease in the United States, it is, in fact, a natural part of the life cycle for those of us lucky enough to live long enough. Attitudes toward aging vary greatly cross-culturally. In most cultures, people who have passed the childbearing and childrearing years are treated with great respect. Their wisdom and experience can be of great value to the community.

On December 26, 2004, a tsunami caused by an earthquake of greater than 9.0 magnitude killed nearly 300,000 people and devastated regions along the northern and eastern coast of the Indian Ocean. Waves also smashed into the east coast of Africa. But people in a village on the Indonesian island of Simelue, near the earthquake's epicenter off the west coast of northern Sumatra, were saved by folklore recounted by an old man. The legend he drew on for cultural knowledge described an earthquake and tsunami that had occurred in 1907, which allowed the old man to recognize the threat posed by the 2004 tsunami. Islanders fled to inland hills after the initial shaking caused by the earthquake had subsided, but before the tsunami hit. No lives were lost. Wisdom acquired through aging can save lives.

Among traditional !Kung foragers of Africa, about 10 percent of those studied by anthropologist Marjorie Shostak reached the age of sixty, compared with 16 percent in the United States at the time of her study. At any age, the cause of death for !Kung was likely to be infectious diseases and accidents. Shostak writes that !Kung "are free of many diseases common to older people in other cultures, including atherosclerosis, hearing loss, hypertension, and diseases that are more obviously stress-related, such as ulcers and colitis" (1981:320). Shostak adds, "Many !Kung at age sixty are vigorous and independent (they have been sturdy enough to resist diseases others have succumbed to), but more than half have some physical problem that makes them dependent on others" (1981:320).

Among these problems are partial loss of vision, walking difficulties, and respiratory diseases, such as tuberculosis, chronic bronchitis, and emphysema. On the other hand, Shostak writes, "Tooth decay is essentially absent, probably because the !Kung eat so little sugar and refined carbohydrates. (They regularly care for their teeth by rubbing them with a plant stem that both cleans and whitens them)" (1981:320). Teeth of older !Kung, however, were worn down because of the abrasiveness of the foods they ate.

!Kung traditionally did not keep track of numerical age, but Shostak notes, they are "acutely aware of relative age. Since age is associated with status, 'who is older'—be it a few years or a few days—is extremely important and affects all relationships" (1981:321). The term of respect *n!a* is a suffix attached to the name of one who has attained full adulthood, usually a male or female forty years old, "a time of great productivity for both men and women" (Shostak 1981:321). The term could also be attached to the name of a younger person who had exceptional achievement in hunting, entering trance,[5] or playing a musical instrument. An individual in his or her late fifties is likely to be addressed by the term *n!a n!a*, which expresses "the greater respect that comes with their advancing age" (Shostak 1981:321).

Cycling for Health

Though aging is often linked to disability, physical activity can reduce the probability of impaired performance. Anthropologist Elizabeth D. Whitaker studied a group of twenty-two Italian cyclists, some of whom continued vigorous activity long after they might be expected to give it up. The youngest cyclist in Whitaker's study was forty-nine; the oldest was an eighty-four-year-old man who had been cycling for sixty-nine years. Four of the cyclists were octogenarians. All of the participants in the study cycled for great distances in difficult terrain, including over the mountain passes covered in the Tour of Italy. Many of the cyclists, including the men in their eighties, regularly rode great distances. The oldest rode sixty kilometers (37.2 miles) on a single trip three to four times a week. Of the cyclists who rode the greatest distances, up to 100 kilometers (62.1 miles) per trip three to four days a week, two were in their sixties and one was in his seventies. Whitaker's study focused on the cyclists' motivations for riding, the aesthetic and social rewards of riding, and the health benefits they accrued from riding.

The primary motive for cycling was that it is fun: "Riding fast in a group, speeding down hills, or challenging oneself over a difficult climb is fun and often thrilling" (2005:21). Cyclists stated that they liked the way vigorous cycling made their bodies feel, and several described the performance of their bodies in almost the same terms as the performance of their bicycles. One said that "the sense of power one feels when riding . . . causes one to marvel and reflect" (2005:21). Another compared his body to a machine: "You have a body, you use it, and it works. A machine that works. You are always amazed at what it can do. You measure yourself. It's a self-check" (2005:21). Still others are fascinated by the machine they ride. One liked working with bicycles so much, he fixed other people's bicycles for fun.

Cyclists liked the feeling of having a body that was lean and strong. They extended this idea to a more general concept, that of *stare bene*, being well in the sense of being alive, happy, and healthy. Another concept used by the cyclists, *sfogarsi*, describes the release of stress that occurs during and after a ride. Yet another term, *reintagrare*, making whole again or reconstituting, describes the experience as restoring a sense of equilibrium. Cycling was described as bringing body and soul together, of intensifying corporal experiences and as a "way to unite the body with the psyche, giving you a somatic/psychological perception à la Zen" (2005:23–24). One cyclist linked the sport of cycling with sexuality and health in older age.

The cyclists extended the aesthetic of the body to the aesthetics of the spirit and the environment. One expressed pleasure in "enjoying nature, the panorama, breathing, training" (2005:24). A cyclist who had once raced preferred cycling for pleasure: "After 540,000 kilometers (335,340 miles), I am having to start over to see the things I missed before when I had my head down all the time. I used to enjoy the competition; now I want to enjoy the surroundings" (2005:25). Another cyclist linked the aesthetics of external surroundings to the aesthetics of internal experience: "Nature, open air, ideal physical surroundings for cycling. It's a pleasure. You see things you wouldn't see otherwise. It's you with yourself. They are intimate voyages; you ask yourself questions, you reflect, you do a little philosophy. It's a whole series of positive values" (2005:25). Cycling also conferred social rewards:

> Many cyclists have been riding with the same friends for years. While these cyclists also enjoy riding alone, they say that it is fun to be in company and to be able to have a conversation during the ride. The more sociable riders are active in their cycling associations, going to weekly meetings, weekend rides, get-togethers for cyclists and their families, and annual cycling trips to other regions or countries. (2005:26)

Whitaker notes that cycling is integral to Italian culture for transportation, sightseeing, and competition. The sense of well-being described by the older Italian cyclists was supported by measures of their blood pressure levels, heart rates, body mass index (BMI), and lung capacity, which tended to be within the normal range for much younger people.

In addition to cyclists, Whitaker interviewed physicians experienced in sports medicine. Rodolfo Rosini, who worked in a public clinic, stated that people who "practice regular exercise have capacities at the level of general physical efficiency and well-being that are superior not just to those of their age cohort but also to those of young sedentary people" (2005:17).

AGING AND MEDICINE

In the youth-oriented culture of the United States, being old is typically described as a medical problem. For example, according to the December 2006 *Harvard Mental Health Letter*, "The older you are, the more likely you are to have a sleep disorder." Research conducted by the National Institute on Aging found that more than 50 percent of people older than sixty-five in the United States report regular sleep problems that trouble them at night or prevent their participation in daytime activities: "They can't fall asleep when they want to, they wake up repeatedly, they wake up too early, their sleep is not refreshing, or they feel drowsy or groggy all day."

One issue is whether the change in sleep patterns is universal or whether it is characteristic of life in the United States. The *Harvard Mental Health Letter* lists medical conditions that could produce sleep loss, such as "overactive thyroid, diabetes, congestive heart failure, high blood pressure, asthma, emphysema, arthritis pain, chronic heartburn and urinary difficulties." Some medications and drugs may also produce sleep loss, including alcohol, caffeine, stimulants, steroids, diuretics, cold and allergy medications, antidepressants, and anti-arrhythmia drugs.

Sleeping pills, often prescribed for sleep disorders, may "do more harm than good," according to the *Harvard Mental Health Letter*. The most effective treatment is behavioral therapy, which involves changing the daily routine. The incidence of sleep loss could be due to behavioral changes associated with aging in the United States, or more generally, the pattern of retirement and loss of social status associated with aging. The retirement age in the United States is sixty-five, which is young compared cross-culturally. Retirement, which involves loss of a regular routine and often a loss of predictable social exchange, may interrupt the circadian rhythm and lead to sleep disorders.

Too Much Medicine?

According to data compiled by the Georgetown University Center on an Aging Society, "More than 131 million people—66 percent of all adults in the United States—use prescription drugs. Utilization is particularly high for older people and those with chronic conditions."[6] The Georgetown study focuses on the cost of prescription drugs; however, it also provides information on the profile of prescription drug use in the United States.

Demographic data indicate that prescription drug use is associated with age, gender, race and ethnicity, income, and health status: "Prescription drug use increases with age. Three quarters of those aged fifty to sixty-four use prescription drugs, compared to 91 percent of those age eighty and older. The average number of prescriptions filled also increases with age, from thirteen for those age fifty to sixty-four to twenty-two for those age eighty and older."[7] Women are more likely than men to use prescription drugs, but the gap closes with age: "Some 40 percent of men and 66 percent of women age 18 to 34 use prescription drugs, . . . some 92 percent of men and 90 percent of women age 80 and older use prescription drugs."[8]

In spite of the high rate of prescription drug use in the United States, people in this country do not have the longest life expectancy. At the time of this writing, the longest life expectancy in the world was that of the people of Andorra, who live in the Aragon region of Spain, with a life expectancy of 83.5 years. Following that region was Japan, with a life expectancy of 80.7 years; San Marino in Italy, with a life expectancy of 81.1; and Singapore, with a life expectancy of 80.1. The average life expectancy in the United States was 77.1. People in Australia, Canada, and countries in western Europe all have longer life expectancies than people in the United States.[9]

The overall life expectancy for Australians is lowered by statistics for indigenous Australians. The average life expectancy for Australian Aborigines is 59.4 for males and 64.8 for females, based on figures made available in 2001. The low life expectancy for Aborigines is attributed to poverty, discrimination, substance abuse, and poor access to health care.

Aging affects people in many different ways. A number of factors have been considered by researchers in explaining why some people live longer than others: genetics, money, lack of stress, a loving family, lots of friends, and other factors that make life worth living. In spite of the abundant research on the subject, however, we still do not know why some people live longer than others.

8

Lifestyle and Health

CASE STUDY
Mountaineering Essays

"I reached camp about an hour before dusk, hollowed a strip of loose ground in the lee of a large block of red lava, where firewood was abundant, rolled myself in my blankets, and went to sleep. Next morning, having slept little before the ascent and being weary with climbing after the excitement was over, I slept late. Then, awaking suddenly, my eyes opened on one of the most beautiful and sublime scenes I ever enjoyed. A boundless wilderness of storm-clouds of different degrees of ripeness were congregated all over the lower landscape for thousands of square miles, colored gray, and purple, and pearl, and deep-glowing white, amid which I seemed to be floating; while the great white cone of the mountain above was all aglow in the free, blazing sunshine. It seemed not so much an ocean as a *land* of clouds—undulating hill and dale, smooth purple plains, and silvery mountains of cumuli, range over range, diversified with peak and dome and hollow fully brought out in light and shade. I gazed enchanted, but cold gray masses, drifting like dust on a wind-swept plain, began to shut out the light, forerunners of the coming storm I had been so anxiously watching. I made haste to gather as much wood as possible, snugging it as a shelter around my bed. The storm side of my blankets was fastened down with stakes to reduce as much as possible the sifting-in of drift and the danger of being blown away. The precious bread-sack was placed safely as a pillow, and when at length the first flakes fell I was exultingly ready to welcome them. . . . Presently the storm broke forth into full snowy bloom, and the thronging crystals darkened the air. The wind swept past in hissing floods, grinding the snow into meal and sweeping down into the hollows in enormous drifts all the heavier particles, while the finer dust was sifted through the sky, increasing the icy gloom. But my fire glowed bravely as if in glad defiance of the drift to quench it, and, notwithstanding but little trace of my nest could be seen after the snow had leveled and buried it, I was snug and warm, and the passionate uproar produced a glad excitement."[1]

John Muir repeatedly explored the glories of the Sierra Nevada mountain ranges and he was well prepared to deal with the storms that arise there. He prepared his shelter, stowed his food as a pillow, and selected firewood that would be easy to kindle. Many contemporary adventurers venture out into these beautiful but perilous mountains ill-prepared. They often need rescue or perish before rescuers arrive.

Muir chose a lifestyle appropriate for his skills and interests. I am perfectly content to sip an excellent glass of wine while watching the sun descend over the Pacific Ocean and contemplating my next book. The Sierra Nevada mountain range is safe forever from my amateurish efforts to explore its treasures. I am content to enjoy its beauty from a distance.

Our choice of lifestyle shapes the trajectory of our lives and health. As the example of Italian cyclists in the previous chapter indicates, a great deal of folk wisdom, as well as scientific evidence, suggests that play is important for psychological and physical health. Lifestyle encompasses varied patterns of activity, including diet, values, concepts of the self, interactions with others, and loci of power, religion, and decision making. In this chapter, we will discuss those issues that have been correlated with health in medical and psychological research or in the cross-cultural research conducted by anthropologists.

PLAY, FLOW, AND HEALTH

The May/June 2007 issue of *AARP: The Magazine* explores the secrets of people who live long, happy lives. Hank Lang, a 94-year-old retired New York City firefighter featured in the article showed no sign of the ailments usually considered "normal" for one of his age. He "has no signs of heart disease, cancer, diabetes, Alzheimer's, or even high cholesterol."[2] Lang's health regime is simple. He always carries birdseed in the event that he encounters birds and squirrels: "The birds and squirrels I feed each day keep me entertained. . . . I have my periods of stress just like everyone else, but feeding the animals takes my mind off of it. It's a nice diversion."[3]

The level of physical fitness Lang was required to maintain as a New York City firefighter no doubt provided the basis for his health, but Lang correctly attributes his freedom from the side effects of stress to his current lifestyle. Firefighters, police officers, and journalists are all subject to high degrees of stress; however, their lifestyles are physically active, and there are major social rewards for the work they do. These social rewards rarely come only in the form of money. Instead, they come in the form of doing important work and being respected by one's peers.

The principle of fulfilling personal goals and performing at high levels is characteristic of many professions and lifestyles. Athletes find intrinsic rewards in competence and competition. Albert Einstein, who is most known for his contribution to physics, lived a full and active life on multiple levels. In addition to pondering the riddles of the universe, he also played the violin, among many other activities.

In Lang's case, as a retired firefighter, he no longer has to undergo the stress of rescuing an incapacitated victim from a fiery furnace, but he is subject to the stresses that plague most if not all members of the human species, including the detritus of everyday life and relationships. In one sense, feeding the birds and squirrels is connected to his life as a firefighter, which involves helping others. Now, however, no one's life is on the line. Feeding the birds and squirrels is an entirely playful activity.

People in all societies play, and play is not restricted to humans. The Swiss philosopher Johan Huizinga asserts: "Play is older than culture, for culture, however inadequately defined, always presupposes human society, and animals have not waited for man to teach them their playing." Huizinga further suggests that all forms of human culture arise out of play. Even war, which is apparently serious and certainly deadly, shares characteristics of play: "Ever since words existed for fighting and playing, men have been wont to call war a game" (1950:89).

There is evidence that the ability to play is linked to psychological and physical health, as well as to productivity in work. The psychologist Mihaly Csikszentmihalyi distinguished between extrinsic and intrinsic rewards. *Extrinsic rewards* may consist of money, power, prestige, and other forms of material rewards. He writes, "The management of behavior, as presently practiced, is based on the tacit belief that people are motivated only by external rewards or by the fear of external punishment" (1977:2).

Csikszentmihalyi suggests that "striving for material goods is in great part a motivation that a person learns as part of his socialization into a culture. Greed for possessions is not a universal trait" (1975:2–3). He notes that some activities, such as rock climbing and playing chess, may convey *intrinsic rewards* to some people because they involve enjoyment. He examines what he calls the "flow" experience:

> In the flow state, action follows upon action according to an internal logic that seems to need no conscious intervention by the actor. He experiences it as a unified flowing from one moment to the next, in which he is in control of his actions, and in which there is little distinction between self and environment, between stimulus and response, or between past, present, and future. (1975:36)

What Csikszentmihalyi calls "flow," professional athletes call being "in the zone." This is an altered state of consciousness that I compare to religious ecstasy (Womack 1982). This state is best described by John Brodie, a quarterback for the San Francisco 49ers, as quoted in George Burr Leonard's *The Ultimate Athlete*:

> At times, and with increasing frequency now, I experience a kind of clarity that I've never seen adequately described in a football story. Sometimes, for example, time seems to slow way down, in an uncanny way, as if everyone were moving in slow motion. It seems as if I have all the time in the world to watch the receivers run their patterns and yet I know the defensive line is coming at me just as fast as ever. I know perfectly well how hard and fast those guys are coming and yet the whole thing seems like a movie or dance in slow motion. It's beautiful. (1977:39)

This altered state of consciousness aids athletic performance by screening out distractions and permitting the athletes to focus on the game (Womack 1982).

Csikszentmihalyi asked subjects of his study to keep track of their activities during a forty-eight-hour period. He found that subjects who enjoyed their work and were regarded as successful introduced play activities into their workday. The psychologist writes, "The many inconspicuous little things that we do during a normal day, the seemingly useless bits of behavior interspersed with our serious instrumental activities, are indeed very useful, perhaps essential to normal functioning" (1975:176). To test this conclusion, he asked his subjects to give up their play activities:

> When people stop noninstrumental behavior, they feel more tired and sleepy and less healthy and relaxed. They report more headaches. They judge themselves in more negative terms, and they especially feel less creative and reasonable. Spontaneous creative performance decreases. Normal daily activities become more of a chore, and they are accompanied by irritability, loss of concentration, depression, and the feeling of having turned into a machine. Subjects report experiences similar in many respects to the disruption found in people who suffer psychotic breaks. (1975:177)

When my children were small we lived next door to a woman determined to turn her children into mega-geniuses. One day, as we were chatting, our combined six children (three each) proceeded to turn one of her planter beds into a city. They constructed houses using whatever materials were available. They built roads in the dirt and used bricks for cars and trucks.

As I was watching this massive construction enterprise, my neighbor pulled out a bag of toys and announced, "These are designed to encourage creativity." She then called the children away from their construction project and sat them down to play with the mass-produced toys designed, no doubt, by "experts in creativity." I cynically call "experts in creativity" those professionals who have been trained in design and marketing. The products they design look good on the shelves, but they may contribute little to creativity. When I was a child on my family farm, my parents bought me a series of dolls suitable for my age. The toys I enjoyed most were the ones I constructed myself using the abundant materials available on a Midwestern farm.

Children are the only real "experts in creativity" because they learn through experimentation. Unfortunately, children are often socialized out of their creative potential because they are socialized out of their potential for experimental play. In the process, they are socialized out of their ability to realize their human potential. Play, though it mimics "real-life," provides an arena within which creativity and experimentation contribute to plasticity, the flexibility and potential for learning that makes human intelligence possible.

AARP: The Magazine lists as its number one requirement for a long healthful lifestyle the ability to laugh. There may well be a physiological basis for the health-giving properties of laughter, in addition to its ability to relieve stress and provide a more positive outlook on life. Michael Miller, an MD at the University of Maryland School of Medicine, suggests that "as little as 15 minutes of laughter daily may help prevent a heart attack by expanding the lining of blood vessels to improve blood flow."[4]

For people who enjoy their work, work is the equivalent of play. David Katz, a preventive medicine specialist at the Yale School of Public Health and coauthor of *Stealth Health: How to Sneak Age-Defying, Disease-Fighting Habits Into Your Life Without Really Trying*, rejects the idea that the "Type A" personality, which emphasizes achievement, is most at risk for heart disease. Instead, he says, indicators for probable heart disease and cancer are characterized by the Type D personality, someone who bottles up his or her emotions.[5] Both "work" and "play" can provide health benefits if they promote enjoyment and a sense of self-worth to the people who indulge in them.

COOPERATION AND COLLABORATION

Humans are **primates**, and as such, we share attributes with our closest relatives, nonhuman primates, which includes apes and monkeys. We have a large brain relative to body size, with an emphasis on the cerebral cortex. The cerebral cortex is the center of abstract thought, which permits us to think about phenomena that exist beyond our senses. For example, as humans, we can draw maps of the earth that have lines where no lines exist in nature. One of these is the equator, the area that is equidistant between the North and South Poles.

In general, primates are social animals. Among chimpanzees, the mother-child bond is the glue that holds the group together. Primates are socialized into what they need to survive by their parents and by peers. Like our primate relatives, humans cannot survive and flourish psychologically or biologically outside the social group.

Negotiating Conflict and Promoting Collaboration

The Netsilik, a hunter-gatherer population occupying a territory above the Arctic Circle, illustrate the importance of collaboration and cooperation in an extreme environment. Netsilik traditionally relied on animals for food, fuel, clothing, and materials for tools, since no plants could survive in this harsh environment. The most important animals were seals, caribou, musk oxen, and salmon. For Netsilik, kinship—including marriage and descent—was the most important marker of group membership. After that, and shaped by kinship, group membership was defined by participation in subsistence activities, especially hunting, and by food distribution. Asen Balikci writes:

> Collaboration is not only an objective necessity related to the technology and strategy of hunting or fishing but a recognized behavioral norm. . . . All should hunt. The elderly Kaiaitok [a key informant for Balikci] added that the most important means of subsistence should be divided among the inhabitants of the settlement according to certain rules. This expresses the norm of food sharing. Collaboration therefore covers both food procurement and food consumption. (1970:127)

Providing food required a continuum of action, ranging from solitary hunting to small groups to cooperation within and between kin groups:

> Both affinal [marriage] ties and consanguineal [descent] bonds were exploited to ensure collaboration. The important consideration was for the hunting group to be of optimal size in order to maximize hunting chances. The residential flexibility so characteristic of Netsilik society allowed for smaller or larger group formations, depending on the availability of the game and the particular hunting strategy adopted. In the case of winter sealing, which was the one situation when a kinship unit could not provide the necessary personnel for a hunt, the Netsilik solution was to join kinship units together. The

vital importance of sealing necessitated the co-operation of the largest possible number of hunters. (Balikci 1970:128)

Economic interdependence was reinforced by social exchange systems. Individuals with identical names shared a social identification with each other, reinforced by exchange practices. They were friendly with each other and exchanged jokes. They also exchanged gifts of identical objects. Balikci writes, "This gift exchange was not carried out to obtain any material benefit, but rather to give expression to a feeling of social solidarity, a sign of enduring friendliness" (1970:139).

Joking relationships also promoted feelings of cooperation and friendship, while providing a means to ameliorate social anxieties. Joking relationships differed from the oft-mentioned "song duels," which were used to settle disputes. Balikci writes: "Joking relationships were established between individuals who were neither indifferent to each other nor very intimate friends. It was a practice that brought people who were casual friends a little closer together, while at the same time allowing for the free expression of ambivalent feelings in a play atmosphere" (1970:140).

It would be a mistake to view the Netsilik as living in a "primitive paradise." The complexities of modern life often lead us to speculate about how much easier life would be if we weren't faced with presidential elections and credit card bills. Some people long for the "good old days." However, life nearly always looks better in hindsight. People may remember their childhood as happy and carefree. They forget about the neighborhood bully who ridiculed them or shook them down for their allowance.

Human social life is always beset with difficulties, as well as pleasures. Typically, the difficulties and pleasures arise from those who are closest to us. Unless they are carrying a gun or other lethal weapon, strangers rarely challenge our sense of well-being, at least not for long. It's those who love us, and whom we love, who challenge our self-esteem. Knud Rasmussen, an early chronicler of the Netsilik, reports an account of a famous shaman who reached an irreconcilable conflict with a hunting associate and rival:

> In this new country I had a hunting companion, and we often had contests. We were equally fast, equally skillful at hunting, but he was the stronger. We were always alone when we practiced our sports, and my companion, who could not run so far as I can, made use of every opportunity to let me know that he was not afraid of me. And so it happened one day that to prove his superiority he rubbed his muck on me, and that was an insult. I could not forget. When a man does that in our country it is an insult that meant that he has an inclination to kill one. The treatment I had received tormented me so much that I could not tell anyone about it. Hatred grew up in me, and every time I met my old companion out caribou hunting it was as if I loathed myself; thoughts that I could not control came up in me, and so one day when we were alone together up in the mountains I shot him. (quoted in Balikci 1970:171)

Such direct solutions are usually not available to people in contemporary societies. Among the Netsilik, however, it is clear that the companion's act of smearing excrement on the shaman is equivalent to a death threat. The two participants in this competition used different means to "kill" each other. One used the symbolic means of killing his opponent with excrement. The other used the literal means of killing his opponent with weaponry.

Most social negotiations are not taken to this extreme. In general, social interactions are aimed at promoting the solidarity of the group, even if that means reducing or elevating the status of some members. Sharing food is an important part of promoting social solidarity and establishing status relationships.

NUTRITION, HEALTH, AND THE CULTURE
OF FOOD PREFERENCE

In addition to sustaining our lives, food also sustains our social relationships. Food is a metaphor for mutual collaboration "Jesus took bread, and blessed it, and broke it, and gave it to the disciples, and said, Take, eat; this is my body. And he took the cup, and gave thanks, and gave it to them, saying, Drink ye all of it." According to the New Testament book of Matthew (26:26), Jesus Christ equated food and wine with his own body and blood. A secular proverb that equates nutrition with the self and wellness states, "You are what you eat."

Whether of divine origin, symbolic inference, or folk wisdom, nutrition is an important component of definitions of self, of well-being, and of social cohesion. Decisions about what constitutes food can also distinguish social status and differences between groups, as Monica L. Smith notes in her article "The Archaeology of Food Preference": "For the individual, food is a basic component of self- and group identification, put into practice every day" (2006:480). She cites Arjun Appadurai's observation that food can "serve two diametrically opposed semiotic functions. It can serve to indicate and construct social relations characterized by equality, intimacy, or solidarity; or it can serve to sustain relationships characterized by rank, distance, or segmentation" (1981:496).

Smith analyzes the sociocultural context of rice production in South Asia, which includes India and Sri Lanka. She notes that the climate of the region made available a wide diversity of crops to be used by humans, including grains, fruits, pulses (lentils and legumes), vegetables, fibers, and medicinal plants.[6] Rice has nutritional benefits and is well adapted to South Asia's monsoon climate, but it is labor-intensive. Smith suggests that rice became a cultural symbol for South Asia as early as the tenth century BC, as recorded in the *Rig Veda*, the earliest known surviving document from South India. Smith writes, "The repetitive trope of rice in these texts [including the Ramayana, Mahabarata and others] shows [rice] to be a food with high moral and social value, and the use of agricultural metaphors shows the recognized relationship between leaders and followers (2006:484–485).

Intensive agriculture, such as that required by rice cultivation, produces a food surplus that permits task specialization giving rise to **stratification**, unequal access to power and resources. Thus, cultivation of storable crops such as rice provides economic support for the power of secular and religious officials. Smith notes:

> More than just serving as a description of consumption, prevailing ideologies of food preference have implications for production and distribution as well. At the level of lived daily experience, households exercise choices in the form and manner of food preparation, and individuals exercise choices in how, whether, and how much they will eat. Households also allocate time and energy in the form of labor for their own needs

as well as to address suprahousehold demands in the form of community projects. Leaders and followers are mutually dependent in these projects, particularly when they involve the production of food items that are of high social value and widely desired but that require considerable amounts of labor investment. (2006:488)

The Value of a Meal

In her book *French Women Don't Get Fat*, Mireille Guiliano, president and chief executive officer of Clicquot Inc., in New York and a director of Champagne Veuve Clicquot in Reims, France, defines the difference between the way nutrition is defined in France and the way it is defined in the United States. She begins her book with a quote from the French poet and philosopher Paul-Toussaint-Jules Valéry: "What is more important than the meal? Doesn't the least observant [wo]man-about town look upon the implementation and ritual progress of a meal as a liturgical prescription? Isn't all of civilization apparent in these careful preparations, which consecrate the spirit's triumph over a raging appetite?"

French and Americans agree that an appreciation of food requires discipline. The difference lies in how the two cultures define that discipline. The French regard a meal as an aesthetic enterprise that requires an education of the senses. Americans demand a numerical index of caloric and nutritional intake. European nutritionists have questioned why Americans do not consider pleasure in evaluating the nutritional impact of a meal. Guiliano describes the pleasure her mother experienced in savoring her daily ritual of consuming chocolate, comparing her mother's approach to Zen meditation: "No one talked. One look at her expressions, her lips, her eyes, commanded a hush in the house. It was a natural way of honoring our mother, allowing her the moment to savor one of her most elemental pleasures" (2005:183).

Michael Coe, an esteemed Mesoamerican archeologist and author of *The True History of Chocolate*, suggests that chocolate was probably cultivated in Central America by the Olmecs, who occupied the region from about 1500 to 600 BCE. He notes that the word "cacao" is Olmec. The earliest known chemical traces of chocolate date to about 460 CE, from the Early Classic period of Maya culture. According to later Spanish reports, the Maya chocolate drink was thick and foamy and was mixed with maize (corn), water, honey, or chili.[7] A common use of chocolate in Mexico today is for Mole sauce, which is typically prepared using a spicy mixture of various kinds of chili peppers. It is a far cry from the chocolate relished by Guiliano's mother. As consumed in Europe and the United States, the tart flavor of chocolate is leavened by mixing it with sugar. For the French, Guiliano observes, the favored chocolate is dark and bittersweet, rather than sugary, as it is normally consumed in the United States.

However consumed, chocolate does have nutritional properties, as Guiliano points out. The purer dark form of chocolate contains more antioxidants than black tea or red wine, as well as magnesium, iron, and potassium. Several theories have been advanced to explain the general feeling of well-being that chocolate generates. The principal alkaloid of the cocoa bean is theobromine, which stimulates the heart muscle and the central nervous system. Theobromine is a less powerful stimulant than caffeine, which chocolate also contains. Chocolate also contains phenethylamine, a precursor to the neurotransmitter phenylethanolamine, which may act as a mood-elevator. In all, chocolate contains more than 300 distinct chemicals, which may interact to raise serotonin levels in the brain. Serotonin is associated with feelings of well-being.[8]

Researchers at the University Hospital of Cologne, in Germany, concluded that cocoa-rich products such as dark chocolate could produce significant reductions in hypertension, enough to reduce the risk of stroke by 20 percent and of coronary heart disease by 20 percent. The findings were based on a survey of ten short-term studies involving 173 participants who regularly consumed polyphenol-rich cocoa products such as dark chocolate.[9] Polyphenols are flavonoids, compounds found in fruits, vegetables, and certain beverages, including tea, coffee, beer, wine, and fruit drinks. Flavonoids have been found to have numerous potential benefits for human health. Various studies have reported on their antiviral, anti-allergic, antiplatelet, anti-inflammatory, antitumor, and antioxidant effects.[10]

Four out of five trials on the effects of eating dark chocolate surveyed by researchers at University Hospital of Cologne found that polyphenol-rich cocoa products reduced both systolic blood pressure (heart muscle contracting) and diastolic blood pressure (heart muscle relaxing). No such favorable results were found for tea in five studies involving 343 participants.[11]

This analysis should not be regarded as a recommendation for eating dark chocolate. The chemistry of the human body is too complex to be reduced to a single variable. Nutrition involves a variety of circumstances, including activity level, age, social relationships, emotions, self-esteem, inherited characteristics, occupation, aspirations, and many other variables that have not yet been scientifically investigated. There is no magic bullet for good health and happiness. Chocolate has absolutely no effect on my feelings of well-being. Nor, fortunately, does cocaine.

In my youth, living in a beach community in Southern California, my friends and associates frequently offered me cocaine. As a scientist, I experimentally accepted their offerings. Cocaine had absolutely no effect on me. "It's a mellow 'high,'" I was told. "It is 'no high' for me," I told them, adding "Save your money." After many occasions when I was offered cocaine, I finally said, "I would rather put my money on my back (buying clothes) than up my nose."

Over several decades, after observing a number of my "friends" offering their bank accounts and livelihoods to the "cocaine god," I finally realized why cocaine had no appeal for me: I have naturally high levels of serotonin. Nor does chocolate appeal to me. I won't attempt to explain it, mainly because I don't understand it myself. As I have stated repeatedly throughout this book, the chemistry of the human body is complex. It cannot be reduced to a single variable or "cause." The most important "cause" is lifestyle, which involves more variables than we could ever explain through laboratory research or clinical trials.

The "French Paradox" Explained

American physicians and researchers have long questioned how the French can indulge in gustatory pleasures that are considered unhealthy by American medical mythology. These include rich or fatty foods and beverages containing alcohol, such as wine.

There are several explanations for this "paradox." The American urban diet consists largely of processed foods, which contain large amounts of refined sugar.

Refined sugar can produce mood alterations. It can also contribute to obesity and diabetes. Americans lead a sedentary lifestyle, such as watching television, whereas the traditional French evening entertainment includes the "promenade," a walk after dinner. Also, for Europeans, a meal is a work of art, to be enjoyed as an aesthetic experience.

There is scientific validity in the European approach of linking food to pleasure and relaxation. Chemically, stress and anxiety interfere with the body's ability to process food. Thus, we do not absorb the full nutrients of food when we eat under stressful conditions. When we experience stress, the energy required to absorb nutrients from food is directed to the need to defend against an invader. Thus, stressful conditions interfere with absorption of nutrition.

Medical anthropologists could easily study the "French paradox" by applying the anthropological approach of holism, which requires that phenomena be studied in their context and in terms of their various components. I described my experiences growing up on a Midwestern farm to a French friend, Jean-Pol Dupin de Franqueuil, an artist who lives and works in New York City. My description evoked Jean-Pol's memories of growing up in the south of France. Like the French, farmers in the American Midwest eat a diet centered on meat, dairy products, and vegetable produce. Typically, they eat five meals a day, in the morning, midmorning, noon, mid-afternoon, and evening. Yet Midwestern farmers—unlike Midwestern urban dwellers—tend not to suffer from obesity. The difference has to do more with lifestyle than with caloric intake.

Both France and the United States developed around agriculture, a way of life that produces a food surplus, giving rise to stratification, population increases, and ultimately, the concentration of populations in cities. Both countries have become industrialized, an economic pattern in which the workplace is separated from the home. This produces a major shift in lifestyles.

Farming requires hard physical labor, which can be conducted at a leisurely pace except during such seasons as harvest time. Though physically demanding, farm work is intrinsically emotionally satisfying. The rewards of work are immediate and aesthetically pleasing, in the form of a beautifully plowed field, newly baled hay, or the smell and taste of home-baked bread. The five daily meals tend to be leisurely events involving the whole family and centering on conversation. The occasions are as much social as nutritional. Even during time-sensitive events such as harvest, farmers have a great deal of control over their schedules, and their meals can be communal, involving the whole neighborhood.

The farm diet loses little nutritional value from transport. Nutrients found in fruits and vegetables are fragile, and their taste deteriorates rapidly. Whereas the urban family relies on produce that has been harvested days or weeks earlier, farmers may consume fruits and vegetables that have been harvested only minutes or hours before the meal, or eaten as snacks straight off the plant. Both French and Midwestern American farmers have the advantage of control over their schedule, leisurely meals, vigorous physical exercise, and access to nutrients at their peak value.

Urban dwellers in the United States are subject to regimentation of their daily schedule, stress due to commuting, a sedentary lifestyle, and degraded nutritional value of the foods available to them. In discussing the "French paradox" with Jean-Pol, I learned that the French lifestyle—urban and rural—is similar to that of my rural childhood. "We took three hours for lunch," Jean-Pol says. "But it was hard on the children," he jokes, "because we had to wait three hours for dessert."

Jean-Pol and I are not the only ones to consider that the lifestyle in rural parts of the American Midwest is similar to those of rural France. Budget-Travel.com ranked Parkville, a ten-minute drive from Kansas City, Missouri, as one of the "10 Coolest Small Towns" in the United States. Based on descriptions of the towns, "cool" refers to a relaxed lifestyle, intellectual companionship, and access to gourmet food and drink. Didier Combe, owner of the restaurant Café des Amis in Parkville, thinks the town is like a village in his native France: "After the last dinner is served, we often sit out on the deck with friends and guests."[12]

Europeans in general prefer quality of food to quantity. Visitors to the United States are often shocked at the large portions served in American restaurants. The Cornell University Food Lab has conducted a number of studies focused on the way people in the United States perceive food portions. In many cases, it is related to visual perception. A food labeled "low fat" is likely to be consumed in larger portions than similar foods not so labeled.

A study conducted by Collin Payne and Pierre Chandon for the Cornell Food Laboratory and published in the journal *Obesity* indicates that French and U.S. eaters respond to different cues about when to stop eating. The 133 French subjects responded to internal cues, such as when they were no longer hungry or when the food no longer tasted good to them. They also stopped eating if they wanted to save room for dessert. The 145 people from the United States relied on external cues of satiety, such as whether they had cleaned their plate, when everyone else at the table was finished, or when the television show they were watching was finished.[13] Whether French or American, the heaviest people were those who relied on external cues to stop eating.

Guiliano writes: "Apart from a brief Jacobin interlude in the eighteenth century, extremism has never been the French way. America, however, gravitates toward different philosophies, quick fixes, and extreme measures. In diet as in other matters, these work for a time, but they're no way to live" (2005:6).

There really is no paradox in the "French paradox." French enjoy life, so they want to live longer. They are healthier than Americans because they eat a greater variety of well-prepared food. They also view walking as a pastime rather than work caused by the lack of a car. It is a simple formula: Pleasure + Nutrition + Exercise + Chemical Processes in the Brain and Body = Health.

Considering the entire context of nutrition—including the values of aesthetic appreciation and relaxed social exchange—can help us to understand why power lunches do not necessarily produce powerful, disease-resistant bodies.

The Chemical Paradox

Researchers in the United States have isolated what they consider to be the explanation for the "French paradox." Typically, this is in the form of a chemical, *resveratrol*, found in grapes, red wine, purple grape juice, peanuts, some berries, beans, and Russet potatoes. Resveratrol is also found in spices such as cloves, cinnamon, and oregano.

The direct biological aspects of resveratrol include its **antioxidant** properties. Antioxidants reduce the damage to living cells caused by bombardment of **free**

radicals, which are derived from **molecules** that no longer have a balanced number of electrons. As the free radicals try to "steal" electrons from molecules that comprise the cells of living organisms, more free radicals are produced, thus destroying the integrity of the cell. This can lead to cell death or alteration of the cell's DNA coding, which can lead to cancer and other disorders.

According to the Linus Pauling Institute at Oregon State University, resveratrol has been shown in the laboratory studies to have anti-inflammatory effects that may protect against atherosclerosis; reduce the formation of blood clots, which may help protect against cardiovascular disease; and maintain cell stability which could provide protection against cancer. Though resveratrol is sold over the counter, it is rapidly metabolized and therefore does not appear to convey the same health benefits as consuming resveratrol through foods rich in this substance.

One drawback to studies that isolate substances is that they do not consider the overall social, psychological, and behavioral contexts. Pleasure is chemical, as is stress, and it may be as important to consider the context within which one consumes foods rich in resveratrol, including with whom one consumes the meal, as well as the chemical properties of the compounds one consumes.

ILLNESS AND AGRICULTURE

Though I have written glowingly of the health benefits derived from the rustic rural lifestyle, the development of agriculture did not eliminate disease. It merely changed its form. Jared Diamond writes that the diet of foragers is typically better balanced than that of agriculturalists: "While farmers concentrate on high-carbohydrate crops like rice and potatoes, the mix of wild plants and animals in the diets of surviving hunter-gatherers provides more protein and a better balance of other nutrients" (1991:73[1987]). As **omnivores**, humans require a varied diet that includes a balance of protein and carbohydrates. Another anomaly in the switch from a forager lifestyle to a lifestyle based on domesticated plants and animals is that meat from domesticated animals contains much more fat than meat from wild animals. One need only compare the lithe form of a wild African gazelle with that of a domesticated bovine raised for beef to bear this out.

The United States has recently witnessed this process in the shift from harvesting wild salmon to domesticated salmon. Wild salmon are recognizable for their "salmon-colored" flesh, leanness, and complex flavor that arise from their need to fend for themselves and their ability to swim freely. Domesticated salmon flesh has wide veins of fat and is gray unless the pink color is added through artificial means.

At the social level, production of a food surplus, which is characteristic of agriculture, permits a high degree of task specialization, which in turn, permits stratification. Stratification associated with agriculture gives rise to illnesses related to social class. People working in agriculture may be exposed to chemicals such as pesticides and fertilizer, as well as diseases characteristic of domesticated animals. People of the upper classes or ruling classes may be subject to chronic illness brought about by rich foods and a sedentary or restricted lifestyle.

Agriculture also supports the rise of cities, bringing people in close contact with each other, permitting the development and spread of new diseases. The trajectory of bubonic plague in the fourteenth century illustrates this phenomenon. An early outbreak of bubonic plague was recorded in China in the 1330s. China was one of the earliest regions to develop agriculture. It was also one of the world's busiest trading nations at that time. The plague had spread by trade routes to Italy by October of 1347 and to England by the following August. The Italian writer Boccaccio provides a vivid image of the rapid progress of the disease. The victims "ate lunch with their friends and dinner with their ancestors in paradise." After five years, the bubonic plague had killed 25 million people, one-third of the European population. Such a rapid devastation of the human population could not have been possible among foragers because of their low population density and dispersed populations.

Industrialization and the Family

A few hundred years ago, large urban populations made industrialization possible. Industrialization has proved to be a mixed blessing for the human species. It is a form of production that separates the workplace from the home. In so doing, it weakens the bonds uniting the family. Throughout much of human evolution, the human family functioned as a cooperative economic unit. As foragers, men typically hunted large game animals, and women "gathered" plants and smaller animals. Children contributed to the family economy. Older children tended their younger siblings, ran errands, and performed other tasks appropriate to their age and maturity. Even very young children could gather sticks for the fire or assist in gathering plants.

With domestication of animals and plants, this interdependency continued. Among pastoralists, women and children could herd cattle; men and boys could herd sheep. This division of labor is pervasive because tending sheep requires the greater upper body strength of males, whereas tending cattle does not. Universally, all members of the family, except infants and very young children, performed tasks appropriate to their age and gender.

Having grown up on a farm myself, I can provide an eyewitness account of the family dynamic of people who both herd animals and cultivate plants, supplemented by information drawn from ethnographies, descriptions of social groups based on studies conducted by anthropologists.

Typically men and boys perform the hard physical labor in the fields. They operate the heavy (and dangerous) machinery when it is required or harvest by hand the crops intended for the market. Men, aided by boys, may also chop wood, maintain vehicles and machinery, and build or repair houses, barns, and other structures. Women and girls maintain the household by cooking and cleaning. They also grow garden produce for the family and raise chickens or other fowl for family use or for the market. Care of larger animals, such as pigs and cattle, varies considerably, depending on tradition and practice. Sheep are typically not grown where there is large-scale production of plants, though goats may be. Sheep and humans are competitors for access to plant materials.

The significance of these forms of subsistence for the dynamic of the family is that all members of the family interact with each other throughout the day. Though social and economic roles are clearly defined, they do not separate family members into discrete units. Separating the workplace from the home, as in industrialization, imposes rigid categories on the basis of age, gender, and class. The modern urban

American conceptual model is that children go to school, fathers travel to work, mothers shop or stay home. In fact, most families in industrialized societies cannot afford this pattern. In most cases, children go to school and parents go to work. Much of childhood socialization takes place in a public setting, often placing children in competition with each other. In industrialized societies, status is not based on production but on how much money one earns.

The industrialization of the family has important implications for psychological and physical health. A child cannot run to a parent or older sibling for help or comfort in a time of crisis. She or he must rely on the generosity of strangers. Husbands and wives occupy separate economic realms. Thus, the organization of the family is based on a shared domicile in which its members spend much or most of their time in groups that do not share kinship relationships.

Industrialization and Health

As a result of industrialization, large numbers of the human animal have been transported from the context in which they evolved—clean air, sunshine, freedom from physical constriction, and the need to make decisions based on the requirements of the moment—to the factory, an indoor atmosphere characterized by pollution, inadequate light, limited ability to move freely, and the need to obey the commands of others. This dramatic change occurred only 300 years ago. If the human species has had difficulty adapting to the changes wrought by agriculture 10,000 years ago, it is even more unlikely that we could have adapted biologically to immobility, artificial light, constricted social and physical environment, and great biological and social pollution in a mere 300 years.

Medicine has made great strides in reducing the spread of disease through the traditional pathogens, bacteria and protozoa, but little or no progress in treatment of illness caused by two highly resistant modern pathogens: viruses and stress. Some severe forms of stress can be linked to industrialization, which includes a restricted and regimented lifestyle, as well as exposure to environmental pollutants, both chemical and social.

A forager, pastoralist, horticulturalist, or agriculturalist could always get away from a hostile social situation by engaging in productive activity. In addition, a horticulturalist or agriculturalist could vent frustration or anger by hacking away at an undesired plant. In an industrialized urban society, it is very difficult to get away from annoying people or frustrating situations. Therefore, the biological condition of arousal, which can promote survival in a nonindustrialized society, can become toxic as stress in an industrialized urban society, where there are no culturally recognized escapes from conflict and frustration.

ASCETICISM AND RITUAL PURITY

An archaeological team including James D. Tabor, chair of the Department of Religious Studies at the University of North Carolina at Charlotte, excavated a site around the caves at Qumran, where the Dead Sea Scrolls were found in a cave. Most scholars consider the Dead Sea Scrolls to be produced by monks who practiced an extreme form of asceticism involving austerity and isolation. Their settlement was located on the northwestern side of the Dead Sea. The archaeological team was able to associate the asceticism with austere toilet practices because the location of the latrine was described in two of the most important scrolls. The archaeological excavation produced valuable information about the relationship between asceticism and the health of these early scholars.

Contemporary scholars consider the settlement to have been occupied by the Essenes, who were described by Josephus, the first century Jewish historian, as being dispersed, having settled "not in one city" but "in large numbers in every town."[14] Similarly, Philo of Alexandria describes the Essenes as being dispersed and numerous. They were generally ascetic and egalitarian. Some groups of Essenes were celibate, but others were married. Some ancient writings and modern people who consider themselves Essenes support the idea that the founders of Christianity, including Mary, Joseph, and Jesus, were Essenes.

Josephus documented Essene toilet practices, an account that greatly aided modern archaeologists. Josephus noted that Essenes dug holes outside the city to bury their bodily wastes. Because they could not leave the city on the Sabbath, they could not defecate on that day. Guided by scrolls providing locations of the latrines, Tabor and Joe E. Zias, of the Hebrew University of Jerusalem and an expert on ancient latrines, took soil samples from areas around the settlement. The most likely site conformed most closely to the location described in the scrolls. As is characteristic of organic matter, soil from that site differed in appearance and texture from other sites around the settlement.

Tabor says the soil from that site "looked different." Zias describes it more specifically: "The earth was so nice and soft, while the rest of the desert was very hard. In fact, I broke my pick collecting control samples for the other areas."[15]

The soil samples were sent to the CNRS Laboratory for Anthropology in Marseille, France, where Stephanie Harter-Lailheugue found eggs and other remnants of human intestinal parasites preserved in the soil considered most likely to be the site of the latrines. No parasites were found in soil taken from other sites around the area, and only a species of animal worms were found in the stable area of the settlement. Zias said, "The evidence shows conclusively that the area was a toilet."

The two scientists compared this data with data from previous excavations of the Qumran cemetery and discovered that fewer than 7 percent of the men buried in the graveyard survived to age forty. Half the men in cemeteries from the same period excavated at nearby city of Jericho lived beyond the age of forty. Zias says, "The graveyard at Qumran is the unhealthiest group I have ever studied in over 30 years."[16]

Ironically, the poor state of health among the men at the Qumran site is most likely due to their emphasis on ritual cleansing. Bedouins in the area defecate on the surface, a practice that would seem "less clean." In terms of health, however, the Bedouin practice exposes human feces to the sun, which quickly kills parasites. Burying the feces, as the Essenes did, would have allowed the parasites to live for a year or more, infecting anyone who walked through the soil. Essenes had to pass through an immersion cistern, or *miqvot*, before returning to the settlement. The water would have provided a warm, moist environment within which parasites would flourish and breed. Zias says the ritual cleansing "is a total immersion, which means that it gets in your ears, in your eyes and in your mouth. It is not hard to imagine how sick everyone must have been."[17]

III

MODELS OF DIAGNOSIS AND TREATMENT

Truth in all its kinds is most difficult to win; and truth in medicine is the most difficult of all.

—Peter Mere Latham, *Collected Works*

In spite of our best efforts, we sometimes get sick. Even if we find the lifestyle that best fulfills our genetic potential, the organisms that cause disease may fight their way past our defences, or we just wear down. Chinese have a saying that people who get the small illnesses don't get the big ones. Whether that is true, it is certainly true that illness is part of the experience of all living beings, including plants and animals. Even stones wear down. Part I of *The Anthropology of Health and Healing* explores the biological, psychological, and social factors that underlie models of health and illness. Part II surveys life cycle and lifestyle issues that shape the maintenance of health. Part III examines the philosophical systems that underlie models of health and treatment of medical disorders.

Anthropologists have studied systems of diagnosis and treatment cross-culturally for more than 100 years, and they have concluded that all these systems have merit. They all address the unique biology and psychology of human beings. In so doing, they are all effective on some level. In most cases, they are effective on multiple levels.

Part III explores a number of healing systems. Limitations of time and printer's ink do not permit us to explore them all. Therefore we will focus on those most studied by anthropologists and most available to individuals seeking treatment in the twenty-first century. We will evaluate these healing systems within their philosophical and social context, rather than with respect to their relative effectiveness. Effectiveness is a multilayered concept. Do we measure "effectiveness" by relief of symptoms, by the patient's satisfaction with the "healing," or by objective measures, such as reduction in numbers of microbes? All of these measures of "success" are important and all have limitations.

The U.S. National Institutes of Health is funding research into the various systems of healing available cross-culturally under the rubric of integrative medicine. This is a major step in an important new direction. Systems of healing need not compete with each other. We can recover from a failed financial venture, but we cannot recover from a fatal medical procedure. Part III of *The Anthropology of Health and Healing* considers the importance of philosophical systems in shaping healing practices.

Chapter 9, "Biomedicine and the Scientific Approach," explores the role of science and the Western focus on the biology of the body in defining biomedicine. It also addresses the role of clinical trials and other cultural models in shaping medical practice.

Chapter 10, "Restoring the Balance: Asian Models of Healing," examines the way in which Asian philosophical models emphasize maintaining health as well as treating disorders. It compares similarities and differences in the way in which Chinese medicine and Indian Ayurveda view health and healing.

Chapter 11, "Calling on the Spirits: Shamans and Mediums," explores traditions that engage the invisible world of spirits in diagnosis and healing. In view of their long history, it would be entirely accurate to include Chinese and Indian medicine as "traditional healing systems." However, traditional healing systems differ in terms of their social organization, their system of transmitting knowledge from one generation to the next, and their beliefs and practices.

Chapter 12, "The Emerging Field of Integrative Medicine," explores the role of the U.S. National Institutes of Health in evaluating medical procedures, a new way of thinking about the practice of medicine, involving medical traditions that have developed outside the Western scientific model. Anthropologists have long noted that some of these non-Western procedures—such as yoga, meditation, and dietary practices—have produced observable health effects. Chapter 12 evaluates the role of nontraditional healing systems and integrative medicine in contemporary healing systems.

9

Biomedicine and the Scientific Approach

CASE STUDY
Emergency Treatment for Ateriovenous Malfunction

In December 2006, U.S. Democratic Senator Tim Johnson was rushed to the George Washington University Hospital in Washington, DC, after becoming disoriented and stammering during a conference call with reporters. It was initially suspected that the senator had suffered a stroke, since his symptoms resembled those of a stroke. Tests ruled out a stroke and the ultimate diagnosis was AVM, arteriovenous malformation, a rare and potentially fatal condition that causes arteries and veins to grow abnormally large and become tangled. The tangles can block blood flow to the brain, and the enlarged arteries and veins sometimes rupture, causing seizures or stroke-like symptoms, as happened in Senator Johnson's case. An AVM is an abnormality of the circulatory system that develops in the embryo. "Although AVMs can develop in many different sites [of the body], those located in the brain or spinal cord can have especially widespread effects on the body."[1] Most people with AVM exhibit few significant symptoms, and the "malformations tend to be discovered only incidentally, usually either at autopsy or during treatment for an unrelated disorder."[2] However, about 12 percent of the population exhibit symptoms that vary greatly in severity. The most common generalized symptoms are seizures and headaches. Medications can alleviate the general symptoms associated with AVM, but the definitive treatments for the condition are surgery and focused irradiation therapy.[3] Surgery can be performed to remove the area affected by the AVM and the resulting blood clot, or a catheter can be used to apply a special glue to close the bleeding blood vessels. Physicians performed surgery to stop the bleeding in Senator Johnson's brain and drained the blood that had accumulated there. An additional procedure was performed later to prevent the formation of blood clots. Admiral John Eisold, a physician involved in the case, reported soon after the intervention: "He has been appropriately responsive to both word and touch. No further surgical intervention has been required."[4]

Senator Johnson's case illustrates the precision of Western medical procedures, as well as their reliance on technological diagnosis and treatment. A preliminary diagnosis is tendered on the basis of symptoms, but a confirmed diagnosis is withheld until the results of tests are received. In the meantime, the condition of the patient is monitored by means of machines that track brain wave patterns, absorption of oxygen, heart rate, and other vital signs. Once a diagnosis is arrived at, physicians, who may be from several disciplines, consult on the appropriate treatment. Though subjective observations may be tendered and considered by attending physicians, the evidence of objective measurements provided by instruments ultimately shapes the course of action, especially in an emergency such as that involving Senator Johnson.

Age, Ethics, and Surgical Intervention

Another case, also widely publicized in media, illustrates more subjective factors involved in treatment decisions. On December 31, 2005, a ninety-seven-year-old man was working in his study when a sharp pain raced through his upper chest and between his shoulder blades, then ripped into his neck. The man assumed he was having a heart attack. When his heart continued to beat, he diagnosed the condition as a dissecting aortic aneurysm, a condition that occurs when blood enters the wall of an aorta, the great artery that carries blood from the heart for distribution by branch arteries throughout the body. An aortic dissection is most common in men between the ages of forty and sixty who have a history of hypertension. The appropriate treatment for such a condition is a quintuple heart bypass operation, among the most demanding surgery for both surgeons and patients.[5]

The patient was the most qualified person to make the diagnosis and decide on the treatment. He was Michael E. DeBakey, who had devised the operation to repair such torn aortas; however, several factors had to be considered. At first, DeBakey refused to surrender to his condition. He refused to be admitted to a hospital and continued to work at home. In medical terms, DeBakey was noncompliant. DeBakey's explanation for his noncompliance illustrates the subjective response of one undergoing a life-threatening event: "It never occurred to me to call 911 or my physician. As foolish as it may appear, you are, in a sense, a prisoner of the pain, which was intolerable. You're thinking, 'what could I do to relieve myself of it.' If it becomes intense enough, you're perfectly willing to accept cardiac arrest as a possible way of getting rid of the pain."[6]

Deciding on treatment for DeBakey involved ethics. Anesthesiologists at Methodist Hospital in Houston, Texas, refused to anesthetize DeBakey because of his age, and the ethics committee debated whether to sanction such a risky surgery on an elderly patient. The decision was made when DeBakey's wife Katrin demanded that the surgery be performed. The patient survived, becoming the oldest patient to survive the operation he devised. He says, "It is a miracle. I really should not be here."[7]

The Efficacy of Western Biomedicine

The case of Dr. Michael E. DeBakey illustrates a number of issues involved in Western medicine: (1) A sophisticated knowledge of science and medicine does not protect us from the ills the human body is heir to. (2) Even those versed in Western biomedicine may choose to avoid treatment. (3) Due to the cost of medical care and insurance, not everyone has access to the kind of attention and treatment DeBakey received. (4) Under certain circumstances, death can be preferable to life. (5) The condition does not always determine the treatment. Life circumstances—such as age and will to live—may be taken into consideration. Yet another consideration is the desire of hospitals and others involved in medical practice to avoid being sued.

These are only a few of the many variables that shape the practice of Western biomedicine.[8] Others include the desire of the patient to pursue traditional remedies and a fear of hospitals among individuals from cultural groups other than the predominantly Western European culture that has shaped biomedicine. In all societies, the practice of medicine is carried out in a social context. The scientific paradigm that underlies Western biomedicine does not protect medical professionals, hospitals, or patients from the many social and psychological responses that illness and the practice of medicine involves.

There is no question that Western medicine has been successful in treating a host of conditions that threaten health and well-being. The efficacy of Western medicine in treating certain medical conditions, especially infections, is recognized by people in many other cultures, as well as the anthropologists who work among them. Anthropologists going to the field take with them a medical tool kit to protect against the diseases they may encounter in conducting their fieldwork.

Typically, the tool kit is intended for the use of the anthropologist and his or her family. Often, however, the role of informal health care provider can become crucial to the anthropologist's success in conducting field work. In evaluating his work among Azande horticulturalists of southern Sudan, Stephen David Siemens (1993) notes that his wife Wendy Rader became especially important because of her involvement with health concerns. Influential older men requested that Wendy conduct a health class, and she was called upon to administer medications, such as aspirin, to suffering villagers.

MEDICAL ANTHROPOLOGY IN THE FIELD

Laura Bohannan, writing under the name Elenore Smith Bowen, describes her emotions as she helplessly watched her friend Amara die in childbirth during Bohannan's fieldwork among Tiv horticulturalists of northern Nigeria. One can almost hear the desperation in Bohannan's voice as she pleads with the Tiv elder Yabo to let her take the suffering woman to a hospital:

> There are doctors who can save both her life and the life of her child. They have stronger medicines than yours to bring forth the child. If those fail, they know how to reach up into the womb. They even know how to cut open the living body, bring forth the child and then heal the mother. I will send a messenger on a bicycle to the hospital and another for a truck. I will pay carriers to carry Amara up to the road and on it, until the truck meets them. I will write a paper to the hospital, asking them to give her the best medicine and telling them that I will pay. I have always spoken truth to you, Yabo, and I speak truth now. Give my friend Amara to me, that she and her child may live. (1964:185)

Midwives came from other villages to brew herbal mixtures and administer them to Amara. Though Bohannan doubted their efficacy, they may have contained pain-relieving or inflammation-reducing ingredients. Traditional herbal treatments often contain ingredients that are effective medically, but Western medicines have more concentrated ingredients and contain higher dosages. From the description provided by Bohannan, it appears likely that there was structural incompatibility between Amara's pelvis and the size of the infant's head.

Tiv Beliefs and Social Relationships

Tiv believe that childbirth is natural. If it fails to take its natural course, it is because some human agency, typically in the form of witchcraft, has blocked the birth. One of the midwives told Bohannan: "There is magic in this, perhaps witchcraft. The world was so created that, as the field brings forth its fruit, so does a woman bear her children. Only evil willed by man [humankind] can prevent it. Unless the elders seek out this evil and remove it, no medicine can help her [Amara]" (1964:184).

Witchcraft results from disrupted social relationships. As the day passed and Amara grew weaker, Yabo sent for diviners to determine the source of the witchcraft, but the diviners refused to come because Yabo had insulted them on other occasions by not heeding their advice. In an effort to save Amara's life, men tried to stave off the effects of witchcraft by reconciling their differences. As the woman neared death, it became imperative to Tiv men to determine which among them was the witch.

The diagnosis of Tiv pertained to the social relationships among them. For Bohannan the significant variable was the life of her friend. Bohannan writes, "The sun sank lower, thrusting yellow fingers of light through the dilapidated thatch of Yabo's reception hut, but Amara still lived, her hand held in her husband's" (1964:196).

Bohannan and Amara's husband kept guard over the suffering woman, and were joined by Yabo's senior wife. As the three maintained their mournful vigil, they would occasionally hear owls hooting outside at a distance. At one point, Amara's husband said to Bohannan, "It is well that you're here, Redwoman.[9] The witches are abroad tonight."

"What do you mean," Bohannan asked, in a barely steady voice.

The answers came from Amara's husband and Yabo's senior wife: "Can you not hear the witch owls calling? They smell death and are gathering for the feast of ghouls. . . . She [Amara] is struggling with death" (1964:198).

Shortly after they spoke, Amara died, but her husband, still clasping her hand, refused to believe it. He insisted that a feather be brought to hold under her nostrils to see if she were still breathing. But the feather did not stir.

> Then, quite close, we heard the call of an owl. Amara's husband tore out of the hut, grazing his shoulder on the low doorway. We heard him shout, "What have I ever done to you that you rob me of my wife and child? I have never eaten human flesh. You have killed. . . ." But even as he shouted, the women broke into a terrible wailing, a banshee lament torn from soul and body. Standing, hands clasped behind the head, body arched and shaking with the cry that began in a high scream and sobbed itself slowly down the scale into silence. (1964:199)

The Social Cost of Illness

It is common in the United States to assume that relations between women and men are antagonistic. Bowen's (Bohannan's) description, along with many other anthropological ethnographies, refutes this characterization. A human life is precious in all societies for many reasons. It takes many resources to sustain a human life and to prepare the helpless human infant for survival in the complex social relationships characteristic of human groups. In a village, where everyone knows each other and has developed economic and emotional ties, the loss of a single human life threatens the entire group. Just as there are disagreements in all groups, there are close emotional attachments that are difficult to understand at a distance. From a distance, we cannot understand the intricate social bonds that cause humans to invest in each other. From a distance, it might appear that Western medicine is soulless. Both of these characterizations would be wrong.

We will never know whether Western biomedicine could have saved Amara had she been taken to the hospital in time. She survived for a long time after her condition seemed hopeless; however, it is difficult to measure the effects that a long ride in a truck over dusty rutted roads might have had on her condition. In the process of deciding the best course to take, Tiv social relationships were placed on trial along with Amara's life. Death can never be defeated; it can only be held at bay. We cannot say with certainty that Amara would have survived under any circumstances.

A common assumption is that modern medicine can work miracles. Contrary to American popular opinion, the United States is not the only country in the world to work medical "miracles," nor is it the leader in certain types of medicine. For example, the United States does not have the lowest maternal death rate in the world because of inequities in access to medical care. In countries where systems of **universal health care** are in place, the rates of maternal death rates are much lower. The disparity in maternal deaths in industrialized nations is due to poverty, lack of access to birth control and the resultant high fertility rates, and lack of access to medical care. The high rate of maternal deaths in parts of Africa is due to extreme poverty, malnutrition, lack of access to medical care, and lack of access to birth control and the resultant high fertility rates.[10]

According to a United Nations report released in 2003, women giving birth in the United States were almost three and one-half times more likely to die during childbirth than their Canadian counterparts. The death rate during childbirth for Canadian women was one in 8,700; for women in the United States, the death rate was one in 2,500. The U.S. maternal death rate was higher than the average in all the industrialized regions of Europe, North America, and Australia. In sub-Saharan Africa, one in 16 women does not survive a pregnancy at some point during her lifetime, the highest rate of maternal death in the world.

WESTERN MEDICINE: A BRIEF HISTORY

A student in one of my medical anthropology classes asserted that Chinese medicine and Ayurveda, a medical practice developed in India, have a long history, whereas Western medicine does not. I corrected that view by stating, "Western medicine also has a long tradition, but we rejected our history with the rise of scientific medicine a little over 100 years ago."

It is true that the medical traditions of China and India have written traditions dating back thousands of years,[11] and that their oral traditions date back even further; however, it is also true that Western medicine has a long written and oral tradition. An important difference between Western medicine and Asian traditions is that the theory and practice of Western medicine underwent a major paradigm shift in the nineteenth century. In this transition, the practice of medicine changed from a profession based on observation to a science, also based on observation, but guided by different standards. The prevailing paradigm of Western medicine is **empiricism**, the idea that science can address only those phenomena that can be observed and measured.

In 1837, the nineteenth-century English physician Peter Mere Latham was appointed physician extraordinary to Queen Victoria, a position he held until his death in 1875. His writings, available in his *Collected Works*, illustrate the complexities of being a physician in the nineteenth century amid conditions that are no less complex than today. In book I, chapter 25, Latham notes, "The practice of physic is jostled by quacks on the one side, and by science on the other." He adds, in the same book, chapter 173, "The diagnosis of disease is often easy, often difficult, and often impossible."

Latham also discusses the subjectivity of medical diagnosis and treatment. In book I, chapter 389, he writes, "Common sense is in medicine the master workman." And in chapter 408, "Faith and knowledge lean largely upon each other in the practice of medicine." In chapter 474, Latham expresses his frustration at the limits of medical practice: "It would be a great thing to understand pain in all its meanings."[12] Even as a physician and as a human subject to pain, Latham could not reduce the universal human experience of pain to a simple formula.

Physicians are witness to the most extreme expressions of the human experience: birth, trauma, illness, and death. At the same time, they may undergo these extreme experiences themselves. The rigors of science cannot erase, or even ameliorate, the subjective indignities of what it means to be human. It is a tribute to the human spirit that throughout our history and prehistory, we have tried to ameliorate our own suffering, as well as that of those with whom we have a shared investment. The record of Western medicine in caring for others begins long before the development of science and the written word. Our earliest record of nursing dates from the Neandertals, who lived from around 130,000 years ago to perhaps as late as 30,000 years ago.[13]

Neandertal Nursing

In contemporary usage, the word "Neandertal" has become virtually synonymous with "savage" or "primitive." The popular image is that of a grunting beast wearing a bearskin slung over one shoulder, carrying a club, and dragging women by the hair. The simplest logic would paint this picture as false. A bearskin slung over one shoulder will provide little protection against cold European winters, and Neandertals crafted stone tools of the Mousterian style, which allowed them to hunt and butcher large game animals.

Evidence in the fossil record suggests that Neandertals cared for each other both in their infirmity and after their deaths. In the summer of 1999, researchers from the

University of Pennsylvania Museum of Archaeology and Anthropology studied radiographic images of the Krapina Neandertal fossil bone collection. The site includes the largest collection of Neandertal bones found to date and provides a sample of variability in Neandertal morphology within a single site.[14]

The University of Pennsylvania study was organized by Alan Mann, curator in physical anthropology at the University of Pennsylvania Museum and professor of anthropology at the University of Pennsylvania, and Janet Monge, keeper of the Physical Anthropology Collection at the University of Pennsylvania Museum and a professor at Bryn Mawr College. They worked with Morrie Kricun, of the Departments of Radiology and Anthropology and other colleagues at the University of Pennsylvania. The research team was looking for signs of pathology, disease, and weakness. Ultimately, they concluded from their study of x-rays of 884 bone fragments from the Krapina Neandertal cave site that these Neandertals were, in large part, a robust, healthy people.[15]

Monge notes that, while the overall picture of Neandertal health, based on the radiographs, was good, not all the specimens showed perfect health: "We were able to document one of the earliest benign bone tumors ever found, one individual may have had a surgical amputation of his hand, and several individuals had examples of osteoarthritis—which may have made them a little stiff in the morning."[16]

Research on Neandertal fossil remains has not produced a consistent body of interpretation. One interpretation of fossil evidence for Neandertal is that they were displaced by early modern humans, as suggested by the fact that Neandertal skeletons showed a higher degree of trauma than those of early modern humans. Another interpretation is that Neandertals formed close social bonds, since they could not have recovered alone from some of the traumas recorded in their fossil remains.

In spite of the fossil evidence indicating that Neandertals cared for each other's health, we should not rush to construct an image of the Neandertal as the original noble savage. European researchers, led by Christoph Zollikofer, a biologist at the University of Zürich, used a computer to reconstruct a skull of a Neandertal man who lived about 6,000 years before the species became extinct, at about 36,000 BP (before present). Virtual reconstruction indicated that a hole in the skull was probably caused by a blow from a weapon crafted and wielded by another Neandertal; however, the St. Césaire skull, named for the site in southwest France where the skull was located, also indicates the practice of nursing. The individual suffering the blow could not have survived without care. Yet a close examination of skull fragments indicates "telltale signs of the healing process."[17] The individual who suffered the blow was also cared for by people who invested their time and energy in ensuring his survival.

Early Brain Surgery: Trepanning

Trepanning—also called trepanation, trephination, trephining, or burr hole—is the earliest known form of brain surgery. It involves drilling or scraping an opening in the skull as a means of treating health problems related to intracranial conditions. Surgeons today continue to use trepanning as a means of relieving pressure on the brain due to epidural and subdural hematomas (tumors or swellings from accumulation of blood). It can also be used to provide access for other surgical procedures, such as intracranial pressure monitoring. The earliest unequivocal evidence for trepanation is from a 7,000-year-old burial at Ensisheim, in the French Alsace region.[18] By this time, Neandertals would have been displaced by biologically modern humans. Healing of the bone surrounding these openings of the skull indicate that many, if not most, of these early surgical operations were successful, in that the patient survived the operation for significant periods of time.

A disadvantage in understanding the history of early Western medicine is that this took place before the development of writing. We know these early physicians only from the results of their work, as recorded in the preserved bones of their patients. We cannot know, for example, whether the practice of medicine was specialized, or whether it was practiced by females or males; however, based on the results of their medical practice, we know that opening the human brain required skill and training.

We also know that childbirth in humans is a difficult enterprise, given the ratio of the human skull to the ratio of the human pelvis. As noted earlier, 70 percent of human brain development occurs after birth. Almost all of this brain development occurs in the form of synapses, the electrochemical reactions that convey information from on neuron to another. At birth, the infant's skull is collapsible, so that even in its undeveloped form it can pass through the birth canal. It appears likely, based on fossil and contemporary evidence, that females played a significant role in early medicine as midwives, almost certainly as herbalists, and perhaps, as surgeons.

With the rise of **stratified societies**, primarily associated with agriculture, males assumed public prominence whereas female life became centered on domestic matters. Typically, in forager societies, the human pattern until about 10,000 years ago, the division between public and domestic realms was fluid, and both females and males contributed greatly to the domestic economy. With the development of cities, which are dependent upon the surplus produced by agriculture, boundaries between public and domestic life became more definitively drawn. Writing systems developed to keep track of possessions, something that was not necessary when humans had equal access to environmental resources. With the rise of writing systems, we now have a record of the thinking of early physicians. Because this chapter focuses on Western medicine, we will examine some of the writings of two early physicians, Hippocrates and Galen, both of whom perfected their skills in Greece.

Early Western Medicine: A Written Record

Hippocrates of Cos (also Hippokrátēs of Kos), who lived from about 460 BC to 370 BC, is considered to be the "father of Western medicine." He is credited with being the first physician to reject the idea that disease is caused by supernatural or divine forces. In so doing, he discredited the belief that illness is a punishment inflicted by the gods, an early form of "blame the victim." Hippocrates considered illness to result from environmental factors, diet, and living habits. In his practice and in his teachings, this early Greek physician made the practice of medicine a profession.

Hippocrates taught his revolutionary form of medicine to his students and wrote down his thoughts on how medicine should be practiced. Hippocrates was the first to categorize illness as acute, chronic, endemic, and epidemic. "Acute" refers to the rapid onset of a disease that is potentially life-threatening. "Chronic" refers to a condition which may not be life-threatening, but may not respond to treatment. Treatment of chronic conditions may consist of alleviating symptoms rather than eliminating their causes. An "endemic" disease is characteristic of a particular locality, and "epidemic" refers to a disease that affects many members of a population at the same time.

An epidemic may both be contagious and of rapid onset. Hippocrates also contributed the terms exacerbation, relapse, resolution, crisis, paroxysm, peak, and convalescence.[19] "Exacerbation" refers to a situation in which an illness suddenly becomes more aggressive and life-threatening. "Relapse" refers to the reappearance of symptoms that had previously been modified or eliminated. "Crisis" refers to an illness phase that could be life-threatening if not treated immediately. "Paroxysm" refers to a sudden increase or recurrence of symptoms, or a convulsion, which involves a violent and involuntary contraction of the muscles. "Peak" refers to the period in which symptoms are most intense, and "convalescence" refers to the time in which a patient is recovering from the illness.

Contemporary medicine has departed from Hippocratic medicine in two key areas: (1) Hippocrates attributed illness to an imbalance of the four humors: blood, black bile, yellow bile, and phlegm; and (2) Hippocrates believed that the body has the power to heal itself, so Hippocratic medicine was aimed at promoting the body's ability to heal itself by restoring the balance of humors. Contemporary Western medicine has drifted away from the model of humors and from the idea that, under certain conditions, the body can heal itself.

Approximately 500 years after Hippocrates died, Claudius Galen was born in Pergamum, in what is now Turkey, where he began his practice of medicine. He practiced later at Smyrna in Greece and Alexandria in Egypt. Galen dissected and observed many animals, including the Barbary apes. This allowed him to describe such structures as the nervous system, the kidneys, and other internal organs. While in Rome, Galen worked as physician to the gladiators, which provided an opportunity for observing trauma to the human body. Galen's philosophy of medicine was based on Hippocrates' concept of humors, but his ability to observe the internal organs of animals permitted him to more accurately describe the inner workings of the human body.

Galen forestalled criticism of research conducted on healthy animals by drawing on Christianity. He suggested that studying Barbary apes promoted God's purpose. This allowed him to continue his work as a physician and promoted his work among Christians throughout the Middle Ages. Galen's distinction between invasive research conducted on healthy animals, but not healthy humans, continues to pervade Western medical research practices.

WESTERN BIOMEDICINE AND SCIENCE

In his book *The Limits of Medicine: How Science Shapes Our Hope for the Cure*, the immunologist Edward S. Golub explains how paradigms shape our understanding and experience of medicine: "How we define disease and understanding how we have brought it under control have special implications in this time of AIDS, because if we do not understand science and medicine, we make unreasonable demands on them that can only lead to disappointment and disillusion" (1997:6).

As Hippocrates observed more than 2,000 years ago, disease results from environment, diet, and lifestyle. A more contemporary view of illness suggests that illness may also result from genetics; however, the precise relationship between the genetic potential for a disease and the development of that disease in individuals has yet to be determined. Some diseases, such as sickle cell anemia and Tay-Sachs disorder are determined by genetics. Other disorders, such as breast cancer and autism, appear to result from the interaction of genetic potential and the environment.

The medical anthropologist Cassandra White (2005:311) suggests with others (Foucault 1994; Hahn and Kleinman 1983) that the biomedical paradigm is itself a folk model of health and illness and that this folk model is subject to political and sociocultural influences. As White indicates, medical anthropologists have observed that medicine does not exist independently of its cultural context. Like other forms of science, it is embedded in the cultural models within which it operates.

What Is Science?

The predominant philosophical system underlying Western biomedicine is science. But what exactly is science? Earl Babbie, a pioneering author of books on social science research, states: "It is difficult . . . to specify exactly what science is. Scientists would, in fact, disagree on the proper definition" (1989:2). Still, he adds, a scientific assertion must be supported by two pillars: **logic** and empiricism: "It must make sense, and it must align with observations in the world" (Babbie 1989:6).

Science does not have a monopoly on either logic or empiricism. In the course of our daily lives, we base our decisions on logic and empiricism. If I throw a ball up in the air ten times and it returns to earth all ten times, I may reasonably conclude that balls return to earth after being thrown up into the air. The results of this "experiment" will permit me to make predictions, such as: "If I throw this particular ball up into the air, it will return to earth." There are many possible variables that may affect the outcome of this experiment. For example, the ball may get stuck in the branches of a tree, so that I might have to climb up after it.

This everyday course of reasoning is similar to that of science, with the important difference that scientific experimentation typically involves more complex phenomena and **variables** that may not be so easy to observe or predict. Babbie notes that both everyday life and scientific research are based in **causal reasoning** and **probabilistic reasoning**. Probabilistic reasoning is based on the idea that a given set of circumstances are likely to produce a predictable result. Causal reasoning is based on the idea that two events occurring together may be the result of one event causing the other. In scientific research, determining causality is much more difficult than observing that a given set of circumstances will produce a predictable result. Two phenomena can occur together without one causing the other. It may be that a third or more variables have produced both phenomena. Thus, one can get a **correlation** that is not based on causality.

A basic flaw in both science and Western biomedicine is the assumption that complex variables, such as health, can be reduced to a single variable. The quest for a "magic bullet" to explain complex variables takes on a moralistic value that shortchanges medical researchers, health care providers, and the public as a whole. Issues involved in maintaining health and promoting healing cannot be reduced to a single variable. In addition, it is a well-known tenet of science that statistics, however accurate, cannot predict individual cases.

Water boils at a temperature of 212 degrees Fahrenheit or 100 degrees centigrade. When the boiling point of water is reached, individual molecules will detach themselves from the water and evaporate into the air. No one can predict which individual molecule will make this hazardous journey. Similarly, in the practice of medicine, we can calculate probabilities that a certain number of patients will survive a particular condition or procedure given a particular set of probabilities. Even the most experienced among us cannot predict which patient that might be. In spite of scientific precision, medical practice still holds many surprises, both for the physician and for the patient.

This brief discussion illustrates the skeletal material of science. In actual research, the variables, and the relationships among them, can become highly complex. One example is the debate over whether certain illnesses, such as cancer and heart disease, are caused by genetics, lifestyle, emotions, or other factors. As anthropologists have noted, it is difficult to sort out the effects of these variables because both genetics and culture are transmitted within families.

Clinical Trials: Medicine by the Numbers

The practice of Western medicine is guided by the principles of science, which tend to be defined in terms of statistical reliability. If a significantly higher proportion of the population benefit from a particular medicine or procedure than would be predicted by random chance, that medicine or procedure would be considered to be effective. The possible 2 percent of the population for whom that medicine or procedure would be harmful would not be taken into account. On a personal level, being part of that 2 percent would be highly significant, even though it would not be statistically significant.

Science is based in careful control of all the variables involved in a particular research situation or medical condition; however, humans are not laboratory rats. Therefore, the clinical conditions that can be controlled for in laboratories cannot be controlled for in everyday life. The apparently random nature of human life is not subject to control. If I am taking a particular medicine to regulate my heart rate, and if I am then involved in a potentially fatal automobile accident, the medication I am taking may be my enemy rather than my friend. It may either prevent me from responding rapidly to an emergency situation, or it may cause me to respond inappropriately.

Statistically based experiments are essential for defining the value of a specific medicine or procedure for large populations. Today, all recognized forms of medical treatments are validated by statistical procedures. There are too many variables involved in the practice of medicine, however, to determine whether a particular medicine or medical procedure would be beneficial for a particular individual in a particular social context.

ENVIRONMENTAL SELECTION AND HUMAN VARIABILITY

Though the statistical emphasis characteristic of Western biomedicine provides a useful overall look at populations, it is of limited use in diagnosing particular cases because it does not consider individual differences in genetic coding, behavioral patterns, diet, attitudes, and lifestyle choices. It also does not consider relative stress levels, values, socialization, economic and social pressures, and individual goals. As Charles Darwin noted a century and a half ago, there is variability in species. In terms of medical practice, this variability can be of immense importance.

Darwin did not view the interrelationship of humans with nature in prosaic terms. He writes, "we see beautiful adaptations everywhere and in every part of the organic world" (1964:61[1859]).

The statistical measures of Western biomedicine do not consider the process of human evolution that has produced such a high degree of variability in the human species, which differs in height, body form, skin color, and other characteristics. In general, populations whose ancestors evolved near the equator tend to have dark skin, an advantage in areas where ultraviolet light is intense. Populations whose ancestors have evolved in more northern climes tend to have lighter skins, an adaptation to low levels of ultraviolet light.

Adaptation to Variation in Ultraviolet Light

Anthropologists have suggested that the range of skin color from the poles to the tropics is related to production of vitamin D. Vitamin D is essential for human health and is available from two sources: diet and exposure to sunlight. Good dietary sources of vitamin D are fortified cereals and dairy products, as well as fish liver oils and fatty fish.[20] Vitamin D is essential for formation and maintenance of bones because it promotes the absorption of calcium and phosphorus from the intestine.

A deficiency of vitamin D may result in bone disorders, including rickets among children and osteomalacia among adults, especially pregnant women. Osteomalacia is a condition that produces soft curved bones. The risk is especially high in individuals who lack the capacity to metabolize vitamin D normally or who do not have sufficient exposure to sunlight. Some anticonvulsants increase the risk of vitamin D deficiency. Symptoms of vitamin D deficiency include muscle spasms, which may occur at any age, and bone deformity, which is characteristic of childhood:

> Older infants may be slow to sit and crawl, and the spaces between the skull bones (fontanelles) may be slow to close. In children aged 1 to 4 years, bone growth may be abnormal, causing an abnormal curve in the spine and bowlegs or knock-knees. These children may be slow to walk. For older children and adolescents, walking is painful. The pelvic bones may flatten, narrowing the birth canal in adolescent girls. In adults, the bones, particularly the spine, pelvis, and legs, weaken. Affected areas may be painful to touch, and fractures may occur.[21]

Overdoses of vitamin D can be toxic. Early symptoms include loss of appetite, nausea and vomiting, followed by excessive thirst, weakness, nervousness, and high blood pressure. Calcium may be deposited throughout the body, particularly in the kidneys, blood vessels, lungs, and heart: "The kidneys may be permanently damaged and malfunction. As a result, urination increases, protein passes into the urine, and the level of urea (a waste product) increases in the blood. Kidney failure may result."[22]

Since vitamin D production in the body is stimulated by sunlight, an excess of vitamin D is most likely to occur in societies near the equator, where ultraviolet light is intense. The melanin found in dark skin is useful in screening out excessive amounts of ultraviolet radiation. Thus, dark skin is selected for in populations that have evolved near the equator. On the other hand, populations that have evolved nearer the poles are subject to inadequate production of vitamin D. Not only is the degree of ultraviolet light less intense, but these populations are likely to wear multiple layers of clothing to protect themselves from the cold. Therefore northern populations are also likely to be subject to bone disorders, unless they are fishing populations able to compensate for inadequate sunlight by fish liver oils and fatty fish.

The Inuit Paradox

Anthropologist Patricia Gadsby studied "the Inuit paradox," which refers to the idea that populations dwelling in the northernmost regions of North America appear to flourish on a high-fat, high-protein diet. Her Inupiat consultant, Patricia Cochran, describes the diet of her childhood:

> Our meat was seal and walrus, marine mammals that live in cold water and have lots of fat. We used seal oil for our cooking and as a dipping sauce for food. We had moose, caribou, and reindeer. We hunted ducks, geese, and little land birds like quail, called ptarmigan. We caught crab and lots of fish—salmon, whitefish, tomcod, pike, and char. Our fish were cooked, dried smoked, or frozen. We ate frozen raw whitefish, sliced thin. The elders liked stinkfish, fish buried in seal bags or cans in the tundra and left to ferment. And fermented flipper, they liked that too. (2007:81[2002])

Gadsby notes that contemporary medical lore in the United States would predict that such a high-protein and high-fat diet would lead to heart disease and stroke. She adds, however, that the life of a forager requires hard physical work, unlike that of contemporary urban dwellers in the United States, where food is abundant year-round and work requires the ability to tolerate enforced immobility. Under circumstances of contemporary urban life, people eat a great deal and exert themselves too little: "Dieting is the price we pay for too little exercise and too much mass-produced food. Northern diets were a way of life in places too cold for agriculture, where food, whether hunted, fished or foraged, could not be taken for granted. They were about keeping weight on" (Gadsby 1007:84[2002]).

Adaptations in Human Body Form

Typically, in contemporary urban contexts, nutritional intake and level of physical activity are dictated by daily routine and cultural attitudes rather than by the biological needs of the body. A significant factor in medicine in the United States is the idea that there is an "ideal" body form that can—and should—be achieved through diet and repetitive exercise. The U.S. Center for Disease Control defines this ideal form according to a statistical measure, the Body Mass Index (BMI). According to the CDC BMI is "a number calculated from a person's weight and height. BMI is a reliable indicator of body fatness for people."[23]

The CDC notes that the BMI is not a direct measure of body fat, but suggests that the BMI correlates with other measures of body fat, including underwater weighting. The CDC website adds:

> BMI is used as a screening tool to identify possible weight problems for adults. However, BMI is not a diagnostic tool. For example, a person may have a high BMI. However, to determine if excess weight is a health risk, a healthcare provider would need to perform further assessments. These assessments might include skinfold thickness measurements, evaluations of diet, physical activity, family history, and other appropriate health screenings.[24]

The same formula is used to calculate BMI for both children and adults. When calculated in pounds and inches, the formula is as follows: weight (lb)/[height (in)]^2. When calculated metrically, the formula is: weight (kg)/ [height (m)]^2. In calculating the BMI for adults twenty years old and older, standard weight status categories are the same for all ages and for both men and women. For children and teens, the interpretation of BMI is both age- and sex-specific. The BMI is not a precise measure because it does not account for individual factors:

- At the same BMI, women tend to have more body fat than men.
- At the same BMI, older people, on average, tend to have more body fat than younger adults.
- Highly trained athletes may have a high BMI because of increased muscularity rather than increased body fatness.

Muscle weighs more than fat, so that the activity cycle of an individual is a factor in whether an individual is likely to be subject to such diseases as hypertension, diabetes, coronary heart disease, or stroke.[25]

Though the CDC lists diseases that may be correlated with being overweight and obese, it does not address conditions associated with underweight, which may indicate a cultural bias. In a videocast sponsored by the UCLA Center for the Study of Women, Abigail C. Saguy, an assistant professor of sociology at UCLA, notes that "Normal or ideal weight is increasingly being defined through a medical and public health lens, in which only 2 percent of the U.S. population is defined as too thin while two-thirds is being defined as too fat" (2007:11).

She adds that the definitions of overweight and obesity are gendered categories, and that the gendering of weight has medical implications: "Medical expertise about ideal weight has gendered implications: women are more likely than men to try to lose weight and to be advised by their doctors to lose weight"[26] and that "strikingly, over 80 percent of weight-loss surgery patients in 2002 were women"[27] (2007:22). The United States produces an overabundance of food, and in light of its puritanical tradition, it could be said that it also produces an overabundance of feelings of guilt.

GENETICS AND MEDICINE

In 2006 a national team of researchers headed by Tobias Sjöblom at Johns Hopkins University analyzed 13,023 genes in eleven breast and eleven colorectal cancers, two common tumor types, that were removed from patients during surgery. The researchers identified 189 genes that were mutated at significant frequency in tumors, a number greater than expected. Mutations in the breast tumors differed from those in the colorectal tumors, indicating that the genetic coding of tumors differs depending on the organ in which they occur. This is a significant finding because it helps to illustrate the mutation process whereby tumors develop in organisms.

Under normal circumstances, every cell in our bodies—except for gametes, that is, sperm and ova—have the potential to shape our bodies. The expression of that coding in a particular part of our body is controlled by regulatory genes. As the name indicates, **regulatory genes** regulate or circumscribe the activity of structural genes. **Structural genes** code for proteins that make up body cells. In multicellular organisms, such as humans, only a limited portion of the genetic coding is expressed in each body cell. Were it otherwise, our bodies would be composed of millions of little humans. Instead, regulatory genes permit the expression of only a small segment of the human **genome**—the total genetic endowment of the human organism—in a single cell. Thus, for example, an epithelial cell—a cell that separates the organs from each other and the skin from the surrounding atmosphere—contains the complete genetic coding of the human organism, but expresses only a small segment of it.

The Johns Hopkins study is significant for a number of reasons. Among them is the discovery that cancer cells have, through mutation, evolved a different genetic coding than is characteristic of normal human cells. A fanciful description of this process would suggest that tumors are a mutated organism that forms a parasitic relationship with its host. This is an important step in preventing and treating cancers because it helps to identity the conditions under which particular cancers might occur. It also helps to explain the difficulties in treating cancers. Researchers have long noted that cancer is not a single disease. It arises from multiple causes and is expressed in a number of manifestations. Tracing this disease to multiple origins and multiple genetic blueprints is a major step in preventing cancer, in identifying the disease in early stages, and eventually, in eradicating its symptoms. Breaking the genetic code of the different cancers that afflict humans is a major step in developing specific treatments for cancer that are both effective and less invasive for other body tissues.

WHY WESTERN BIOMEDICINE IS NOT A CURE-ALL

Western biomedicine is a miracle of science and technology. In just more than 100 years, humans have lengthened their expected life span, lifted themselves off the ground through aerospace, learned to peer into the workings of other solar systems, and probed the genetic code that gives rise to the human form. Yet all the genius that has transformed human life within a dramatically short period of time has not been able to challenge that one implacable foe: death. Western biomedicine has been so successful at preserving human life that many people in the United States have come to view death as a medical failure. But is this view accurate?

At one time, physicians in the United States referred to pneumonia as "the friend of the elderly" because it conferred a relatively quiet and painless death compared to many other medical conditions. This perspective on death focuses on the personal level. It considers the well-being of the patient based on the physician's experience of having been witness to many deaths over the course of his or her career. This is especially personal for medical personal because, unlike most of us, they cannot avoid awareness of how their own lives will end.

At the level of the human species, death clears space for those who are born. This harsh truth is characteristic of all living organisms, animal and plant. At the time of this writing, there were nearly 7 billion people living on earth. Were all the **hominids**, animals most closely related to humans, still alive on earth, this biomass would stifle all other forms of life. We would have nothing to eat and insufficient oxygen to breath. Dying is part of the life cycle for all living organisms, plants and animals. The life cycle characteristic of living beings has been **selected for** during many billions of years. Science does not have the technology to conquer death, a characteristic of all living species for the following reasons:

1. **Scientific empiricism has limits.** Science's strength—empiricism—is also its weakness. Just about all human experience is subjective, shaped by a perspective unique to the individual. This experience cannot be objectively observed or measured, and a large part of this experience consists of emotions and motivations. Emotions and motivations play an important role in health and illness, and these subjective factors can be resistant to the best efforts of medical personal to provide treatment. An individual can court illness, and even death, to punish others for presumed slights or wrongs. The tools of Western biomedicine—surgery, medications, and even psychotherapy—cannot excise the roots of emotions and motivations.

   The experimental techniques of science are based in the ability to sort items into neat categories, to explore complex situations in terms of its variables, its limited and observable components. Human experience and behavior do not come in such neat categories.

2. **Science is based on the ability to control variables.** Only a few variables in a patient's life are accessible by health care workers, and these are measurable primarily by the use of technology and questioning techniques. Medical personnel may be able to tell a great deal about a patient's condition, both physical and psychological; however, decisions made on the basis of these observations must ultimately be substantiated by courts and insurance providers. People make lifestyle choices that are not subject to the control or observation of medical personnel.

3. **Science does not predict individual cases.** Science is based on the principle of **probability**, the statistical likelihood that an event will occur given a specific set of circumstances. In medicine, scientists can predict that certain behaviors and environmental conditions are likely to give rise to particular medical disorders, but they cannot predict exactly who will succumb to those disorders. Avoiding certain behaviors does not guarantee that we will not be subject to the medical conditions associated with those behaviors. Thinking we can avoid illness by singling out and avoiding a particular substance or behaviors is a form of magical thought. Illness occurs as a result of many interrelated variables, and even a medical professional—or scientist—cannot say that a particular illness was caused by a particular behavior or condition.

4. **Because of advances in science, people in the United States have been led to expect miracles.** In his book *The Second Sin* (1973), the psychiatrist Thomas Szasz wrote, "Formerly, when religion was strong and science was weak, men mistook magic for medicine; now, when science is strong and religion weak, men mistake medicine for magic." This is a dangerous perspective for patients to take. People make choices that can affect their health and ability to survive. As a product of science, Western biomedicine does not have the power to prevent an individual from making a bad survival choice or a choice that negatively affects health. And, in many cases, medical personnel cannot reverse the effects of these bad choices.

Related to this is the fact that individuals do not take responsibility for their own health. Writing in the January 2008 issue of *UCLA Magazine*, doctors Andrew W. Seefeld and Adam Landman describe the case of an elderly woman who came to the UCLA Emergency Department "complaining of nausea, vomiting and weakness. She told the physician that she had 'high sugar and heart problems'" (2008:16). She told medical personnel she took medications for those conditions, but didn't remember the names of the medications. "All she knew was that she takes one white pill in the morning and a blue pill at night" (2008:16). Results of her physical exam and electrocardiogram revealed that her symptoms were due to a dangerously slow heart rate, a condition likely to have been caused by an overdose of one of her medications, but the attending physician had no way of knowing which medication had caused the overdose: "So he was forced to treat a patient with a life-threatening condition with an incomplete medical history. Regrettably, that's the rule, not the exception, in today's health-care system" (2008:16). After the patient was stabilized, lab results indicated that she had taken a potentially fatal overdose of the cardiac medicine digoxin, for which there is an antidote. The woman could have been effectively treated much sooner had she known the names and dosages of her medications. Seefeld and Landman note that, according to "a 2003 Yale University study of 94 underserved patients found that only 42 percent could accurately cite their medication names, 13 percent knew their medication doses and 29 percent were able to identify their medication frequencies" (2008:17).

5. **There is a high degree of specialization in the healing professions.** Seefeld and Landman note that due to the high degree of specialization in Western biomedicine, patients may routinely visit multiple specialists, sometimes in completely different health-care facilities: "This makes it difficult to ensure that any single provider has access to a patient's complete medical record, including clinical notes, lab results for such things as blood work, or imaging results such as X-rays. A universal electronic medical record would help, but that's years, if not decades, away from becoming a reality" (2008:17).

Although Seefeld and Landman do not address this issue, having a patient's medical records scattered among multiple health-care facilities increases the probability that medications prescribed in these different facilities might result in overdoses due to an overlap in ingredients. On the other hand, a universal electronic medical record system could result in privacy issues, which would have to be addressed in the process of setting up such a record system. Another issue involved in setting up such a system is ensuring that reports from the different health-care facilities are standard-ized, so that all medical professionals involved in a patient's health care know what treatments have been recommended and/or provided. In the absence of such a system, Seefeld and Landman state, "for now, it's up to the patients themselves to make sure their doctors have all the information they need. Whether you're visiting a local clinic or entering a nearby Emer-gency Department, the ability to communicate accurate knowledge of your medications, medical/surgical history, allergies and much more is invalu-able to any health-care provider" (2008:17).

6. **Medicine in the United States is driven by the consumer market.** A 2007 case in Los Angeles illustrates this often-tragic principle. A 17-year-old girl suffering from leukemia remained in intensive care due to complications after a successful bone marrow transplant. These complications would require a liver transplant, and doctors treating the girl advised her parents that patients in similar circumstances have about a 65 percent chance of liv-ing for six months if they have a liver transplant. At first, the family's insurer declined to cover the transplant, and as the case was debated, the patient remained on life support systems. In despair over the girl's condition, the family gave permission to remove her from life support systems. At approx-imately the same time, the insurance company reversed its decision and agreed to pay for the procedure.

There are many medical issues involved in this case, and none of them is clear or simple. One issue is whether another patient, with more optimistic chances for surviving more than six months, might have been better served by the liver transplant. Another is whether this patient would have had adverse reactions from the immune suppressant drugs necessary to prevent the patient's body from rejecting the transplant. Yet another issue is quality of life: What kind of life might this patient and her family have had if the transplant had been successful?

Regardless of these issues, any of which might have mediated against a transplant, the deciding factor was economic. Someone has to pay for such an expensive medical procedure. In the United States, it could be the family, the insurer, or the hospital. Because the medical system in this country is consumer-driven, the more affluent, or those covered by some kind of insur-ance or medical payment plan, have greater access to medical care than those who are poor or uninsured. In countries that have universal health care, decisions about which procedures are appropriate still have to be made, but they may be made on the basis of medical priorities, rather than on the basis of cost.

It can be argued that high-risk procedures serve the community as a whole, since they may lead to breakthroughs in medical treatment. This is a valid argument. It is also true that no one, even medical professionals, can predict which life can by saved by which particular medical treatment. Medical proce-dures are precise, but medical judgments are still subject to the fact that humans—not even scientists—can predict the future. We can only speculate on the basis of probability.

7. **The human body is not designed to last forever.** The human life span is short, compared with the durability of mountains, rocks, and some kinds of trees, such as redwoods. But all organic life ends at some point. Humans, and some other primates, may choose to sacrifice or endanger their lives for what they consider a good cause. According to the apostle John, "Greater love hath no man than this, that a man lay down his life for his friends" (15:13). Anthropologists have noted that macaques, monkeys that live on the African veldt, will give alarm calls when a predator appears, even though warning other members of the group increases the probability that the macaque who gives the call will be the one picked off by the predator.

Western biomedicine is organized around the principle that its goal is to preserve human life. As noted in earlier chapters of *The Anthropology of Health and Healing*, it is not always easy to determine when life begins and ends. Throughout human history, that decision has been made by a counsel of peers (family, friends, and neighbors) based on observable signs. In recent decades, the ending of life is often based on the output of machines, which measure the body's ability to respond.

10

Restoring the Balance

Asian Models of Health and Healing

CASE STUDY
The Legendary Monks of the Shaolin Monastery

The Shaolin monastery, built at the foot of Mount Songshan in Dengfeng county in the province of Henan in 495 AD, has long been revered as the birthplace of Zen Buddhism and kung fu, both believed to be developed by the Bodhidharma, who is said to have introduced Buddhism into China. According to legend, a monk associated with the Shaolin monastery was able to heal the mother of the emperor of Shu, Wang Yan, who was viewed by the monks at the monastery as debauched, ruthless, and cruel, who had "no sense of human sympathy and his subjects lived in abject poverty." This is a serious indictment, since the role of a Chinese emperor is to mediate the balance between heaven and earth. An emperor's failure to sustain this balance results in wars, famines, poverty, and natural disasters. When Wang Yan's mother became seriously ill, the emperor called in a series of famous doctors. None was able to cure her, so Wang Yan put them to death. Soon, no doctor was willing to treat her. Zhan Zhi, a monk from Shaolin who was traveling to find out more about life outside the monastery, entered a village where an esteemed physician feigned death to avoid healing the emperor's mother. Zhan Zhi took the place of the doctor and went to the emperor's palace to heal the dowager empress. After arriving at the palace, the monk put down the bundle of silk gauze curtain he was carrying and felt the Queen mother's pulse.[1] When he had finished asking all he needed to know about her illness, Zhan Zhi replied, "As the Queen mother will not take medicine or acupuncture as treatment, if you wish to cure her you must do as I suggest." The monk ordered that a house with nine empty rooms was to be found and that each room was to be painted to cover any cracks in the walls. Thick cotton curtains were to be hung over all the doors and windows. Three charcoal fires were to be placed in each room, making a total of twenty-seven in all, and on each fire a large earthenware pot was to be placed. A bag of the doctor's medicine was to be placed in each pot along with a lot of water, and the fires were to be kept burning continuously. The patient was to be taken into the house and, with only silk gauze draped over her shoulders, she was to sit quietly inside for three days and nights. After this she was to be brought out to rest for a day, and then put back into the house for another three days. This was to be done nine times, after which she would be totally cured (Wang Honjun 1988:59).

The Queen Mother was healed by this technique, and the monk posing as a physician was allowed to live. The tale was told to demonstrate the spiritual power of monks at the Shaolin monastery, which still exists. It is also clear from the description that the cure could have been based on the healing power of herbs administered by means of steam.

The treatment also called on the symbolic value of multiples of three. The number of rooms required was nine, three times three. The number of smoking pots in each room was three. The total number of fires was twenty-seven, three times nine. The sequence of rest and treatment was also based on a multiple of threes, or twenty-seven. According to the I Ching, the Chinese Book of Changes, the number three is associated with heaven. In general, uneven numbers are associated with heaven, and even numbers are assigned to earth.[2]

Monks living at the Shaolin monastery at the time would have attributed the cure to the monk's ability to manipulate *qi* (pronounced "chee"). Chinese view qi as the energy which comprises the universe. Chinese medicine, whether it involves herbal treatments, acupuncture, or various other forms of manipulation, is based on the idea that health is maintained by a balanced flow of *qi*, whereas illness is caused by stagnant *qi* or by *qi* that is either too hot or too cold. Illness, poverty, and bad luck in general are caused either by blocked *qi* or by *qi* that flows too fast. Blockages of *qi* are treated by a number of means, including acupuncture, herbs, and *qi gong*, a form of exercise and meditation.

Energy Models

Chinese medicine is a medical system based on the idea that humans exist within energy fields that define the universe. In Asian models of health and healing, all phenomena are comprised of energy. Thus, numbers—as well as emotions, attitudes, and objects—consist of energy and interact with other energy fields. By itself, energy is neither good nor bad; it is part of the overall cycle of life.

In Hindu cosmology, the ebb and flow of energy is expressed in all aspects of life, as well as in three important deities: Brahma, Vishnu, and Śiva, who represent the cycle of human life, agriculture, and the universe. Brahma, the Creator, presides over the beginning of life and the universe. In Hindu iconography, Brahma has completed the creation of the earth-world and, therefore, is no longer active in its maintenance or destruction. He will return again after the present universe ceases to exist. Today, his worship is largely confined to Rajasthan, in northwest India. Vishnu originated as a solar deity, associated with fire, lightning, and the sun. His avatar Krishna represents the playful manifestation of the universe. In Hindu iconography, the manifest universe is the play of the gods. Śiva, the destroyer, expresses dual imagery. He both dances the universe into destruction when it has completed its cycle and plants the seed that will emerge as the next cycle of creation.

The Western scientific discipline of physics is also based on the idea that the dynamics of the universe are based in energy. One of my assignments as a journalist was to write a story on Stanford University's linear accelerator, an assignment that sparked my interest in the energetic properties of atoms and subatomic "particles." The linear accelerator "smashed" positively charged protons and negatively charged electrons together through the use of positively and negatively charged bipolar magnets.

It is no longer a matter of scientific debate whether "energy" is the elemental force underlying the universe. The question is whether physicists and Asian philosophers are talking about the same kind of energy.

ENERGY MODELS AND SCIENCE

The U.S. National Institutes of Health (NIH) identifies energy medicine as a domain in its National Center for Complementary and Alternative Medicine (NCCAM). The position of the NIH with respect to Complementary and Alternative Medicine (CAM) represents a significant departure from previous NIH positions. Earlier NIH positions were based on a model that assumed a diagnosis or treatment was not effective if it could not be measured through empirical procedures. This assumption was embraced even though human powers of perception and scientific measuring devices are known to be limited. NCCAM continues to adhere to the empirical model characteristic of science, but it holds open the idea that energy models not currently verifiable may at some point be empirically verifiable.

Some energy models listed by NCCAM, such as "intercessory prayer, in which a person intercedes through prayer on behalf of another," may never be scientifically verifiable because human motivations are complex. Scientists studying these phenomena would have to inquire into a variety of subtle and unacknowledged relationships. For example, would an individual who could expect to inherit a great deal of property from a seriously ill patient be able to set aside motives of personal gain? Similarly, could a religious official who knows the patient has generously endowed his or her institution be entirely free of conflicting interests?

How exactly could one identify and measure the conflicting emotions that characterize the human mind? A limitation of science is that it seeks to be objective, but human experience is inherently subjective. NIH has taken a bold and courageous step in acknowledging that science cannot currently address all the variables that define health and healing. Further, some healing systems are effective in relieving symptoms or providing greater quality of life, though they may never be subject to scientific verification. NCCAM addresses issues related to energy models of healing by identifying them as "veritable" (i.e., subject to scientific verification) or "putative" (not scientifically verifiable using current measurements).

Veritable Energy Models

Veritable energies, those that are subject to scientific measurement, "employ mechanical vibrations (such as sound) and electromagnetic forces, including visible light, magnetism, monochromatic radiation (such as laser beams), and parts of the electromagnetic spectrum."[3] Radiation therapies used to treat cancer are in this category. These energy therapies "involve the use of specific, measurable wavelengths and frequencies to treat patients."[4]

The NCCAM website notes: "There are many well-established uses for the application of measurable energy fields to diagnose or treat diseases: electromagnetic fields in magnetic resonance imaging, cardiac pacemakers, radiation therapy, ultraviolet light for psoriasis, laser keratoplasty, and more."[5]

Many kinds of energy influence our lives. Wind in the form of cyclones, hurricanes, and tornadoes are invisible forces that have the power to destroy homes, public buildings, and other structures designed and built by mere humans. In the United States, wind is now being used to produce electricity. Electricity lights and heats our homes, and powers the sophisticated electronic devices that hospitals now rely on. It would be absurd to deny that energy exists, even if we can see it only in the form of results it produces.

Putative Energy Models

Putative energies, which "have defied measurement to date by reproducible methods,"[6] include Asian medical traditions, as well as some other forms of energy healing models. The NCCAM website notes: "This vital energy or life force is known under different names in different cultures, such as qi in traditional Chinese medicine (TCM), ki in the Japanese kampo system, doshas in Ayurvedic medicine, and elsewhere [under other names]. . . . Practitioners of energy medicine believe that illness results from disturbances of these subtle energies."[7]

NCCAM does not suggest that "putative" energy fields do not exist. The NCCAM position is that they cannot be measured with contemporary technology or that it is not currently possible to distinguish them from surrounding energy fields, such electricity or radar. At this point, the "efficacy" of non-Western systems of medicine based on "putative" energy models is defined in terms of alleviation of symptoms as reported by patients. In spite of skepticism expressed by NCCAM, the organization notes: "Energy medicine is gaining popularity in the American marketplace and has become a subject of investigations at some academic medical centers."[8]

Energy models are aimed at addressing the relationship of the microcosm (the human patient) with the macrocosm (the total energy of the universe). Biomedical models are typically aimed at eradicating a particular disease or condition, whereas energy models target the underlying "cause" of the disorder, which may be the "disorder" of the patient's lifestyle and/or world view.

Asian "Science"

In putting quotation marks around the word "science" with reference to Asian science, I do not suggest that scientific observations associated with the development of Asian medicine are less important or factual than those that have shaped Western biomedicine since the late nineteenth century. Rather, I am indicating that the validity of Asian science is not based in statistical analysis, but in the skill and reputation of the physician.

Asian medicine does not rely on the Western scientific method of verification through isolation of variables believed to be healing and comparing their results to results that might be expected of placebos. However, that does not rule out the idea that Chinese and other forms of non-Western healing might be based on less formally controlled and strictly defined experimentation and observation.

As noted in chapter 3, taxonomies of healing may be based on long experience in observing illness and the results of treatments. Hausa of northern Niger in Africa effectively treated nightblindness with foods that were rich in vitamin A, which has been identified by Western researchers as significant in causation and treatment of nightblindness. A lack of sufficient sources of vitamin A can cause nightblindness. Administration of vitamin A can quickly reduce symptoms, whether delivered in medication by Western-trained medical personnel or in the form of "good foods" that are rich in vitamin A by indigenous caretakers.

Whereas Western models of medicine are based on cells and organs, Eastern models of medicine are based on the flow of energy and on types of energy. Disease is believed to be caused by a disruption in the flow of energy, as opposed to the malfunction of a specific organ or part of the body. In traditional Chinese medicine,[9] however, organs may be loci for specific kinds of energy. It may never be possible to identify and measure the precise components of Asian energy models according to Western empirical standards.

An important difference between biomedicine and Asian models of healing is that the latter are holistic, not only in treating a particular illness but in considering the context within which illness occurs. Health and illness are seen as resulting from the relationship of the individual to the family, the local group, the environment, and the universe, which includes the social, physical, and spiritual universe. The health of an individual is viewed as being a matter of alignment between the individual, his or her social relationships, and the universe as a whole.

Arthur Kleinman, a professor of social medicine at the Harvard Medical School, is considered "one of the world's leading medical anthropologists."[10] He has conducted research in both Taiwan and China. He compares the principles of Chinese medicine with the practice of Western medicine:

> Classical Chinese medicine regards most diseases to be caused by disharmony to man, while Western medicine regards most diseases in terms of the organ-specific lesions they produce. Classical Chinese medicine speaks in a "functional" language of imbalances in the body's *yin/yang*, of disharmony in the systematic correspondences of the Five Evolutive Phases (*we-hsing* [*pinyin, wu xing*], also rendered Five Elements (wood, fire, earth, metal, water), including the integrated functioning of the five interrelated internal organ systems (*we-tasang* [*we chang*]. Five body Spheres), and of blockage of the balanced circulation of *ch'i* [*qi*] (vital essence)." (1980:91)

This embeddedness of the patient within a social and universal flow of energy contrasts with patients' experiential issues characteristic of Western biomedicine. In Western medicine, once an individual is labeled by a particular disease, the "patient" becomes viewed as a disease or disorder, rather than as a human being. The label, and the treatment associated with that label, isolates the patient from his or her social and contextual environment. If the diagnosis is terminal, friends and relatives begin to view the patient as a potential dead person, a zombie.

This was brought home to me by the experience of a friend who was diagnosed with terminal colon cancer. Over lunch with two mutual friends, one of my companions bemoaned, "We have lost this wonderful man."

Startled, I replied, "He's not dead yet." I then compounded my companions' shock by stating, "We could die before he does."

In fact, our friend lived long enough to finish writing his eighth book, *Living Buddha Zen*,[11] published shortly before his death.

Asian medicine addresses the health of an individual through a variety of means, including diet, herbs, manipulation of the body, and lifestyle. Though there are many variations on energy medicine, this chapter will focus on two important Asian traditions: Chinese medicine and the Ayurvedic tradition of India.

Both Chinese medicine and Ayurveda are embedded in the philosophical traditions of their respective nations. In both Chinese medicine and Ayurveda, there are many lineages, all of which can be traced back to a philosophical origin. In Asian medical practice, the reputation of lineage replaces the reputation of medical schools in shaping the career of practitioners. The importance of lineages in Asian medical traditions reflects the importance of lineages and extended families in Asian social life. The Western emphasis on medical schools, which transmit knowledge through public institutions rather than familial relationships, is due to the emergence of science as the dominant biomedical paradigm in the West. Both traditions have much to learn from each other.

THE *YIN* AND *YANG* OF CHINESE MEDICINE

The two forms of *qi* are *yin* and *yang*. Harmony in the universe is maintained by the balance of female (*yin*) and male (*yang*) energy. Yin energy is dark, moist, and receptive; yang energy is light, dry, and penetrative. An excess of yin energy causes illness and misfortune because it is too moist and cold; it produces illnesses related to dampness, such as influenza and pneumonia. An excess of yang energy causes illness and misfortune because it is too dry and hot; it produces illnesses related to heat, such as fevers. All illnesses are produced by unbalanced energy.

Since energy is in a constant state of ebb and flux, every phenomenon in the universe is subject to change. According to the *Nei Jing*, the leading classic of Chinese medicine: "Yin and yang are the *dao* of heaven and earth. They are the principles of the myriad matters of the universe and the father and mother of change."[12] This philosophy is reflected in the title of the Chinese classic, the *I Ching*, roughly translated as the Book of Changes. Energy should never be blocked, nor should it be forced. In practice, change occurs on multiple levels.

The concept of energy flow is based in Taoism, and the classic text on this philosophical school is the *Tao Te Ching*. The *Tao Te Ching* is reputed to have been written by Lao Tzu, which is an honorific title meaning "Old Master." The identity of Lao Tsu is in doubt and his works may have in fact been compiled by many authors.

Chapter 29 of the *Tao Te Ching* compares the roles of the yang and the yin, especially with respect to the balance of these two energies, the masculine and the feminine. This philosophical work advises the reader to comprehend the thrust of yang energy, but to model one's thoughts and behavior on the receptiveness of yin energy. Yin energy allows one to accept the inevitable changes that are thrust into our lives and circumstances.

When I diagram the yin and yang symbol for some of my classes, I explain that the yin and yang are complementary, not oppositional. It is hard for students raised in the United States to understand this principle. They have been taught by media to think that "women are from Venus and men are from Mars." Based on this oppositional view of gender, Westerners fail to comprehend the perspective that females and males complement and complete each other in Asian philosophy.

The idea that females and males are antagonistic to each other would undermine the philosophical and practical basis of Asian forms of healing. This would violate the concept of energy balance in the human body. In Chinese medicine, every human body contains centers of feminine and masculine energy. If the feminine and masculine aspects of energy were at war with each other in the same body, that would be a prescription for disease, just as a war between wife and husband would be a prescription for disharmony in the Chinese household. Chinese medicine is aimed at aligning the body's feminine and masculine energies so that health can be maintained and illness can be avoided.

The psychologist C. G. Jung writes, "The method of the *I Ching* does indeed take into account the hidden individual quality in things and men, and in one's own unconscious self as well" (1967:xxviii). Jungian psychology bridges the traditional gap between Western biomedicine, which deals with observable and measurable phenomena, and Eastern universalism, which considers health and illness to be manifest at multiple levels, and as resulting from multiple levels of experience.

The Chinese energy model is based on the philosophical model of "as in heaven, so below." There is continuous energy flow throughout the universe and throughout the human body. The body is not considered as distinct from other aspects of the universe. Chinese systems for maintaining health and treating illness are based on a model of the relationships between the body and the universe as a whole. In Chinese tradition, the universe that most directly affects our health and well-being is the family.

Energy and the Family

Chinese are traditionally agricultural, and economic resources, such as land, are held in families. Family relationships are codified in the I Ching as the eight trigrams, groups of three lines that, when combined, represent forms of energy underlying the universe:

Ch'ien (the Creative): its attribute is strength, its image is heaven, and its family relationship is father.

K'un (the Receptive): its attribute is devoted and yielding, its image is earth, and its family relationship is mother.

Chên (the Arousing): it incites movement, its image is thunder, and its family relationship is first son.

K'an (the Abysmal): its attribute is dangerous, its image is water, and its family relationship is second son.

Kên (Keeping Still): its attribute is resting, its image is mountain, and its family relationship is third son.

Sun (the Gentle): its attribute is penetrating, its image is wind or wood, and its family relationship is first daughter.

Li (the Clinging): its attribute is light-giving, its image is fire, and its family relationship is second daughter.

Tui (the Joyous): its attribute is joyful, its image is the lake, and its family relationship is third daughter.

These symbols accurately emphasize the importance of relationships within the traditional Chinese agricultural family and explain the dynamics of these relationships. The first son has the duty of assuming leadership of the family when the father dies; therefore, he must prepare himself for this duty. The second son is dangerous because he may challenge the position of the first son (according to one of my Chinese informants, this has happened). The third son is resting because he has little possibility of claiming the rights of the first son, and therefore is distanced from the transition of leadership from father to son. The first daughter is gentle but penetrating because she will leave her household of birth and make her way in the household of her husband. The message of this image is that she must carve out her role in her new household, but her strategy must be gentle. The second daughter (light-giving) is not required to fulfill the social obligations required of the first daughter;[13] and the third daughter is joyous because she has few responsibilities to fulfill. She is a belated gift from the universe.

Richard Wilhelm, author of the introduction to the Princeton University Press edition of the *I Ching* (Bollingen Series XIX), writes: "The sons represent the principle of movement in its various stages—beginning of movement, danger in movement, rest and completion of movement. The daughters represent devotion in its various stages—gentle penetration, clarity and adaptability, and joyous tranquility" (1969:li). Because of the importance of the family in Chinese social life, it is not surprising that lessons learned from these relationships should be incorporated into their vision of the universe.

Chinese Philosophy and the Practice of Medicine

Sun Si-miao, the great Tang Dynasty master of medicine has said: "If you do not study the *I Ching*, you cannot understand medicine at all."[14] In his foreword to the Wilhelm translation of the *I Ching* (the Chinese *Book of Changes*) the eminent psychologist Carl Jung writes:

I can assure my reader that it is not altogether easy to find the right access to this monument of Chinese thought, which departs so completely from our ways of thinking. In order to understand what such a book is all about, it is imperative to cast off certain prejudices of the Western mind. It is a curious fact that such a gifted and intelligent people as the Chinese has never developed what we call science. Our science, however, is based upon the principle of causality, and causality is considered to be an axiomatic truth. (1950:xxii)

Jung draws upon Immanuel Kant's (1787) *Critique of Pure Reason* to suggest that the Western model of empiricism does not explain all of our understanding of the universe. Kant writes:

> There can be no doubt that all our knowledge begins with experience. For how should our faculty of knowledge be awakened into action did not objects affecting our senses partly of themselves produce representations, partly arouse the activity of our understanding to compare these representations, and, by combining or separating them, work up the raw material of the sensible impressions into that knowledge of objects which is entitled experience? In the order of time, therefore, we have no knowledge antecedent to experience, and with experience all our knowledge begins. But though all our knowledge begins with experience, it does not follow that it all arises out of experience. For it may well be that even our empirical knowledge is made up of what we receive through impressions and of what our own faculty of knowledge (sensible impressions serving merely as the occasion) supplies from itself.[15]

As Kant notes, experience is not the only source of human knowledge. There is a priori knowledge that is not derived entirely from experience, but from "a universal rule" which is "borrowed by us from experience."[16]

For example, we may believe in a beneficent or punitive God without ever having experienced that entity through our senses. We may also believe in a moral order or form of government that is not subject to sensate experience. We may believe in love without submitting that subjective experience to empirical verification. Some people kill for what they call "love" or "patriotism"; others risk their lives for it. Empiricism cannot fully account for these phenomena, but empires have been built upon them.

At the risk of presuming to understand precisely what Kant is saying, I will attempt to apply his ideas to medical anthropology in general and, specifically, to Asian energy models. We may not be able to confirm the objective effectiveness of Asian forms of healing by direct empirical methods. We can, however, acknowledge that they alleviate symptoms that are distressing in the subjective experience of patients. More simply, we may not understand precisely why some medical procedures do not conform to scientific verifiability, but some patients feel better because of them. Alleviation of symptoms is a part of medicine in all traditions. Pain and other adverse symptoms can prevent people from engaging in lifestyles that could promote their health.

One way in which Asian energy models differ from Western biomedicine is that the Asian emphasis is on promoting health and preventing illness, rather than waiting for illness to occur. In addition, Asian models of healing are aimed at promoting harmony in the individual's lifestyle and physical space.

Health and the Conceptual Environment

Chinese models are organized in the concept of *feng shui*, literally "wind/water," which implies a balance of the five elements: wood, fire, earth, metal, and water. These elements are integral to an agricultural society. Earth is essential for cultivating plants, and water is essential for promoting their growth and keeping them alive. Agriculture makes permanent or semipermanent dwellings possible. Therefore, wood is an important component of agricultural balance and lifestyle. Fire is important for heating the home and for burning the detritus of fields to prepare them for the next cycle of production. Metal can be shaped into tools for planting and harvesting.

Having studied the Chinese models of space as expressed in the practice of *feng shui* and also having experienced the pleasant vistas available during my childhood on a farm in the Midwest, I have incorporated the principles of harmonious surroundings in my home and work. I have set up my computer so that, on a clear day, I can enjoy the vista of the entire Santa Monica Bay from the Palos Verdes Peninsula to Point McGoo. The view both draws me to my computer when I don't feel like writing and gives me a pleasant perspective when I pause to compose my next sentence. The vista increases my productivity and improves my mood, so that a routine I could interpret as work becomes play. Both work and play are important for psychological and physical health, and both conform to the Chinese principle of *feng shui*, the balance of natural energies.

This balance can also be explained in medical terms. Our bodies naturally release endorphins, hormones that can be found in the pituitary gland, in other parts of the brain, or in distribution throughout the nervous system. Endorphins interact with the opiate receptors in the brain. Medically prescribed opiates can produce this effect, but so can events in our daily lives. When I am writing or teaching, occupations that require intense occupation, my body feels no pain. My conscious awareness of my body is of gratitude and enjoyment.

As agriculturalists, Chinese have long been aware of the importance of the balance of *feng shui* for their economic well-being, as well as for their general well-being. My childhood home backed onto the side of a hill, with a vista overlooking our fields. Three thirty-foot-tall tall cedar trees, in a row about twelve feet from our house, dominated our small front yard. One day, my mother and I came home from a trip to the market and found the northernmost cedar tree twisted off at its base. There was no damage to the house or to the other trees. My mother diagnosed the cause of the event as a tornado, a powerful wind that must have bounced off the hill behind the house, leaving the house intact.

According to traditional Chinese beliefs, a house should be built south of a mountain to fend off the ravages of winds that typically come from the north. Our particular wind came from the west, but the hill served the purpose of protecting our home. Significant empirical truths may be derived from subjective experience. The significant scientific measure for Chinese agriculturalists did not rely on statistics. It was a lesson learned through the long experience that harsh north winds generally cause harm and that gentle warm winds from the south are generally beneficial.

Change and Healing

As noted earlier, the idea of change is integral to Chinese philosophy. It is also integral to the practice of Chinese medicine. Miki Shima, a practitioner of Chinese medicine and the Japanese author of *The Medical I Ching*, bases his healing practices on the *I Ching*. He suggests that casting the *I Ching* diagnoses the pattern of change operative at a particular point in time:

> The practice of traditional Chinese medicine is based on the recognition of patterns of change within one's patients. When these patterns of change or *zheng* are harmonious and foster life and well being, we say the patient is healthy or recuperating. But when these patterns of change are disharmonious or tend to foster death and dissolution of the body and mind, we say the patient is ill and seek to remedy their disease with appropriate therapies and medications. Such therapies and medications do nothing more or less than nudge the patient's pattern of change from a disharmonious and life-negating trend to a harmonious and life-promoting course." (1992:2–3)

Shima notes, "Chinese medicine recognizes that the *qi* or life functions of the individual are not distinct from the *qi* or functions of the macrocosmic whole" (1992:3). He adds, "Chinese medicine, it is said, is easy to study but difficult to master. It is not so much a science in the Western sense as an art" (1992:4):

> Modern Westerners are used to thinking in a linear and diachronic way, but the language of the *I Ching* is symbolic and synchronic. We tend to think of time and space in a linear way as if things happen as a chain of cause and effect phenomena. But this is not the world the *I Ching* describes. The world of the *I Ching* is more like a web of numerous patterns which are organically and synchronically intertwined without clear-cut cause and effect relationships. This is the world of interdependent arisings. (Shima 1992:5)

Agriculturalists understand that the yield of their crops is dependent on the vagaries of weather. People who live in cities live largely in controlled environments. In urban environments, cold can be conquered by heating systems; heat can be conquered by air conditioning systems. It is not possible, however, to heat or air condition entire fields. Farmers can control the flow of water through irrigation, but they cannot control the temperature or course of air. Concomitantly, health is sustained through one's daily life, which includes adequate nutrition, exercise, and meditation.

A Chinese Model of Energy Flow

Just as the Chinese form of Buddhism, Chán, has given rise to the Japanese form of Zen Buddhism, Chinese medicine has influenced the practice of medicine in other parts of Asia. Chinese medicine has also been adapted to other cultural contexts. Further, since Asian medicine is based on lineages, it has given rise to different "schools" of practice. The *wu-hsing* system links the five evolutive phases or elements with particular internal organs, orifices, tastes colors, and moods, as shown in table 10.1.

Diet and Maintenance of Health

As table 10.1 indicates, food is integral to the Chinese emphasis on maintaining balance. However, there is no single presentation of food that could be said to represent Chinese food, which varies according to region and available resources. People in

Table 10.1   The Five Evolutive Phases and Their Associated Internal Organs, Orifices, Tastes Colors, and Moods

Five evolutive phases	Internal organs	Orifices	Tastes	Colors	Moods
Wood	Liver, gall bladder	Eye	Sour	Blue	Anger
Fire	Heart, small intestine	Tongue	Bitter	Red	Happiness
Earth	Spleen, stomach	Mouth	Sweet	Yellow	Desire
Metal	Lung, large intestine	Nose	Spicy	White	Worry
Water	Kidney, urinary tract, bladder	Ear	Salty	Black	Fear

Source: http://www3.niu.edu/acad/psych/Millis/History/2004/easternpsychology.china.htm

the United States are most familiar with Cantonese food characteristic of southern China. The historical reasons for this have to do with the California Gold Rush. In 1848, gold was discovered in northern California. Since transportation was limited at the time, and in view of the ongoing war between Mexico and the United States, the news traveled more quickly down the west coast of North and South America and to China than to the U.S. government on the East Coast and to Mexico City, which is inland. This is because seagoing vessels carried news more quickly than horse-drawn vehicles or travelers journeying by foot. Early Chinese immigrants to the United States were from Canton in southern China, and for more than a century, Cantonese cuisine dominated the view of what constitutes Chinese food in the United States.

However, China is a large country with many ecological niches containing a variety of exploitable resources. This is reflected in the food styles of the five main regions of China. The Cantonese region of southeast China is noted for roasted and grilled meat and fried rice, as well as bird's nest soup and shark's fin soup. This is a largely agricultural region with access to marine resources. The access to natural and cultivated food sources produced a highly varied diet. In a visit to a seafood market in Hong Kong, my daughter and I observed marine species that we did not know existed on this planet.

On the east coast, Fukien is noted for its soups and seafood. The Beijing/Shantung area is noted for the subtle and artful use of seasonings, as exemplified in the dish Peking duck. The Beijing/Shantung region has long been the political and artistic center of China, so it is not surprising that it would also be renowned for the elegance of its cuisine. The central Hunan region is noted for combining sweet and sour tastes. The Szechuan-Hunan school is known for its hot, spicy dishes. None of these forms of cuisine is nutritionally "better" than any other. Each depends on local resources. A great value of the Chinese meal is the variety of nutritional sources integral to each meal.

Contrary to advertising in the United States, Asians (including Chinese) do not live on rice alone. Rice is a staple of the Chinese meal in many parts of the country, but wheat serves this role in parts of northern China. Wheat is typically served as noodles or steamed buns. Also contrary to Western advertising, most Asians do not eat brown rice. I have traveled to Canton in southern China, Hong Kong, Macao, Japan, Korea, Taiwan, Thailand, Malaysia, Indonesia, and Singapore, and I have never seen brown rice served or eaten.

Both brown and white rice are good nutritional sources. White rice is the endosperm (generative source) found beneath two types of protective coating, the hull and layers of bran. The hull protects the grain of rice during harvesting. The bran, which is the outer coating of brown rice, protects the endosperm. Both the bran and the endosperm provide important nutrients.

There are many varieties of rice, but the most aromatic and flavorful is Basmati rice, which has been cultivated for centuries at the foot of the Himalayas. The Hindi term "basmati" means "queen of scents" or "pearl of scents." At one time when I was cooking Basmati rice, the scent was so enticing, I could barely wait for the rice to cook. I had planned to serve it with dal tadka, a type of lentil curry. In the end, I ate the Basmati rice straight from the pan. This was a direct—but extremely tasty—violation of the principles of Asian cuisine.

Whereas high-protein dishes—such as meat, fish, or poultry—constitute the major portion of the Western diet, in Chinese cuisine these typically are served alongside and equally with vegetables. I have rarely seen these high-protein dishes served alone. Contrary to some Western assumptions, most Chinese are not vegetarians. Each meal typically includes a variety of dishes, so that every meal is balanced according to flavors, textures, and methods of preparation. It is also balanced according to types of energy each component represents.

Meals are social occasions, involving the entire family. Sharing of food occurs on multiple levels. It unites the *qi* of the earth's abundance with the *qi* of human social relationships. If this exquisite balance of *qi* is disturbed, it can be restored through a variety of means, including herbs, and techniques such as cupping and acupuncture. In this volume, we have space to deal with only a few. In general, herbs will be discussed in Chapter 14. In this chapter, we will deal only with the redressive technique of acupuncture and the balance of Ayurvedic medicine.

CHINESE HEALING TECHNIQUES—ACUPUNCTURE

Evelyn Y. Ho, who specializes in medical communications at the University of San Francisco, describes the traditional goals of acupuncture: "Acupuncture aims to restore the smooth flow of 'Qi.' With the insertion of needles at one or more of the almost 400 acupuncture points on the body, it brings the body back to a balanced state of health."[17]

The objective of **acupuncture** is to balance the flow of energy in the body. It follows the principles integral to Chinese philosophy in general. Energy should not flow too fast, nor should it be blocked. Health results from a balance of *yin* (feminine) energy with *yang* (masculine) energy. Yin energy is cold, slow, and passive, while yang energy is hot, excited, and active. A predominance of either of these forms of energy can cause illness.

The National Center for Complementary and Alternative Medicine describes acupuncture as "a family of procedures involving the stimulation of anatomical points on the body using a variety of techniques. The acupuncture technique that has been most often studied scientifically involves penetrating the skin with thin, solid, metallic needles that are manipulated by the hands or by electrical stimulation."[18] NCCAM notes, "Relatively few complications from the use of acupuncture have been reported to the FDA [Food and Drug Administration], in light of the millions of people treated each year and the number of acupuncture needles used.[19]

NCCAM has supported a number of research projects involving acupuncture, including the following:

- Whether acupuncture works for specific health conditions such as chronic low-back pain, headache, and osteoarthritis of the knee.
- How acupuncture might work, such as what happens in the brain during acupuncture treatment.
- Ways to better identify and understand the potential neurological properties of meridians and acupuncture points.
- Methods and instruments for improving the quality of acupuncture research.[20]

NCCAM adds that acupuncture is widely used in the United States by physicians, dentists, acupuncturists, and other practitioners "for relief or prevention of pain and for various other health conditions."[21] An estimated 8.2 million people in the United States have used acupuncture.

Acupuncture and Traditional Chinese Medicine

The practice of **Traditional Chinese Medicine (TCM)** in mainland China has been greatly influenced by policies of the Communist Chinese government established under Mao Zedong. Traditional Chinese Medicine was standardized and codified by Mao in the 1950s.

Mao rejected the traditional philosophical models underlying the practice of Chinese medicine in favor of secular verification of its contribution to maintaining health and healing. The Communist influence shifted the emphasis of traditional Chinese medicine to what is now known as Traditional Chinese Medicine, which emphasizes subjecting traditional Chinese medicine to scientific verification and practice.

This form of Chinese medicine has not found universal acceptance. Some practitioners consider that the scientific approach "excludes the more spiritual, mental, and emotional components of an older Chinese medicine that still exists in Taiwan, Korea, Japan, and elsewhere" (Ho 2006:415; see also Eckman 1996).

There is validity to this perspective; however, the scientific approach has also eliminated a great deal of superstition that had accrued to the earlier approach. I do not use the term "superstition" lightly. One of my professors had told me "superstition is someone else's religion." I held this opinion until a brief experiment with a traditional acupuncturist who connected my "illness" with my specialization as an anthropologist. She associated anthropology with old things and diagnosed my condition as having been caused by invading ancient spirits. She described her treatment as "closing [my] chakras" so that the "old spirits" could not continue to invade me. Since I had spent many years in meditation trying to open my chakras, I was reluctant to pay someone to close them again.

In scientific verification experiments conducted at the UCLA Center for East-West Medicine and at other scientific research centers, acupuncture has demonstrated efficacy in treatment of such conditions as pain. At the time of this writing, the UCLA Center for East-West Medicine was collaborating with other UCLA Centers and other universities to study the role of TCM in treating a variety of medical conditions, including neck pain, "the improvement of eye health and quality of life through the integration of acupressure massage into standard medical care,"[22] and "the potential of the integrative East-West approach to improve the outcomes of breast cancer survivors with disabling symptoms."[23]

Ho notes: "In the United States, acupuncture and TCM practices vary greatly due to state licensing and educational institutional differences" (2006:415). Ho conducted her research in the state of Washington, where acupuncture licensing covers only the practice of acupuncture. In California, an acupuncture license also requires knowledge and experience in prescribing herbal remedies.

The Neurobiology of Acupuncture

The paradigm underlying acupuncture is that it acts on meridians. In the practice of Chinese medicine, the term "meridian" refers to linkages among various energies in the human body. In their book *Acupuncture Meridian Theory and Acupuncture Points* (1991), Li Ding et al. describe the essential functions of the meridian system as transporting *qi* and blood, maintaining conductivity and resisting the "invasion of exogenous pathogenic factors."[24]

Sung S. Kim, a physician specializing in acupuncture, describes both the traditional Chinese explanation for the efficacy of acupuncture in relieving symptoms and his own explanation based on contemporary Western research involving neurotransmitters. Kim does not reject the traditional Chinese explanation for the efficacy of acupuncture. Instead, he translates it into contemporary medical terminology:

> Stimulating the acupuncture point with a needle transmits a signal to the portion of the brain, especially the hypothalamus, where signals by acupuncture are interpreted and decoded. Newly found messages are sent to Mother Nature, that is, our own body's defense mechanism, through the autonomic nervous system. This in return enhances the natural healing process of the body to relieve pain and help cure the disease.[25]

Kim's explanation conforms to contemporary research findings, though his explanation takes them a step further. According to a study published in 2005 in the journal *Neuroscience Letters*, inserting a needle into acupoint L14 on the hand—traditionally used to treat pain—is effective in reducing pain because it deactivates parts of the brain involved in processing pain. John Farrar, a pain researcher at the University of Pennsylvania School of Medicine, notes that imaging research has shown that people who get better with acupuncture have clear changes in brain function at the level of the thalamus, a region that processes information from the senses, including touch and pain.

Acupuncture also affects activity in the brain region called the cingulate gyrus, as well as other brain structures that make up the limbic system. Regulating emotion is an important function of the limbic system. The cingulate gyrus, a fold in the brain located above the corpus callosum, is involved in coordinating sensory input with emotions, emotional responses to pain, and in regulating aggressive behavior.

The limbic system in general is involved in emotional reactions and motivated behavior. Terry Oleson is a board member of the Society for Acupuncture Research and a director at Emperor's College of Traditional Oriental Medicine in Santa Monica, California, which trains acupuncturists and offers degrees in Asian medicine. Oleson suggests that because acupuncture deactivates the brain's limbic system it "diminishes the emotional part of the pain experience," such as anxiety or that "woe-is-me feeling."

Other processes relating to the brain could be key to the efficacy of acupuncture in relieving symptoms. Thirty years ago, about the same time acupuncture started to pique the interest of people in the United States, Chinese medical researchers began studying acupuncture in animals. They showed—and subsequent Western researchers confirmed—that acupuncture increased the body's production of its own natural painkillers, known as **endogenous opioids**, or endorphins. People experienced no pain relief from acupuncture if they were first injected with a drug that blocked the opioids' activity. John Longhurst, director of the Susan Samueli Center for Integrative Medicine at UC Irvine, notes that most Western researchers agree that acupuncture's stimulation of endorphins plays a large part in explaining how the practice works to relieve pain.

Though there is agreement that acupuncture effectively blocks the experience of pain, there is less agreement among researchers about whether points along the meridians as defined in Chinese medicine correspond to particular functions or parts of the body. In many cases the acupuncture point is located far from the targeted area or function. For example, nausea and pain are treated by inserting a needle in the front right leg just below the knee joint. Urinary and reproductive conditions, as well as lower back pain, are treated by inserting a needle along the meridian in the inner right ankle. Other meridian points are more logical from the Western medical model. For example, headache and neck pain are treated by inserting a needle in the back of the neck.

Oleson's research as a graduate student and postdoctoral candidate at UCLA and UC Irvine in the 1970s demonstrated a link between tenderness or sensitivity in ear acupuncture points governing a certain organ or body part, and the corresponding health of that part of the body. For example, if a patient had foot pain, a foot-specific acupoint on his ear was also likely to be tender and inflamed. Chinese researchers linked pain or sensitivity at acupoint L18 during acupuncture and severity of disease in the liver, which L18 governs.

Still, it is difficult to perform such correlations objectively and in conformity with scientific guidelines demanded by Western researchers. Pain is subjective, and pain experienced in one part of the body may actually be caused by a condition in a nearby region. Further, even though Western researchers have come to accept the idea that acupuncture relieves pain, they are still working to identify the precise mechanism.

Acupuncture and the Nervous System

Some researchers, such as John Farrar at the University of Pennsylvania School of Medicine, have noted that diagrams of the meridians display similarities to the nervous system. In a study published in the scientific journal *Anatomical Record* in 2002, Helene Langevin, an associate professor of neurology at the University of Vermont

College of Medicine, demonstrated that about 80 percent of the acupoints on the arm correspond to areas of connective tissues between muscles.

This might be why practitioners and patients alike often notice a distinct feeling when an acupuncture needle is inserted into the skin, says Langevin. Patients sometimes describe the feeling, called *de qi* in Chinese, as pressure, a nick, something akin to a mosquito bite. To the practitioner, the grip on the needle feels like catching a fish on a line, or a "tightening" of the skin around the needle.

Langevin is examining what implications this might have for how acupuncture sends messages to the brain. She has published data showing that when needles are inserted into acupoints, the underlying connective tissue winds around the needle "like spaghetti around a fork," she says. This doesn't happen when a needle goes into a non-acupoint area. Langevin has also shown that the winding action causes the cells in the area to change shape, a process that she theorizes might send a signal to the central nervous system. At the time of this writing, she was testing the theory in a series of animal experiments.

Other, older studies conducted and published in Asia and Europe during the 1970s and 1980s produced evidence suggesting that acupoints might be areas of very low electrical resistance, might be slightly more sensitive to touch, or might lie near major nerve pathways. But scientists have not known the significance of these characteristics.

In more recent years, brain imaging has been used to clarify the relationship between acupoints and the functions they represent. The practice was pioneered by Zang-Hee Cho, an imaging expert and UC Irvine professor of radiological sciences. Cho's interest in acupuncture and pain was stimulated when, just over a decade ago, he took a spill while on a hike in South Korea. Plagued by the pain that later radiated from his back, he eventually gave in to his wife's suggestion to see a local acupuncturist—who made his pain (F7) disappear in fifteen minutes.

Pain is an important part of inducing healing and preventing trauma. For example, the pain associated with a broken bone alerts us to the danger of continuing to exert pressure on that part of the body. On the other hand, pain can be caused by overtense muscles, in which case we need to follow a different course of treatment, which may involve gently relaxing and releasing the tension of the muscles involved.

AYURVEDA: AN ANCIENT HEALING
TRADITION WITH NEW ADVOCATES

As of this writing, the University of Maryland Medical Center was one of an increasing number of educational institutions conducting research on Ayurveda. The word **"Ayurveda"** is derived from the Sanskrit word *ayus*, which means life or lifespan, and *veda*, which refers to knowledge. The literal meaning of the term Ayurveda is understanding life. The University of Maryland website writes:

> Considered by many scholars to be the oldest healing science, Ayurveda is a holistic approach to health that is designed to help people live long, healthy, and well-balanced lives. . . . It has been practiced in India for at least 5,000 years and has only recently became [sic] popular in Western cultures. The 'contemporary' form of Ayurvedic medicine is mostly derived from several sacred Indian texts which were written in

Sanskrit between 1500 BC and 400 AD. The basic principle of Ayurveda is to prevent illness by maintaining balance in the body, mind, and consciousness through proper
drinking, diet, and lifestyle, as well as herbal remedies.[26]

The U.S. National Institutes of Health considers both Traditional Chinese Medicine
and Ayurveda to be **Whole Medical Systems**. That is, they are complete systems of
theory and practice that have evolved independently from allopathic (conventional
Western medical systems) medicine. According to the NIH, **Ayurvedic medicine** "is
a comprehensive system of medicine that places equal emphasis on the body, mind,
and spirit, and strives to restore the innate harmony of the individual. Some of the
primary Ayurvedic treatments include diet, exercise, meditation, herbs, massage,
exposure to sunlight, and controlled breathing."[27] In their book *Ayurvedic Cooking
for Self-Healing*, Usha and Vasant Lad write, "Ayurveda is a way of healing and a way
of life that always takes into consideration the whole person. According to the teachings of Ayurveda, every aspect of life contributes to overall health. Poor health seldom has a simple or single cause" (1997:25).

The focus of NIH policies is that every medical procedure, regardless of its social or
philosophical origin, must be validated through controlled scientific experiments
before the NIH conveys its imprimatur. As noted earlier, Traditional Chinese Medical
practices, such as acupuncture, are being subjected to rigorous experimentation, and
in the case of acupuncture, have been demonstrated to be effective in treating certain
conditions, such as pain. The NIH has issued the following advice on Ayurveda:

- The aim of Ayurveda is to integrate and balance the body, mind, and spirit. This
  is believed to help prevent illness and promote wellness.
- In Ayurvedic philosophy, people, their health, and the universe are all thought
  to be related. It is believed that health problems can result when these relationships are out of balance.
- In Ayurveda, herbs, metals, massage, and other products and techniques are
  used with the intent of cleansing the body and restoring balance. Some of these
  products may be harmful when used on their own or when used with conventional medicines.[28]
- Before you seek care from an Ayurvedic practitioner, ask about the practitioner's
  training and experience.[29]
- Tell your health-care providers about any complementary and alternative practices you use. Give them a full picture of what you do to manage your health.
  This will ensure coordinated and safe care.[30]

Ayurveda is a holistic medical practice organized around lifestyle and the unique characteristics of individuals. Ayurveda has two philosophical sources: Hinduism, "one of
the world's oldest and largest religions,"[31] and "ancient Persian thoughts about health
and healing."[32]

Ayurveda and the Hindu World View

The Ayurvedic tradition is based in the holistic world view of Hinduism. The
world view underlying Hinduism is that the manifest universe arises from

Brahman, the creative energy underlying the universe. Words in other traditions defining this creative energy are "God" and "Allah," among many others. Cross-cultural studies of religious systems indicate that concepts of the creative energy underlying the universe are virtually identical. This energy is manifest in all things available to the senses. The Bengali poet Rabindranath Tagore, a Nobel laureate, expresses the relationship between human and divine existence as a mutual inter-dependency: "In my life thy will is ever taking shape. And for this, thou who art the King of kings has decked thyself in beauty to captivate my heart. And for this thy love loses itself in the love of thy lover, and there art thou seen in the perfect union of two."[33]

The energy model underlying Ayurveda shares similarities with the energy model underlying the practice of Traditional Chinese Medicine. The universe is not viewed as being composed of discreet objects, as is the case with Western medicine. Instead, the human body is considered to be a part of the energy comprising the universe. Similar to the Chinese model, the Hindu world view expresses the idea that harmony requires a balance between masculine and feminine energy; however, this is expressed in different symbolism. All but one of the Hindu gods and goddesses have consorts, a balance of masculine and feminine energy expressed through the marital and sexual union of males and females.

The English term "consort" has several meanings, most of which apply to the relationship of Hindu deities and their consorts. Among these meanings are to "share," "accompany," "unite," "make harmony," "play" or "harmonize." As noted earlier in this book, illness is experienced as disorder or chaos. Health is experienced as order. Some medical anthropologists have noted that healing is a process of restoring order to the human body or mind.

Harmony and Human Relationships

The symbolic relationships expressed in the pantheon of Hindu deities, as well as in Hindu myths and legends, reflect the importance of maintaining harmony in the universe, as well as harmony in human relationships. The story of Rama, Sita, Lakshmana, and Hanuman provides a moral lesson illustrating the chaos that ensues when the balance of normal human relationships is disrupted. Rama is an avatar (manifestation) of Vishnu, the sustainer, the Hindu deity who maintains the world in the form of play, or illusion. In human form, Rama was a prince, heir to his father's throne. Sita, Rama's wife, was an avatar of Lakshmi, wife of Vishnu and goddess of prosperity.

To save his father's honor, Rama left his father's home and went to live in a forest. Sita and Rama's brother Lakshmana were inconsolable without Rama, so they joined him in exile in the forest. Sita was kidnapped by the demon king Ravana. Despite Ravana's attempts to seduce her, Sita remained virtuous and loyal to her husband. Accompanied by Hanuman, the monkey god, Rama, entered into battle against Ravana and his armies. Ultimately, Rama slew Ravana and returned to claim his throne; however, Rama's victory was blighted when he refused to believe that Sita had maintained her virtue while Ravana held her captive. In an effort to prove her virtue, Sita walked through flames but Rama's followers still did not believe her. Sita fled the castle and went to live with a sage in the forest. Though Rama became King of the Universe, he lost the true center of his universe, his wife Sita.

The story of Rama and Sita illustrates the complexity of human relationships with respect to balance and imbalance, order and disorder. The relationships involve father/son, husband/wife, elder brother/younger brother, emperor/subject, and friend/friend, much like the Five Relationships in the Confucian[34] model of harmonious social relationships. The Hindu story of Rama extends this relationship into the divine realm. Chinese also incorporate the divine/human relationship into their model of the universe in the role of the emperor as mediator between heaven and earth. As noted above, the Bengali poet Tagore draws on the metaphor of lover and beloved to express his relationship with the divine.

There are two significant differences between Western medicine and Asian energy models of healing: (1) Western physicians focus on treating illness, rather than sustaining health. (2) Western physicians focus on the patient, whereas Asian systems of healing focus on the social context. According to Usha and Vasant Lad, authors of *Ayurveda Cooking for Self-Healing*, an important ingredient in the Ayurvedic lifestyle is relationships, "both the relationships we have with one another and the one we have with ourselves":

> Ideally, clarity, compassion and love should characterize these relationships. It is often easier to love and respect others than one's self. Relationships are mirrors to use for self-learning, inquiry and investigation. Through that very learning, radical transformation of one's life can take place. If our relationships are unclear, confusion and conflict will affect our well-being. (1997:28)

For Lad and Lad, preparing and sharing food is a basic component of forming and sustaining relationships.[35] Robert E. Svoboda, an American scholar with a BS in chemistry from the University of Oklahoma and formal training in Ayurveda in India, describes the relationship of the divine to the health-giving properties of cooking and eating:

> Like many Indians, Usha Tai [Lad] genuinely loves to cook for guests, because every guest, indeed every living being, bears the spark of divinity. That I had arrived in her home meant that I should be fed, not as some grudging obligation but from the love of cooking and feeding. Every morsel fed to that visiting incarnation of God is a morsel fed back to the Creator as an offering of gratitude for nature's bounty; and since the scriptures remind us that "food is indeed God," to feed the hungry is to serve God to God. (1997:9)

Food is energy. In preparing and sharing food, we participate in the life-giving energy of the universe. Svoboda notes, "Food creates the *rasa*, that juicy nutritional essence which nourishes the body's hungry tissues and pleases and satisfies the mind and the senses" (1997:9).

Vasant Lad served as a house physician in the departments of medicine, surgery, gynecology, and pediatrics at the Ayurvedic Hospital in Pune, in western India. He suggests that the holistic Ayurvedic lifestyle begins with diet. He writes, "At that time I observed over and over again how the correct diet, combined with proper herbal medicine and lifestyle, can play a vital role in healing. I became increasingly aware that illness provides an 'invitation' to change one's habitual patterns related to thinking, feeling and feeding ourselves properly" (Lad and Lad 1997:11).

The biological components of food form the cells of our bodies. The appearance, smell, taste, and texture of food feeds our senses. That is the true nutritional value of food. It is not simply a matter of calories and other chemicals. It forms the basis of our biological, social, and emotional chemistry. It feeds our souls as well as our bodies. When we ingest good food and drink, we share in the essential flow of energy in the universe. When we share the experience of choosing, preparing, and consuming good food, we promote harmony in our social relationships. If we extend the paradigm of Ayurveda further, by choosing, preparing, and sharing good food, we promote harmony in our bodies and in the universe.

Energy and Health

In Ayurveda, just as each human has a unique fingerprint, every human has a unique pattern of energy, "a specific combination of physical, mental, and emotional characteristics."[36] These energies are based in the tridoshas, three basic energy types called *doshas*. Each of the doshas makes specific contributions to human life; however, one or more of the doshas are likely to predominate in a particular individual. The doshas and their functions are as follows:

1. **Vata** energy regulates bodily functions associated with motion, including blood circulation, breathing, blinking, and the beating of the heart. When vata energy is balanced, there is creativity and vitality. When it is out of balance, vata energy produces fear and anxiety. Vata is associated with the element air.
2. **Pitta** energy governs the body's metabolic systems including digestion, absorption, nutrition, and body temperature. In balance, pitta promotes contentment and intelligence. Out of balance, pitta can cause ulcers and arouse anger. Its element is fire.
3. **Kapha** energy controls growth in the body. It supplies water to all body parts, moisturizes the skin, and maintains the immune system. In balance, kapha is expressed as love and forgiveness. Out of balance, kapha leads to insecurity and envy. Kapha is associated with the element earth.

In balance, these elements promote health and reduce the effects of illness. To my Western eye, the concept of balance appears to be more complex in Ayurvedic medicine than in Traditional Chinese Medicine. The Ayurvedic doshas, or energy fields, are associated with the time of day, the process of digestion, the seasons, relationships and emotions, types and times of exercise, meditation, and overall lifestyle. Lad and Lad write of meditation and well-being:

> Meditation plays a most important part in daily life and is a powerful tool to help maintain health. While the dictionary says that the term meditation means to think, to ponder, to go through and examine, this definition does not impart the profound meaning of the word. Meditation is an action of clear perception, an observation with total awareness and without any conclusion, judgment or criticism. Meditation demands that you be utterly one with the moment. In this oneness, there is radical change in one's psyche. In this moment-to-moment awareness, there is a cleansing of the body, mind and consciousness. This cleansing will bring one to that state of peace which is joy, bliss and enlightenment. At that point, life becomes a movement of spontaneous meditation. (1997:29)

The Ayurvedic approach allows the essential energy of the universe to express itself in our bodies and consciousness. It transcends isolation and anxiety. We do not have to make war or impose our will on our social and physical surroundings. This does not imply that we should live in blissful ignorance of the distressing events that take place around us. Hindu cosmology suggests that conflict is an essential component of the human experience. Conflict and illness are teachers that help us better understand our biological, social, and spiritual needs. In so doing, they help us avoid circumstances and people that make no contribution to sustaining our health and promoting our healing.

Western medical research has identified some health benefits of Ayurveda, including relief of stress, which promotes the ability of the body to resist illness. Western research has also indicated that Ayurveda lowers blood pressure and cholesterol, slows the aging process, and speeds recovery from illness.[37] Herbs used in Ayurvedic medicine often have antioxidant effects, which means they protect against free radicals, by-products of the body's normal metabolism. The herbs may also protect against long-term illnesses such as heart disease and arthritis. Ayurveda has also pioneered in some forms of surgery.

Paradigms and Medical Procedures

The philosophical **paradigm** underlying a particular form of medical diagnosis and healing affects the way in which diagnosis and healing occur. If we view the human body as a biological object distinct from other objects, as is the case in Western biomedicine, we are less likely to consider the social and psychological contexts of illness and healing. If we become aware that individual manifestations of health or illness occur in social contexts, we can consider those contexts in making diagnoses and developing healing regimens. In energy models such as Traditional Chinese Medicine and Ayurveda, individual manifestations of health and illness are considered within the overall context of relationships and social positioning. In both healing traditions, the particular is framed within the context of the infinite, as the role of humans interacting within a universe of interrelated energy.

11

Calling on the Spirits

Shamans, Sorcerers, and Mediums

CASE STUDY
The Healing Song of a Kuna[1] Shaman of Panama

A Kuna shaman of Panama used a long incantation to successfully escort a woman through a difficult and potentially fatal childbirth.[2] He accomplished this feat without touching the woman's body. Among Kuna, who live on islands off the east coast of Panama, childbirth is typically accompanied by a **midwife** rather than a **shaman**. A shaman is called if a childbirth outcome appears likely to be fatal for mother or infant. The shaman's song describes the midwife's confusion and her visit to the shaman, as well as the shaman's visit to the hut of the woman in labor. Once there, the shaman fumigates the hut, invokes his spirit helpers, and breathes life into his carved images, which represent tutelary spirits who will guide him on his journey into the spirit world. On this journey the shaman must confront Muu, the female power responsible for shaping the spirit of the fetus. In this difficult birth, Muu has not only refused to release the spirit of the fetus, she has also captured the spirit of the birthing mother. Without a spirit, which is the life force, neither the infant nor the birthing mother can survive. In his song, the shaman describes his long and difficult journey into the spirit world, his encounters with wild beasts, and his defeat of Muu and her daughters. After persuading Muu to release the two spirits, the shaman describes in song his preparations for his return to the world of humans. The shaman's description of his return from the spirit world also describes the descent of the infant through the birth canal:

The (sick) woman's body lies weak,

. . .

Her exudations drip down below the hammock all like blood, all red.
The inner white tissue extends to the bosom of the earth.
Into the middle of the woman's white tissue a human being descends. (1983:190)

The French anthropologist Claude Lévi-Strauss suggests that the shaman's ability to conduct the woman through a difficult labor draws on the woman's unconscious awareness that the shaman is symbolically describing the birthing process. As the woman follows the shaman's story of his treacherous journey, she associates it with her own perilous journey. When the shaman describes his success and return, the woman's tense muscles relax, allowing the birth to take place.

The shaman's visible body does not leave the room. He or she evokes aid from the spirit world through his incantations. His negotiations with Muu were not hostile. They were much like those of a vendor in the marketplace. Both parties sought to benefit from the transaction. "The fight is not waged against Muu herself, who is indispensible to procreation, but only against her abuses of power. Once these have been corrected, relations become friendly" (Lévi-Strauss 1973:187).

Songs are an important part of Kuna political and spiritual life. The leader of each community informs and educates the people of his village by singing about the group's sacred history in a traditional dialect. *Voceros* translate the songs into the group's contemporary dialect or into Spanish. Thus, the singing tradition transmits knowledge and history about Kuna social life. A healing song performed by a shaman, who is able to journey into the spirit world, exerts a compelling influence on his patients and other members of the community. The role of the shaman is to establish and maintain harmony both within the group and with the spirit world.

Asian energy models discussed in the previous chapter emanated from highly stratified societies based on agriculture, the production of a large food surplus using a plow. The large food surplus permitted stratification, as well as the emergence of cities and the development of writing systems. Thus, we know a great deal about early Asian philosophy and lifestyle through writings and archaeological records. We can also link their philosophies and lifestyles to their healing practices. In this chapter we will deal with healing systems, and the philosophies underlying them, that are primarily recorded in the minds of the healers and are difficult to document in the historical record.[3]

Anthropologists have been studying shamans for more than 100 years, documenting both shamanic practices and relationships within the groups of which shamans are a part. These studies have been based both on observations of shamanic healing and on interviews with shamans. In general, both historically and in the present, most anthropologists have concluded that these healing practices are effective because of shamans' skills in understanding psychology and social relationships, as well as the psychobiology of the human body. Treatments are enhanced by the shamans' knowledge of **herbal medicine**.

Shamans, Mediums, Sorcerers and Witches

In this chapter, we focus on healers who call on spirits to aid them in their work. In so doing, we will distinguish between **shamans** and **mediums**, as well as between **sorcerers** and **witches**. Shamans and mediums differ in their procedures and the philosophies underlying their practices. Shamans summon spirits through rituals that conduct them on a journey into the spirit world, as in the case of the Kuna shaman. Mediums heal through **spirit possession**. They enter into a **trance** and allow the spirits to take control of their bodies. Typically, shamans remain conscious of their surroundings, whereas mediums do not. Shamans undergo a long period of training that allows them to control the spirits.[4] Mediums undergo a period of training and initiation in which they learn to invite the spirits to control them.

A survey of the vast literature on forms of healing calling on the spirits indicates that the categories of shamans and mediums become a little fuzzy in actual practice. A primary reason is that those who have studied these forms of healing have approached it from different perspectives. Some observers have dismissed the practices as "superstition" or trickery. Shamans and mediums do use theatrical devices in their healing practices, much as Western medical doctors use placebos. Both the theatrical devices and placebos can be effective in alleviating symptoms. On one level, theatrical devices and placebos are effective because they reassure the patient that his or her illness can be controlled by the shaman or physician. As noted earlier in this book, illness is experienced as disorder. In all traditions, the healer works to restore order in the mind of the patient and in his or her experience of illness.

One problem in drawing on the voluminous literature on healing systems that rely on spirit intervention is that the terminology has become standardized only within the past few decades. Prior to this standardization, observers lumped together a variety of healing and other ritual interventions. Some early accounts refer to shamans and mediums as "witch doctors" or "magicians." They did not distinguish among the techniques and philosophies underlying these practices. In drawing on the literature in this area, I am relying primarily on accounts that describe with a high degree of precision methods used by the healer. Most are written by anthropologists, but some are written by missionaries and other adventurers.[5]

Sorcerers and witches differ from shamans and mediums according to their philosophies. Sorcerers, shamans and mediums all seek to enlist the aid of spirit beings in their enterprises. They differ in their goals. Shamans and mediums use the aid of spirits in healing; sorcerers enlist the aid of spirits to cause harm to others.

As defined by the eminent British anthropologist E. E. Evans-Pritchard (1976[1937]), witches are disgruntled individuals who cannot attain their goals through ordinary social relationships. Typically, a witch might be a cowife of a more socially powerful first wife. Because of her more powerful social position, the primary wife can shift her more irksome responsibilities to her subordinate cowives.

The term "witch," as used by anthropologists, refers to individuals who do not have the power to fulfill their social goals. The philosophy underlying the concept of witches and sorcerers is that evil spirits are attracted to human groups. However, they cannot enter without invitation. Witches invite them into the groups through their own jealousy and anger. Sorcerers invite evil spirits into the group through manipulation of ritual symbols. In this chapter, we will focus on **shamanism**, with a brief side trip into the social and psychological world of sorcery.

THE HISTORY AND PSYCHOLOGY OF SHAMANISM

The term "shamanism" has been applied to a variety of healing practices that may have developed independently around the world. They are remarkably similar in their form and practices. If there is a single original source, that source would have been in

Africa, since this is the where humans evolved. An original hominid species, Homo erectus, spread out from Africa sometime after two million years ago. We have no direct evidence that shamanism developed this early. Our only evidence derives from the similarities in shamanism wherever it is practiced, and shamanism is practiced on every continent and every known island. Wherever it is practiced, shamanism is a complex that involves calling on the aid of the spirits.

The word "shaman" comes from the Tungus/Evenki people of central Siberia,[6] and is used as both a noun and a verb. Thus, in the Evenki language, a person who demonstrates extraordinary powers can be called a "shaman," or a person who is especially trained in the magical arts can be said to "shaman" someone or some thing. In the latter use of the term, to "shaman" someone or a thing is to work magic.

Shamanism and Healing

Anthropologists have long noted that shamanic practices are effective in diagnosing illness and bringing about healing. The only debate rests in how they go about it. In practice, shamans are psychologists, social analysts, and herbalists. They produce cures; they address problematic social relationships. They concoct potions that cure life-threatening conditions. This has all been observed by anthropologists and others. There is no argument among anthropologists about whether shamans can heal. Shamans have even proved efficacious in treating illnesses that resist Western medicine. The World Health Organization has recommended that Western physicians work in tandem with shamans. This unites the biological efficacy of Western medicine with the efficacy of shamans in understanding the source of disorders, which may arise from social conditions.

There has been some dispute among anthropologists about whether shamanism could be described as **religion** or as **magic**. Both religion and magic are symbolic systems, in that they draw on multiple levels of meaning, conscious and unconscious. Because **symbols** draw on unconscious associations, they are powerful in evoking emotion and compelling action:

> No one can escape the power of symbols. If we are not involved in the symbolic complexes of religion and magic, we observe symbolic dramas on television, at the movies, or on the sporting field. If we manage to evade the influence of symbols in our daily lives—which is virtually impossible—we will still encounter symbols in our dreams. (Womack 2005:1)

In psychological terms, the power of symbols arises from the emotions and from unresolved conflicts that are stored in the unconscious. That is why symbols are effective in healing, both in contemporary psychological practice and in the traditional practice of shamanism.

Shamans typically use symbols to describe a medical condition to their patients, on psychological, social, and biological levels. Medical practitioners now know that stress can produce biological illnesses. Shamans do not rely on symbols alone, however. They are the traditional pharmacologists. Shamans were the first to use pharmacological preparations to treat biological disorders, and many of their recipes have formed the basis of Western medicines. Shamans use psychological, social, and herbal means to treat illness and redress social relationships.

Shamanism: Religion, Magic, or Mysticism?

The eminent French sociologist Emile Durkheim noted that both religion and magic are composed of beliefs and rituals. He distinguished magic from religion by stating that magic is aimed at "seeking technical and utilitarian ends, it does not waste its time in pure speculation" (1965:57). Durkheim writes of religion:

> The really religious beliefs are always common to a determined [specifically defined] group, which makes profession of adhering to them and of practicing the rites connected with them. They are not merely received individually by all the members of this group; they are something belonging to the group, and they make its unity. The individuals which compose it feel themselves united to each other by the simple fact that they have a common faith. (1965:59)

For Durkheim, the defining characteristic of a religion is the social group, which is organized around a church: "In all history, we do not find a single religion without a Church" (1965:59). According to Durkheim, the church defines the spiritual realm in terms of its own social organization, a view that has been translated as "Religion is social organization projected into the heavens."

The anthropologist Michael Harner asserts that "Shamanism . . . is not a religion." Harner rejects the idea that shamanism is a religion on the basis that religions define spiritual reality for their members in negative terms. Shamanism is egalitarian. As it is practiced today in stratified societies, religion is hierarchical:

> The spiritual experience usually becomes a religion after politics has entered into it. So the renewed interest in shamanism today can be viewed as democratization, returning to the original spiritual democracy of our ancestors in ancient tribal societies where almost everyone had some access to spiritual experience and direct revelation. We are now restoring ancient methods to get our own direct revelations, without the need of ecclesiastical hierarchies and politically influenced dogma. We can find out things for ourselves. (Harner, in Bowie 2000:190–191)

Harner's approach to the spiritual experience is known as **mysticism**, which is the attempt to find direct communion with God or other forms of spiritual awareness. Mysticism is a part of religious experience in many parts of the world, even in hierarchical religions that emphasize conformity to church beliefs and practices over personal spiritual transformation. Mysticism emphasizes direct experience over religious dogma. The Sufi poet Rumi describes mysticism as direct experience rather than dogma.

In a sense, the experience of the shaman is similar to that of the mystic. Though the shaman's body is still visible in the room where the healing ritual is held, his mind is journeying into the world of spirits. Anthropologists and psychologists call this an "altered state of consciousness."

Harner fails to specify exactly how people in contemporary stratified societies are "restoring ancient methods" to gain "direct revelations," but one "ancient method" is the use of hallucinogenic drugs. Use of **hallucinogens** by shamans is not the same as recreational drug use. Traditional shamans undergo years, or even decades, of instruction from experts who have demonstrated their ability to negotiate with spirits. This expertise is demonstrated by the shaman's ability to heal. Shamans must acquire a number of skills, including the ability to diagnose psychological disturbances and physical illnesses. They also typically have expertise in diagnosing social relationships. Cross-culturally, shamanic healing techniques include practices that restore social relationships or alleviate the negative consequences of disturbed social relationships.

Cross-cultural research on shamanism indicates that neophytes imbibe hallucinogenic drugs under the guidance of experienced members of the group. They do not undertake unguided journeys into the spirit world, or as anthropologists put it, into the unconscious. There are "demons" (unresolved problems) in our unconscious, and there are "demons" in unresolved social relationships. An unguided journey into the unconscious using hallucinogens can produce psychosis.

Shamans and Sorcerers

Anthropologists distinguish between shamans (healers) and sorcerers, who use their manipulative powers to cause harm. In his classic work on the Murngin, an Australian aboriginal group described by W. Lloyd Warner, the anthropologist writes: "All deaths, sicknesses, certain types of bad luck, and, in general, all those occasions on which the individual is seriously out of adjustment with his community, physically, mentally or socially, are looked upon as the effects of black magic; and in almost every case except that of soul-stealing[7] the white magician is called in to remedy the situation" (1969:183). Warner describes the relationship between what he calls the "black magician" (sorcerer) and "white magician" (shaman) as a battle:

> There is a kind of warfare between the forces which do good and those which do harm to man. The latter are related to an organized set of concrete techniques embodied in the person of the black magician, while an entirely different set gives practical expression, in the personality of the white magician, to those forces which control the effects of black magic. The struggle then becomes a warfare between these two types of magical personalities. (1969:183)

Shamans practice their craft in public, and people go to them to be healed. Typically, sorcerers hide their craft. Of the Azande of southern Sudan, E. E. Evans-Pritchard writes, "It is not advisable at court [the higher ranks of Zande[8] society] to know much about medicines, other than a few old-established ones, because a man who is found to possess a strange medicine may be suspected of sorcery" (1976:182–183). Among the Azande, men who are suspected of sorcery are likely to be killed. Further, all their male relatives may be killed because Azande believe that sorcery is inherited through patrilineages.

A Zande Initiation Ceremony

Contrary to what some Westerners presume, Azande do not live in a world of magic. They are well aware that all successful enterprises involve a degree of labor; however, they recognize that some results cannot be explained by effort alone: "Azande do not suppose that success in an empirical activity is due to use of medicines, for they know that it is often attained without their assistance. But they are inclined to attribute unusual success to magic" (1976:187).

Evans-Pritchard describes a Zande healing ceremony and instruction of a neophyte. The ceremonies begin with preparation of herbal medicines by boiling a mixture of plants previously gathered by the presiding shaman, or host. The host is usually the owner of the homestead at which the ceremony is held. At first, the mood of the ceremony is jovial and playful. When the water in which the plants are boiled becomes colored from the herbs, the presiding shaman "takes the pot off the fire and pours out the liquid into a second pot, which he places on the fire for further boiling" (1976:91). The roots used for the mixture are saved and stored for further ceremonies.

Evans-Pritchard writes: "At this point the [shamans] . . . rivet their attention upon the business in hand, drop their secular conversation, and develop a noticeable degree of concentration on the medicinal juices now boiling on the fire. This is the first sign in their behaviour that they are dealing with magical forces" (1976:91–92). At this point in the ceremony, the presiding shaman begins chanting invocations for protection.

The aid of all the shamans present, and recognition of their skills, is symbolically represented when the presiding shaman gives a portion of a paste made from oil-bearing seeds to all attending shamans, who then consign the paste to the boiling mixture. Thus they demonstrate their commitment to the enterprise of gaining the aid of spirits. The presiding shaman then stirs the mixture and intones, "May no evil fall upon me, but let me rest in peace. May I not die. May I acquire wealth through my professional skill. May no relative of mine die from the ill-luck of my medicines; may my wife not die; my relatives are animals, my relative is a [religious mystery], may my [religious mystery] be fruitful" (1976:92).

Through this incantation, the presiding shaman acknowledges the danger of his profession. The shaman pronounces a similar protective incantation over any novice who may be present: "May your home be prosperous and may no witchcraft come to injure your friends. May none of your relatives die" (1976:92). He then tells the novice that his relatives are bush animals. The renouncing of relatives appears to be aimed at protecting the shaman's relatives and the novice's relatives from any malice that may be directed against them as a result of the shaman's magical powers. The shaman adds: "If witchcraft comes here to my home let it return whence it came. If a man makes sorcery against me let him die. If a man bears ill-will towards my home let him keep away, and may disgruntled fellows who come to show their spite in my home receive a nasty surprise. Let my home be prosperous" (1976:92).

Each of the shamans at the ceremony stirs the mixture and makes similar incantations. The mixture is then measured out to the participating shamans, who eat what has now become a paste. The presiding shaman then cuts incisions into the faces and chests of the attending shamans. He also makes incisions above their shoulder blades. He rubs some of the liquid he has earlier decanted into the incisions while chanting incantations of protection over them. Thus, the power and protection of the sacred potion is "imbibed" though the incisions.

Limitations of space prevent me from describing the full ritual Evans-Pritchard has recorded; however, symbolism of the ritual appears to be aimed at establishing a fellowship among the shamans that provides them with mutual powers and protection.

THE "SHAMANIC CAREER": BECOMING A SHAMAN

In his book *Religion*, the anthropologist Anthony F. C. Wallace describes the process of becoming a shaman as "the substitution of one identity for another" (1966:145). In other words, the body and consciousness of a potential shaman must be deconstructed and rebuilt. Wallace writes, "[The shaman] usually undergoes . . . a . . . dramatic and radical religious experience, one to which he does not subject his clients" (1966:126). Wallace cites what he calls "a classic description of the process [of becoming a shaman] among the Zulus of South Africa" from an account by an early missionary, Canon Henry Callaway:

> The condition of a man who is about to become an inyanga[9] is this: At first he is apparently robust; but in process of time he begins to be delicate, not having any real disease, but being very delicate. He begins to be particular about food, and abstains from some kinds, and requests his friends not to give him that food, because it makes him ill . . . and he is continually complaining of pains in different parts of his body. And he tells them that he has dreamt that he was being carried away by a river. He dreams of many things, and his body is muddled and he becomes a house of dreams. And he dreams constantly of many things, and on awaking says to his friends, "My body is muddled today; I dreamt many men were killing me; I escaped I know not how. And on waking one part of my body felt different from other parts; it was no longer alike all over." (Wallace 1966:145–146)

The man's dream reflects the idea that the shaman must die to his previous life before taking on the obligations of a shaman. His obvious psychological distress now becomes apparent to the people who know him. Because of their concern, his relatives and cohorts consult with diviners, who divest the initiate of his material possessions. When the destruction of the potential shaman's material possessions is complete, a true inyanga appears and guides the potential shaman into a new phase of his initiation. He tells the villagers that they have consulted false izinyanga [plural of inyanga] and that the man has become possessed by the Itongo, a spirit. The inyanga adds:

> If you bar the way against the Itongo, you will be killing him. For he will not be an inyanga; neither will he ever be a man again; he will be what he is now. If he is not ill, he will be delicate, and become a fool, and be unable to understand anything. . . . Just leave him alone, and look to the end to which the disease points. Do not give him any medicines. He will not die of the sickness, for he will have what is good given to him. (1966:146)

Throughout a period of years, the condition progresses from psychological discomforts to physical discomforts. His hair falls out, and his body becomes dry and scaly.

He has lost a great deal of weight and has become nothing but "skin and bones" (1966:147). At this point, the man begins to sneeze and yawn, which indicates that he is about to be possessed by a spirit. He then begins to have slight convulsions. The people of the village think that he will die, but he enters another stage: "He habitually sheds tears, at first slight, and at last he weeps aloud, and in the middle of the night, when the people are asleep, he is heard making a noise, and wakes the people by singing; he has composed a song, and men and women awake and go to sing in concert with him" (1966:147).

From this point, the potential shaman takes instructions from the spirits, at first while he is asleep. He is introduced to ancient inyangas. Then he is instructed to go to a contemporary inyanga, who administers an emetic-ubulawo. This marks the final stage in destroying the man's previous personality. He returns to his village, "and he comes back quite another man, being now cleansed and an inyanga indeed" (1966:148).

The cross-cultural literature is consistent in describing the shamanic career. In general, shamans do not volunteer to become part of the exclusive shamanic religion/medical practice. They must undergo a special selection process and a long period of intense training. The shaman undergoes five stages or conditions:

I. **Possessing innate ability.** The innate ability to become a shaman is believed to run in families.

II. **Receiving a "call from the spirits."** Not everyone in a family that has a shamanic tradition receives the requisite "call from the spirits." The "call" may vary, depending on the shamanic tradition or the particular circumstances. The call may come in a dream, through what Western psychologists would call a "psychotic episode," or through a severe illness that is not treatable through ordinary means. This "call" must be answered. An individual who does not answer the "call" dies or becomes psychotic.

III. **Diagnosis by a shaman.** In societies where shamanism is practiced, the condition must be diagnosed by one who has already undergone the initiation required of a shaman, as illustrated in the case of the Zulu, described above. In the case of Haitian *vodou*, the shamanic diagnosis will name the specific *lwa*, or spirit, possessing the individual. Thus, the individual undergoing the psychological "trauma" acquires a new spiritual and social identity (Womack 1993, 2001).

IV. **Apprenticeship to a shaman.** Cross-culturally, it is believed that an individual who receives the "call from the spirits" must undergo the training necessary to become a shaman. Individuals who do not receive this training "go crazy" because they do not understand what the spirit voices are telling them. They may be misled by false shamans, who only seek power over others rather than the insight required to heal others. The apprenticeship to a recognized shaman typically takes years, often as long as twelve to fifteen years. This is approximately how long it takes to get a PhD or MD. In the process of acquiring the skills to be a shaman, the individual takes repeated journeys into the spirit world, or as anthropologists describe it, "journeys into the unconscious." In this process, the initiate acquires spirit helpers that guide him or her through the dangerous landscape of the unconscious. In this sense, undergoing the training to become a shaman is similar to the process of undergoing psychotherapy. It takes a long time to rout the "demons" in the unconscious.

V. **Becoming a shaman.** After a long period of apprenticeship, the initiate acquires skills that allow him or her to heal others. These skills must be demonstrated to the satisfaction of others in the group. Shamans typically do not single themselves out by announcing their "calling." They acquire shamanic status by relieving the symptoms of distress experienced by other members of the group. When this occurs, shamans acquire the status of "healer." E. E. Evans-Pritchard writes of the Azande: "Azande insist that magic must be proved efficacious, if they are to employ it. They say that some magicians[10] have better magic than others, and when they require a magician's services they choose one whose magic is known to be efficacious" (1976:187).

The process of becoming a shaman involves a long period of instruction, both from the spirits and from acknowledged shamans. A shaman is not self-declared. He or she must submit to the judgment of the most demanding court of appeal, the opinion of others in his or her social group.

SHAMANISM COMPARED TO PSYCHOSIS

In teaching anthropology in Los Angeles, I often encounter students who are part of a subculture in which a significant component use recreational drugs. Some experience such pleasant feelings they consider it a religious experience. I have also encountered students with such neurological damage they cannot sit still long enough to take an exam or listen to a lecture. They may be happy when they take instant mood elevators, but they can't control their own lives, much less control or negotiate with the spirits. The spirits they encounter are the projections of their own unconscious impulses. In one incident (not in my classroom) that made the news media because it caused the deaths of several people, a young man declared, "I am the angel of death."

In traditional societies, such bizarre behavior would quickly lead to ostracism. Margery Wolf describes the "uproar and agitation" in a small Taiwan community as it considered the behavior of a young mother of three who "lurched out of her home, crossed a village path, stumbled wildly across a muddy rice paddy. The cries of her children and her own agonized shouts quickly drew an excited crowd out of what had seemed an empty village" (1993:279). For a month, the community debated whether the woman was simply crazy or had received a call from the spirits to become a shaman.

Ultimately, based on the advice of a senior male, the woman was considered to be insane, in part because she was a outsider but also because her behavior did not conform to that expected of a shaman or *tang-ki*: "A good *tang-ki* must be able to separate his or her behavior as a *tang-ki* from his or her everyday behavior" (Wolf 1993:293). Both psychotics and shamans may undergo experiences not available to ordinary members of their communities. The difference between them is that psychotics disrupt the community. Shamans gain the ability to analyze relationships within the group and use that understanding to diagnose and heal social and psychological disruptions.

Shamans are not self-declared. They must be validated by the social group in which they practice. In 1965, the psychiatrist Ari Kiev compiled seventeen articles written by anthropologists who had studied shamanism in indigenous groups on six continents. In his preface, Kiev writes:

> Several years ago I had an opportunity to study the healing practices and beliefs relating to psychiatric disorders among the Vodun[11] groups in Haiti. These people, although uneducated and impoverished—in fact living on a marginal subsistence level—have developed a therapeutically effective form of psychological treatment centered around certain religious beliefs and rituals. Most striking was my finding that the relationship between healer and patient in this culture appeared to parallel in a number of ways the psychiatrist-patient relationship in Western society, despite the absence of scientific methods and knowledge of the discoveries of modern psychiatry. (1964:xiii)

Kiev describes some common elements of traditional shamanic healing and modern psychiatry that affect the outcome of treatment:

> This finding suggested the possibility that certain general features of therapeutic relationships in various cultures—for example, the hope, expectation, and faith of the patient in the designated healer, coupled with the healer's use of meaningful symbols and group forces—might contribute more in therapeutic results than is ordinarily recognized in contemporary theories of psychodynamic psychiatry. (1964:xiii)

Since Kiev wrote those words, modern psychiatry (but not modern psychology) has shifted to a predominantly biological paradigm. The patient is labeled as having a biochemical "disorder" and then treated with drugs that target a specific neurological pathway. The "condition" is considered to be chronic and responsive only to drugs. This paradigm ignores the behavioral and social context of mood states.

The Psychology of Shamanism

In his foreword to Kiev's book, the psychiatrist Jerome Frank contrasted shamanic diagnosis and healing with that of Western biomedicine:

> In nonindustrialized cultures, illness is believed to have a variety of causes, both natural and supernatural. These causes include noxious environmental agents, the enmity of other persons, and the disfavor of the gods, incurred perhaps by unwitting offenses against them. All illness, therefore, arouses fear and self-doubt in the victim and disturbs his relations with his compatriots. (1964:vii)

Frank suggests that fear and self-doubt generated by an implied offense against powerful spirits may adversely affect the patient's relationship with others, and as a result, aggravate his condition. Therefore, the shaman must draw on a variety of interpersonal skills to alleviate the patient's distress:

> The shaman's role may thus involve aspects of the roles of physician, magician, priest, moral arbiter, representative of the group's world-view, and agent of social control. His

success may often depend more on his ability to mobilize the patient's hopes, restore his morale, and gain his reacceptance by his group than by his pharmacopoeia. (1964:viii)

According to Frank, Western physicians may also draw on many of these mechanisms, but they operate under a different paradigm, that of the machine:

> Industrialized societies hold quite a different concept of illness and healing. We fondly expect someday fully to comprehend the human being as a complex machine controlled by a computer in the skull. Disease will then be merely a derangement of the machine's functioning produced by noxious environmental agents in interaction with inborn or acquired vulnerabilities or errors of metabolism. . . . In this view, the physician is an expert scientist-technician whose job is to get the body into good running order again, and many psychiatrists dream of the day when they too can obtain triumphant cures with pills and injections. (1964:viii)

The day that Frank asserts psychiatrists dreamed of more than forty years ago has arrived, but it has failed to produce the "triumphant cures" Frank envisioned. Instead, it has spawned an entirely new hierarchy of disorders: (1) environmental factors that produce illness; (2) the manifestation of illness in individuals; (3) the social disruption that manifestation of physical or psychological disorders produce; (4) the social discomfort that increases an individual's discomfort; (5) the side effects of medications used to treat the primary and secondary symptoms of illness; and (6) treatments required to address the social, psychological, and physical side effects of medical interventions.

Writing in the halcyon days of the 1960s, Frank did not consider that illness causes fear and self-doubt in all those who experience it, especially if the illness seems life-threatening. Illness also challenges our relationships with others. As noted earlier in this book, illness is experienced as disorder, whether it is attributed to the work of spirits or to "little animals too small for the human eye to see," as one of my students put it. Invisible agents of harm, whether spirits or microbes, are frightening. They challenge our sense of order and well-being. This is why, as Kiev and Frank observe, the essential processes of healing are similar for both the shaman and the physician. In some cases, contact between Western medical personnel and shamanic healers result in partnerships that benefit both.

INTEGRATING MEDICAL SYSTEMS

As Yanomamö of Venezuela and Brazil have become acclimated to interaction with people who now occupy their region of the Amazon—through contact with missionaries, gold miners, and government workers—they have integrated their explanation of shamanism with that of health-care workers from outside. The *Faces of Culture* television series notes that Yanomamö shamans believe that Western health care professionals treat the symptoms of disease, but Yanomamö treat the causes, which are spirits. In one scene, the public health care nurse calls on a Yanomamö shaman to treat her malaria.

Shamans do not behave like people we regard as "normal." "Normal" people do not go into trance or speak with beings no one else can see. And, unless they are trained as shamans, there is no reason "normal people" should. In his book *Ecstatic Religion*, the noted scholar I. M. Lewis considers whether shamanism is a form of psychosis. Based on his studies of Tungus shamans, S. M. Shirokogoroff (as quoted in Lewis) "was careful to point out that while he judged some Tungus shamans to be insane, many were in perfect psychological health" (quoted in Lewis 1971:182). Lewis adds, "Similarly and more recently, the Soviet ethnographer Anisimov reports of Evenk shamans that although some revealed hysterical neurotic characteristics, there were also many who were extremely sober individuals" (1971:182). Other writers, both anthropologists and physicians, have noted that, on the whole, shamans tend to be "unusually mentally healthy" (quoted in Lewis 1971:182).

The situation is clarified by P. M. van Wulfften Palthe, former head of the Dutch psychiatric service in Java, in his distinction between "schizophrenic and 'normal' hysteric possession, classifying all the Balinese material in the latter category" (quoted in Lewis 1971:182 and Belo 1960:6). In his study of the Nuba of Africa, the anthropologist Siegfried Nadel took the concept further:

> Neither epilepsy, nor insanity, nor yet other mental derangements are in themselves regarded as symptoms of spirit possession. They are diseases, abnormal disorders, not supernatural qualifications. . . . No shaman is in everyday life an "abnormal" individual, a neurotic, or a paranoic; if he were he would be classed as a lunatic, not respected as a priest. . . . I recorded no case of a shaman whose professional hysteria deteriorated into serious mental disorders. (Nadel 1946: 25–37)

Though people who do not have access to biomedicine do not share the linguistic categories of biomedical personnel, they can observe the cause-and-effect relationship of behavior, circumstances, and disease, such as in the case described earlier in this book of the relationship between lack of vitamin A and night blindness. Healers not trained in Western biomedicine may attribute disease to spirits, sorcery, or **witchcraft** (concepts alien to biomedicine) but their evaluation of cause-and-effect can be highly accurate.

During the 1960s and 1970s, psychologists and anthropologists in the United States began to note that shamans and other traditional healers were sometimes able to alleviate symptoms that resisted the ministrations of physicians trained in Western medicine. The World Health Organization has recommended that Western medical personnel working in areas where the traditional medical practice is shamanism establish partnerships with the shamans. This can provide a means of bringing biomedicine to underserved populations. It can also recognize the healing contribution of shamans, who are likely to be more familiar than foreign physicians with the social and psychological conditions that contribute to the health care outcome.

Perhaps one of the greatest contributions that studying shamanism can contribute to the practice of medicine is the recognition that health, illness, and healing are intricately bound up in social relationships, psychological dynamics, and the experiences that people encounter in their everyday lives. No medical practice yet known can reverse the ravages of an unhealthy lifestyle.

12

The Emerging Field of
Integrative Medicine

CASE STUDY
The UCLA East-West Center

Though Asian energy models and Western organic models seem to contradict each other, there has been an emerging consensus among both factions that the two medical systems are complementary, rather than contradictory. In 1993, Ka-Kit Hui, MD, succeeded in persuading UCLA administrators to establish the UCLA Center for East-West Medicine. The stated purpose of the center is to establish "the theoretical and scientific construct of a new model of medicine based on findings from the latest scientific research on the integration of modern western medicine and Traditional Chinese Medicine (TCM)." TCM was formulated by the government of the People's Republic of China (PRC) from traditional Chinese medical practices based in Taoism, Confucianism, and Buddhism. A goal of the UCLA East-West Center is to develop a "system of comprehensive care with emphasis on health promotion, disease prevention, treatment, and rehabilitation through the integrated practice of East-West medicine." The mission of the center also aims to "stimulate interest and collaboration with UCLA and other institutions worldwide to address multidisciplinary issues relating to integrative East-West medicine," and to offer "professional and public education programs on TCM and integrative East-West medicine."[1] The center collaborates with the UCLA Medical Center and other research centers. These projects include collaboration with the UCLA School of Public Health and the University of Toronto on a study of neck pain, focusing on its implications for quality of life. The center also collaborated with the UCLA Department of Psychiatry and Behavioral Studies in applying the integrative approach to improving the outcomes of breast cancer survivors with disabling symptoms. The center has also worked with the UCLA Jules Stein Eye Institute on integrating acupressure into standard medical treatment for patients with dry eye syndrome.

Until recently, some Western scientists and physicians scorned healing systems that were not based in the biomedical paradigm. Conversely, many practitioners working in alternative healing traditions scorned Western medicine. In recent years, there have been efforts to bring these approaches together in what the U. S. National Institutes of Health call **integrative medicine**. Medical anthropology has contributed greatly to this developing trend.

For more than 100 years, anthropologists working in small-scale societies noted that shamans and other non-Western healers often brought about cures that could not be explained by the biomedical paradigm. During the 1960s and 1970s, anthropologists such as Jerome D. Frank (1963) and Ari Kiev (1964) explained the apparent efficacy of non-Western healing techniques as being due to the shamans' skillful manipulation of psychological and social factors.[2]

Even as scientists and biomedical practitioners dismissed them, so-called alternative medical practices flourished in the United States and around the world. Some forms of alternative medical treatments, as identified by the U.S. National Institutes of Health's National Center for Complementary and Alternative Medicine (NCCAM), are **homeopathic medicine** and **naturopathic medicine**, as well as traditional Chinese medicine and other traditional medical practices. Since 1995, when a National Institutes of Health (NIH) conference organized by the Office of Alternative Medicine (OAM) was held, alternative medical practices have achieved greater recognition among many members of the biomedical establishment.

NCCAM analyzes and studies the many forms of nonbiomedical treatments. The NIH defines complementary and alternative medicine as "a group of diverse medical and health care systems, practices, and products that are not presently considered to be part of conventional medicine."[3]

NCCAM distinguishes between *complementary* medicine, which is "used together with conventional medicine" and *alternative* medicine, which is "used in place of conventional medicine." *Integrative* medicine, as defined by NCCAM, "combines mainstream medical therapies and CAM (complementary and alternative) therapies for which there is some high-quality scientific evidence of safety and effectiveness."[4] NCCAM defines *conventional* medicine as "medicine as practiced by holders of M.D. (medical doctor) or D.O. (doctor of osteopathy) degrees and by their allied health professionals, such as physical therapists, psychologists, and registered nurses. . . . Some conventional medical practitioners are also practitioners of CAM."[5]

NCCAM's position is necessarily a conservative one because it is affiliated with NIH and some people may take the highly regarded institute's recommendation as law. Some treatments that may eventually be recognized as effective could be excluded from NCCAM's designation as a component of integrative medicine because they do not yet meet the scientific experimental standard of being more effective than a placebo. This conventional experimental standard may exclude many forms of alternative medicine that meet another criterion, that of making the patient feel better. In experiments and clinical trials, empirically measurable results take precedence over the patient's subjective experience.

NCCAM's position makes sense when cautioning against unproven substances taken internally and forceful forms of manipulations because these treatments may cause damage over the long term or have side effects not recognized by the patient;

however, insisting upon scientific rigor in evaluating complementary and alternative medicine may err on the side of caution, especially if the patient's condition prevents him or her from engaging in health-promoting behavior or life-affirming pursuits. As many biomedical practitioners have noted, placebos can be effective in relieving symptoms, which can promote the overall well-being of the patient.

Emotions play an important role in a patient's sense of well-being, and consequently, can affect the outcome of a medical treatment. An underlying theme in *The Anthropology of Health and Healing* is that the human experience is complex and cannot be reduced to a single variable. As Marcel Proust wryly observes in his multi-volume oeuvre, *Remembrance of Things Past*, published between 1913 and 1927, "Happiness is good for the body but it is grief that develops the powers of the mind."

Over a long career—much of which has involved studying the psychological, biological, and social processes involved in maintaining health and treating illness—I have observed and/or participated in a number of systems aimed at healing illness or promoting health. My master's thesis was based on two years of participant observation in a Spiritualist Church in an impoverished area in South Los Angeles. This group practiced laying on of hands. Healers formed a circle and invited an individual seeking healing to become part of the circle. The healers saw their role as channeling energy from a higher source (the energy of departed sages) to a lower source (the patient seeking healing). In my two years of research, I was never able to document a case in which a patient recovered from his or her illness. My research design was not aimed at documenting healing, but rather, understanding the motivation and social relationships of both healers and those being treated.

I have also practiced yoga, jogged, bicycled, and have undergone acupuncture and massage therapy. I have been diagnosed using the Chinese technique of foot reflexology. I have studied shamanism, albeit at a distance. I have also experimented with diets and meditation techniques. None of these is a cure-all and some, such as dietary limitations and ingestion of untested substances, can be dangerous. There are as many means of diagnosing and treating illness as there are human groups on earth. Most of these means have demonstrated efficacy at alleviating symptoms under certain circumstances. The key factor in the efficacy of these techniques is the skill of the practitioner. That is as true of Western biomedicine as of traditional healing systems.

A related factor is the desire of the patient to be healed. Patients are often motivated to seek treatment out of fear; however, fear—and to an extreme degree, panic—can mediate against healing. The chemical side effects of extreme fear can be fatal. Fear can also mediate against following appropriate medical procedures.

The mission of the NIH is to regulate medical potions and practices as a means of ensuring the safety of the American public. Exploring the efficacy of complementary and alternative medical practices is a bold step. It may not be possible to scientifically validate all forms of CAMs; however, the NIH move in this direction can do much to alleviate the competing claims that have divided the practice of Western biomedicine from traditional practices that have been shown to alleviate patients' symptoms. At the time of this writing, NCCAM recognized five types of CAMs:

1. Alternative medical systems are built upon complete systems of theory and practice. These include homeopathic medicine, naturopathic medicine, traditional Chinese medicine, and Ayurveda.

2. Mind-body interventions are based on using a variety of techniques designed to enhance the mind's capacity to affect bodily functions and symptoms, such as meditation, prayer, mental healing, and therapies based on art, music, or dance. The NCCAM definition of mind-body interventions incorporates the traditional Western philosophical assumption, dating back to Plato, that the mind and body are separate and distinct entities. Thus, it ignores the body's physiological response to art, music, and dance. NCCAM notes that some techniques formerly considered CAM, such as patient support groups and cognitive-behavioral therapy, have become mainstream.
3. Biologically based therapies use substances found in nature, such as herbs and foods. Dietary supplements are included in this category.[6]
4. Manipulative and body-based methods involve manipulation or a combination of manipulation and/or movement of one or more parts of the body. These include chiropractic or osteopathic manipulation and massage.
5. Energy therapies involve the use of energy fields associated with the human body. Qi gong, Reiki, and therapeutic touch are attempts to manipulate energy purported to surround and penetrate the human body. Other types of energy therapies "involve the unconventional use of electromagnetic fields."[7]

WHAT IS "EFFICACY"?

"For many centuries and in virtually every society, long before the appearance of evidence-based medicine, people with medical problems have turned to healers" (Mayer and Saper 2000:3). The primary difference between Western medicine and previous healing systems, Mayer and Saper note, is the shift to an evidence-based approach that relies on experiments comparing treatment to placebo. Traditional and non-Western healers also rely on evidence that a particular treatment results in a positive outcome for the patient, but the systematic approach of comparing treatment to placebo helps to rule out more subjective factors, such as the desire of a healer to report improvement in the patient and wishful thinking on the part of the patient.

Wishful thinking on the part of healers in the Spiritualist Church I studied (Womack 1978) played an important role in their assessment of the effectiveness of their healing. In one case, a chronically ill individual who was regularly treated by the healers was often assured that he "looked much better" even though, from my perspective, there was no perceivable change in his coloring or disability.

Though scientific procedures are ostensibly more reliable than subjective procedures for evaluating effectiveness of particular treatments, use of scientific procedures do not guarantee that these treatments will be effective in all cases. Mayer and Saper write: "Many patients and some physicians have come to expect that treatments that meet this standard should be available for all conditions, and that evidence-based medicine should be able to provide cures or at least effective treatment for all ills. Alas, this has not proved to be the case" (2000:3).

When patients believe that scientific procedures can guarantee a cure for a particular condition, they may lose faith in Western medicine and science altogether if such procedures fail to produce a desired result. At that point, people who suffer chronic ailments may turn to alternative healers. Some treatments, such as acupuncture and relaxation therapies, have demonstrated effectiveness in scientific experiments. Others, such as herbal treatments, "high colonics," magnets, homeopathy, prayer, and meditation have not stood up to scientific standards of proof. This does not mean these practices are ineffective. The human experience, including health and healing, involves many factors, not all of which are subject to scientific validation.

Meditation has been proved to alter brain wave patterns and reduce stress, effects which may improve overall health, but meditation has not been linked to improvements in a particular medical condition. As a result, unproven treatments may be scorned by many physicians. However, Mayer and Saper note, "Other physicians have recognized that patients often respond to kindness, human contact with perceived healers and the attractiveness of a 'holistic' view of health and disease as providing benefits, despite the absence of an effective evidence-based therapy" (2000:3).

An individual's health and healing are strongly influenced by the social and physical environment. As noted in Chapter 10, on Asian concepts of balance, and in Chapter 11, on traditional healing such as shamanism, these healing systems include healing the social and physical environment of the patient. This is typically not viable in Western biomedicine because industrialization produces isolated social groups based on class and income. Some psychological disorders are treated in group therapy or other social contexts; however, a limitation of Western biomedicine is that it focuses on the individual displaying symptoms and does not adequately consider the social and environmental factors that produced those symptoms. Even in "holistic" medicine, treatment focuses on the patient rather than on the context that produced the patient.

A "holistic" view is based on the idea that health and disease are influenced by the entire organism, rather than by one particular part. Further, a holistic view includes the idea that systems and social networks may be toxic. Therefore, according to this view, the most effective treatments address the "whole" person, and the person's social and physical environment, not a particular organ or symptom. Being treated as a whole person rather than as a particular condition may produce a more positive response in the patient. It may well be that patients improve because they "feel better." Mayer and Saper write, "These [holistic] views are reminiscent of the historic concepts of health as a state of internal and external harmony, self-healing abilities of the body and the health promoting effects of re-establishing the flow of 'energy' within the body/mind continuum" (2000:3–4):

> The universal concepts of traditional healing practices, ranging from the prehistoric shamans to the practitioners of Western Hippocratic, Chinese, Ayurvedic and Native American Medicine include the following beliefs: (a) the belief in a universal life force (pneuma, chi, prana, animal magnetism, vis medicatrix naturae); (b) the belief in the unity between mind, body and universe; (c) the conceptualization of health as a state of harmony between mind and body, and between the organism and nature; and (d) the conceptualization of disease as a loss of such harmony. The role of the healer was seen as a catalyst who uses subtle interventions to stimulate the body's own healing abilities, with the goal to reestablish harmony and the undisturbed flow of the universal life force. (2000:3)

Mind-Body Research

In addition to establishing an Institute of Comprehensive and Alternative Medicine, the NIH has extended its aegis and funding to establishing national NIH-sponsored Mind Body Research Centers. Mayer and Saper note that this movement of the NIH into research using scientific procedures has been fueled by "an unlikely alliance of forces, including breakthroughs in neuroscience, economic considerations of managed care organizations, a popular demand for more natural healing approaches and a general political concept of self reliance ("self-efficacy") applied to health and disease" (2000:4).

Even if "alternative" healing practices do not meet scientific standards of "evidence," their effectiveness may not be disproved. Mayer and Saper write: "Even though the placebo effect is considered Western Medicine's eternal and most formidable competitor, it is agreed by all that placebo is effective at relieving pain and suffering" (2000:5). Mayer and Saper suggest that the effectiveness of placebos in alleviating symptoms may be "the manifestation of the remarkable self-healing abilities of the organism against a wide spectrum of diseases, ranging from coronary heart disease and cancer to rheumatoid arthritis" (2000:4). They add that placebo has been used effectively in the practice of Western medicine:

> If we are honest with ourselves, practices do not necessarily have to be better than placebo to find a useful place in medical practice, and honest practitioners have used this approach to the benefit of their patients for many years. Conversely, practitioners who eschew the healing arts in favor of only offering their patients scientifically based therapies may be justifiably accused of doing their patients a serious disservice. (2000:4)

Most placebos are relatively benign in that they promote a sense of well-being, which itself promotes health; however, a contemporary use of placebos is prescribing antibiotics for viral infections. Antibiotics are completely ineffective against viruses because viruses invade human cells and replace their nucleus with their own nuclei. Bacteria are independent organisms. They are complete cells. Therefore, they are affected by antibiotics. A medication that could kill a virus would also kill other body cells. This is the dynamic of chemotherapy. Cancer cells are "hungry." They reproduce faster than normal body cells. Chemicals used in chemotherapy are aimed at killing organic cells. Because cancer cells are hungry and absorb more of these toxic chemicals, the medical "gamble" is that the cancer cells will die before the patient dies.

In practice, medicine is an art as well as a science. Machines can only measure a limited range of the factors involved in whether a patient will recover from an illness. A value of integrative medicine is that it considers the multiple facets of being human. It also provides patients with options that might not be available in conventional Western biomedicine.

EFFICACY AND THE PRACTICE OF MEDICINE

In her study of concepts of efficacy among practitioners of American acupuncture, anthropologist Linda L. Barnes was told by the manager of a health food store,

"People just want what works" (2005:258). But of what does "working" consist? How is it defined and who defines it?

Like many medical terms, the word "efficacy" evolved through a series of meanings reflecting their social context. The term derives from the Latin *eficacia*, which seems to have a similar meaning to the English term "effectiveness." But effectiveness against what or for what purposes? According to Barnes, by the sixteenth century, the term "efficacy" meant the power to produce particular results, whether the power behind these results originated from God, the devil, or medical therapies. Hilton P. Terrell, a Christian physician, compares medical efficacy to medical ethics. In so doing, he discusses the pro-life movement, which aspires to save lives at all cost while disregarding factors related to quality of life:

> The pro-life movement has a problem, an undiagnosed illness, as it were, which may cause the movement to self-destruct. It is a problem commonly found among those ardently involved in saving the lives of the unborn, the crippled, the senile and others unable to fend for themselves. The problem is an overvaluation of medical care often taking the form of a valuation of physical life even beyond the great worth God has assigned to it in His word.[8]

Terrell comes from a religious, as well as a medical, perspective. As Barnes notes, religion and medicine are closely aligned in all healing systems, though it is often denied. The anthropologist Byron Good (1994) suggests that Western biomedicine is aligned to the soteriological aspects of medical possibilities. That is, biomedicine practitioners see themselves in the role of *soter* (savior), as epitomized in Christ's sacrifice for humankind. Good asserts that, in biomedicine, "the maintenance of human life and the reduction of physical suffering have become paramount. Health replaces salvation" (1994:86). As a Christian physician, Terrell rejects the exclusively biological emphasis that biomedicine and the pro-life movement place on survival:

> However effective medicine may be, it is clear that the focus in the U.S. is on the material aspects of health and disease. We emphasize bacteria, cholesterol, blood pressure, mammograms, surgical techniques, drugs, etc. Far less importance is granted to such intangibles as the patient's comfort, his relationship with others, the compassion of the medical team or the contributions of the patient's belief system to his condition.[9]

Terrell aims to demonstrate that what he considers the exclusively biological model in biomedicine is not as efficacious in medicine as we generally assume:

> Our fixation upon the material aspects of medical care may actually be retarding both our physical health and our performance of the central duty of medicine—to care for the whole patient, body and spirit. One correction needed by the pro-life movement is more emphasis on the spiritual features of medical care. Without a spiritual focus, medical care loses true caring and becomes mere medicine. With too great a focus upon physical features, medical care risks obedience to God.[10]

Ay, there's the rub.[11] How can mere mortals know what offends God in medical practice? And as Hamlet observes, who knows "For in that sleep of death what dreams may come, when we have shuffled off this mortal coil, must give us pause."[12] It may also give pause to medical practitioners, who must decide to give or withhold treatment. Biomedical practitioners are not trained to diagnose what God may want. Their decisions must be based on conventional medical practice, as well as their training and experience.

Physicians now have the expertise to perform major reconstructive surgery for cosmetic reasons. The world's first partial face transplant occurred in France on a woman who had been attacked and mauled by her dog. As is the case with most other transplants, the partial face had been harvested from a person who had died. After this first successful face transplant, others were performed, including on a Chinese farmer who had been attacked by a bear and a European man disfigured by a genetic condition. Technology does not address the question of why the woman's dog attacked her. This is beyond the reach of conventional medicine.

Late in 2008, the first near-total face transplant was performed on a woman at the Cleveland Clinic. Cosmetic medical transplant procedures, such as facial transplants, are controversial because they are aimed at improving a patient's quality of life rather than saving it. These procedures also require recipients to take immune-suppressing drugs for the rest of their lives. Some effects of transplants can be life-threatening, either because the transplant recipient's body rejects the new tissue or because the new tissue attacks the body of the transplant recipient.

The success of the face transplant procedure depends on suppressing the immune system. The immune system of the transplanted tissue or organ may recognize the DNA of the transplant host as an invading organism or the immune system of transplant host may recognize the DNA of the transplant as an invading organism. In weighing the cost-benefit of a medical procedure, there are great risks on both sides. The patient may lose his or her life; the attending physician may lose his or her livelihood, and with it, the ability to heal other patients.

"Efficacy"—whether in the field of medicine or outside it—is defined by its social context. A similar point is made by Barnes. As the context shifts to traditional medical and healing systems studied by medical anthropologists, meanings of the term "efficacy" become even more fluid. As Barnes notes, "efficacy" can be defined on multiple levels. A patient can experience pain or distress even after his or her medical condition has been "cured." Thus, the treatment may be considered efficacious by the physician, but not by the patient.

AN EXPERIMENT IN INTEGRATIVE MEDICINE

In the gospel of Luke 4:23, the apostle writes, "Physician heal thyself." These words have been in the back of my mind throughout my research and writing of this book. How can one speak authoritatively on a subject one has not experienced personally? Until I began writing this book, I had never suffered from a chronic illness. I have always been blessed with good health. In writing this book, I began an experiment in participant-observation by developing the stress-related condition of acute eczema.

As any astute researcher or scholar would note, I have pushed the envelope in writing this book on both the professional and personal levels. On the professional level, researching and writing *The Anthropology of Health and Healing* required many hours of work and total commitment to the enterprise. My goal was to integrate for the first time the far-flung field of medical anthropology. As one reviewer wrote, "I would recommend this [book] to colleagues as a textbook that contains all of the topics that are typically covered in medical anthropology and [is] thoroughly compiled from a holistic perspective." I approached this task with a missionary zeal. I thought it was time to take an integrative approach to this important discipline.

Because of the magnitude of the task, as well as the time it required, I experienced many changes in my life, both positive and negative. Psychologists have noted that change—whether positive or negative—can produce life-threatening illness. Changing careers, getting a new job, losing a job, getting married, getting divorced, moving, having a child, losing a child can all lead to potentially life-threatening medical conditions. My scholarly research on the biological and psychological effects of stress did not protect me from this profound truth.

Acquiring the Condition

There were times during researching and writing *The Anthropology of Health and Healing* that my stress levels were so high I wasn't sure I would survive to finish the project. As a former journalist, I was used to stress. At the time of my career in this field, journalism was rated one of the top ten high-stress jobs in the United States, along with air traffic controllers and police officers. I was almost always on deadline.

I had also faced a number of life-threatening situations, including being stopped at gunpoint at midnight on a lonely road in northern Chile by Augusto Pinochet's armed soldiers. My sources tell me that a number of journalists who covered the 2005 tsunami that struck the countries around the Indian Ocean had to be treated for potentially debilitating high levels of stress. Not only were they at times in great personal danger, they were forced to deal emotionally with the devastation and high death tolls occasioned by the disaster. To most people listening to or reading about the tragedy, the death toll was a statistic. To survivors, journalists, and rescue workers, the devastation was told in human faces, bloated bodies, and the agony of grieving relatives.[13]

The stress I experienced in researching and writing *The Anthropology of Health and Healing* was of a different kind, more difficult to explain. It was more like that of an explorer traversing previously unexplored and dangerous terrain. Was the effort really worth it? Was I on the right track? Would all my efforts be wasted? When I finally mailed the completed first draft of the manuscript to the publisher, I was shaking. One week later my hands were densely covered with blisters.

Long-term unremitting stress attacks the most vulnerable part of the body. As previously noted, stress produces chemicals that can either promote our survival by giving us the power to act decisively or endanger our survival if blocked activity causes our immune system to turn on our own body. In my case, there was no antelope to stalk and kill for food, and there was no lion from which to flee.

My particular area of specialization is in the analysis of symbols.[14] Symbols are words, images, or behaviors that communicate multiple levels of meanings arising from both the conscious and unconscious levels. Because symbols are rooted in the unconscious—which is a fertile ground for life-affirming and self-destructive impulses—they play an important role in maintaining health and promoting healing. In reflecting upon my own stress-induced medical condition, it amused me to consider that the prolonged stress I experienced in researching and writing this book attacked, not an internal organ, but the skin, the barrier that distinguishes self from other.

In writing *The Anthropology of Health and Healing*, I was transcending many barriers: the Western dichotomy between mind and body, the definition between health and illness, the many stages of the human life cycle, and my sense that I was crossing boundaries among the different healing paradigms. On a psychological level, it seemed fitting that my "disorder" should manifest as the eroding of my skin, the boundary between self and other. It may seem strange to analyze symbols in addressing a disorder that is "clearly" physiological, but this attitude is a relic of the Western mind-body dichotomy, which tends to view psychological and physiological functions as entirely separate from each other. In fact, they work in tandem.

There were pragmatic concerns, however, including how this new medical condition should be treated. I did not propose to spend my life scratching blisters. Nor did I want to pass up an opportunity to explore the psychological, social, behavioral, and physiological bases of my skin condition. As one of my colleagues noted, I experimented on myself. This experiment predated the skin condition. I began with an experiment in diet. I had long disputed the idea that the ideal human diet is vegetarian. The formation of out teeth suggests otherwise. We have incisors for chopping such resources as celery, canines for tearing meat, and two kinds of molars for grinding. This suggests that humans have evolved as omnivores rather than herbivores. Omnivores derive nourishment from both plants and animals. Herbivores eat only plants.

My dietary experiment began with a strict vegetarian regimen, then gradually began to include foods as I felt my body demanded them. The development of my skin condition provided a new opportunity for research. I decided to undertake an experiment in integrative medicine which, as I defined it, included diet, exercise, and appropriate medical procedures described in the previous chapters of this book. The two areas I failed to address were stress reduction and the importance of maintaining appropriate fluid balances. I had always maintained a high fluid intake, but I live in an area—Los Angeles—in which the tap water tastes like the byproduct of various plant and animal secretions. At the same time, the local markets sold fluid products that consisted either of filtered tap water or factory produced products with unacceptably high levels of sugar. I couldn't tolerate the taste of any of these products. As a result, I became dehydrated, thus increasing the negative effects of stress, which itself produces dehydration.

Within weeks after sending the initial manuscript to the publisher, I became afflicted with dangerously high levels of stress and eczema over 90 percent of my body. Eczema is an agitated skin condition characterized by intense itching. Extreme stress is typically its underlying cause. Prolonged stress can cause a hyperactive immune response that causes the body to respond to ordinary environmental conditions as though they were invasive agents. Some common triggers of eczema include the following: soaps, detergents, weather conditions (such as heat, coldness, humidity or dryness), environmental allergens, jewelry, creams containing additives such as perfume, foods, clothing, sweating, gloves, rubbing, and bacteria.[15] All these ordinary environmental conditions can become toxic when an individual is under stress.

Reactions produced by stress are related to allergies. Allergies are typically inherited conditions that produce greater than normal sensitivity to environmental conditions. Allergies can come and go, depending on the degree of exposure to the allergen and the susceptibility of the individual at the time of exposure. Stress produces cortisol which heightens sensitivity to environmental conditions. My extreme reaction to stress was later augmented by a misadventure in Western biomedicine. As a result, I became an interested participant-observer in integrative medicine.

The psychology, biology, and social context of stress are my specializations and have been since my undergraduate training in the UCLA Psychology Department. I would like to have explained my condition as purely medical, perhaps treatable with such reliable drugs as antibiotics. But I knew better. Stress-related eczema is systemic, caused by chemicals released by the arousal response. Had I been fleeing from a lion, these chemicals could have saved my life. Because the chemicals were triggered by a high degree of stress over a long period of time, they were potentially life-threatening.

My PhD dissertation addresses the means by which professional and other high-level athletes deal with the extreme stress of competition. I was aware of the ravages that prolonged stress can wreak on the human body. Under normal or even unusually stressful conditions, the body can promote homeostasis or prepare us for action, depending on what the situation demands. I regularly follow procedures, including rituals that permit me to deal with stress in my everyday life. In this case, I knew I needed help.

Treating the Condition

I was faced with a dilemma. I wanted rapid relief from my symptoms, but I also wanted to address the underlying causes of the condition. My philosophy has long been that Western biomedicine excels at dealing with emergencies, whereas lifestyle conditions are better addressed by ongoing therapies that relieve stress: including yoga, meditation, acupuncture, massage, and physical activities such as walking. My dilemma lay in which path to choose. In the end I opted for both Western biomedicine and complementary treatments, thus giving myself an opportunity to test my theories regarding stress, Western biomedicine, and alternative forms of treatment. This was a risky decision, since ingredients in Western medicines may duplicate those in homeopathic medicines, thus resulting in an overdose. It is also possible that herbal medicines may interfere with the benefits of pharmaceuticals.

Since my health was in a state of crisis, I first sought the counsel of a physician trained in the Western biomedical tradition. The physician I consulted prescribed medication to reduce my dangerously high stress levels. I also began a program of exercise, diet, acupuncture, and massage therapy aimed at reducing my stress levels in a more sustainable way.

I was at first impressed by the physician's approach to my condition. As I had expected, my blood pressure was in the danger zone. Having studied stress among professional athletes (and their means of dealing with stress)—as well as having covered as a journalist many athletic contests, including the first running of the women's marathon in the modern Olympics—I was well aware of the tremendous stress high-level athletics exert on the human body. I had watched runners stagger across the finish line or vomit after running a hard race. I had known that injuries were the price a high-level athlete pays for pushing his or her body to extreme exertion. I had interviewed a physician specializing in sports medicine about the biology and psychology of high-level athletic competition. As I completed the high-stress marathon of writing *The Anthropology of Health and Healing*, I felt a sense of triumph. Like the apostle Paul, who wearily summed up his successes and failures, I thought, "I have fought the good fight, I have finished the race, I have kept the faith" (I Timothy 4.7). I was proud of my accomplishment, while knowing that it had taken a terrible toll on my body.

The physician I consulted saw it differently. He viewed my biological symptoms as a permanent condition. He considered his role to be bringing me back to "normal." He said, "You are a Type A personality. If I brought your blood pressure down to normal levels [about 120], you wouldn't be able to walk. So I am prescribing a mild tranquilizer to bring it down gradually."

I accepted the prescription, but added, "I'm planning to undertake a course of acupuncture and massage therapy."

"Those aren't medically proven," he cautioned.

"Yes, I know," I replied. "But they are part of what the National Institutes of Health considers complementary medicine."

I had previously undertaken a course of acupuncture when I was undergoing a difficult change from a secure job as a journalist to an insecure job as a part-time college professor, and I had found the treatment effective in lowering stress levels.

I accepted the prescription, had it filled, and began to take it as directed. A cautionary note was that the medication could cause drowsiness. Within a couple of weeks, I almost wrecked my car on the way to teach one of my classes. In spite of my best efforts I could not control the car. By exerting extreme concentration, I was able to make it to my class.

I later learned that the medication I had been prescribed was a beta-blocker, which alters the brain-wave pattern. There are four brain-wave patterns associated with levels of activity. The brain generates beta waves when engaged in mental activity, such as making a speech, teaching a class, performing before an audience, conducting research, or writing a book, all of which are integral to my profession. Alpha waves are produced in states of rest, relaxation, and meditation. Theta waves are produced when an individual is daydreaming or engaged in a repetitive task. Delta waves are the slowest, occurring during a deep, dreamless sleep.

Beta waves stimulate the sympathetic nervous system and are therefore associated with states of arousal, which can be experienced either positively or negatively, as excitement or anxiety. By blocking the production of beta waves, beta-blockers reduce both the experience of pleasure and of fear. They also inhibit sexual desire and can cause impotence in males. Beta-blockers block the effects of the hormone epinephrine, also known as adrenaline.[16] Beta-blockers are typically prescribed for heart conditions and migraines because they slow the heart rate and, therefore, reduce hypertension. They also open up blood vessels to improve blood flow. The Mayo Clinic website notes: "Beta-blockers aren't usually prescribed until other blood pressure medications, such as diuretics, haven't worked effectively."[17]

I stopped taking the medication, which I thought was a mild tranquilizer, because driving a car is an essential skill in Los Angeles and I had completely lost interest in teaching classes, conducting research, and writing books.

As I neared the end of my demanding teaching schedule and no longer needed to drive daily to my office, I resumed taking the medication prescribed by my bio-medical physician. I began to experience strange moods, emotions, and puzzling sensations. I was often near tears, which would overwhelm me at unexpected times. I began to consider whether life was worth living and whether I really wanted to live long enough to finish the books I had contracted to write. I also experienced feel-ings of anxiety. I attributed this to the aftermath of the high levels of stress I had pre-viously undergone. My skin irritation had largely abated, but now it returned in full force. There were numerous fresh eruptions of blisters, about the size of pinpoints, all over my body.

One afternoon, as I lay on the acupuncture and massage table, I felt the usual sense of deep relaxation, but I also questioned why it didn't seem as effective against my eczema as it had been earlier in my treatment. The thought entered my mind that there was something toxic in my body. Because my research specialization addresses the psychological, social, and physiological aspects of stress, I considered that my body had not yet sloughed off the chemical aftereffects of stress.

In writing up this experiment on integrative medicine, I looked up the medication I had been given by the physician. I learned that I had been taking a high dosage of a powerful beta-blocker, and its side effects included hives, depression, anxiety, and a number of other emotions and sensations that had previously seemed inexplicable to me. Now I had to confront a new menu of problems and decisions. Ceasing to take such potent medications as beta-blockers can be fatal, but the side effects of the par-ticular medication I was taking was depleting my enjoyment of life and my ability to function.

Fortunately, I came to this realization just before Christmas vacation, when I would have time to relax. Thus, I would not encounter the usual stresses of teaching and grad-ing papers. For nearly a week after discontinuing the medication, I experienced symp-toms similar to those of someone recovering from a morphine addiction. My skin was so sensitive, even the touch of a hair against my cheek was agonizing. I repeatedly questioned my wisdom in deciding to discontinue the medication. I kept the unused pills in case of an "emergency." Listening to Christmas carols moved me to tears. I can-celed almost all Christmas-related events and read escapist novels. I couldn't write. I couldn't think. My world focused entirely on my skin. I spent most of my time count-ing the blisters as they emerged or faded.

Then came the day of reckoning. I had to ask myself why I had followed a regime that violated everything I knew about medical anthropology. The physician followed medical procedures, but he did not consider individual cases. He saw me at a time when I was highly stressed as a result of the important book I had just written He assumed it was a permanent condition, as evidenced by his description of me as a Type A personality. My age also factored into his equation. To him, I was an aging patient, rather than an individual still engaged in the challenges of a stimulating and active lifestyle.

In his evaluation, he followed standard procedures. The error in this type of West-ern medicine is that none of us is standard. Medicine by the numbers (statistics) has conferred great advantages overall, but it may not be effective for particular individ-uals. In the practice of medicine, we cannot predict which individuals will benefit from a particular treatment and which will suffer setbacks.

Regulations governing biomedical practices protect the least capable physicians from malpractice, but they do not necessarily protect patients from inadequately prepared physicians. In a case that made news in Southern California early in this century a physician left his surgical patient cut open on a gurney while he went off to make a bank deposit. He thus exposed his patient to two of the most dangerous conditions of surgery: (1) extending the period in which a patient is under anesthetic and (2) exposing a patient to the bacteria that inhabit all environments, including surgical rooms. This physician lost his license to practice medicine, but the patient on whom he was operating could have lost his life.

My decision to combine Western biomedicine with complementary healing practices was based on decades of research. It is not reasonable to say that one form of medicine is "better" than another. The outcome of a medical procedure, whether based in Western biomedicine or complementary systems, relies on a number of variables: (1) the kind of condition being treated; (2) the skill of the physician with regard to the condition being treated; (3) the aspirations and expectations of the patient; (4) the patient's understanding of what is required to treat a particular condition; and (5) the willingness of the physician to adapt a medical practice to an individual's need for treatment.

Questions not typically asked of a patient in a Western medical diagnosis are: What are your goals? What kind of lifestyle do you want for yourself? Are you undergoing any unusual situation that might have led to this particular medical condition? An ordinary patient in the United States is typically a number, a statistic. The patient's goals and lifestyle are not considered, even though these can shape the outcome of a medical procedure.

Beneficial Practice of Western Biomedicine

It is only fair to recount two of my experiences with Western biomedicine that confirmed my respect for this tradition. One involved a Kaiser Permanente facility in the southern part of the Los Angeles area; the other involved the UCLA Medical Center.

On a remarkable evening when I was convinced that I would live and be healthy forever, my son took me out to dinner at one of my favorite restaurants. I was looking over my shoulder talking to my son, and not looking in front of me, so I tripped and fell down a small flight of stairs. This resulted in what my orthopedist called an "unusual event." I broke both my ankle and my foot at the same time. Upon my arrival at the Kaiser Permanente emergency facility, I was inducted according to standard hospital procedure. My blood pressure and other vital signs were measured, and then I was sent to be evaluated by emergency personnel.

The next procedure involved X-rays. Once the double fracture was diagnosed, I was taken to what I think of as the swaddling room, where I was fitted with a cast. The night duty physician prescribed Vicodin as an emergency pain reliever. He also advised me that bones do not contain nerve endings, so any pain I might suffer would involve the soft tissues surrounding the bone. I was told that, in the event of pain, I should elevate my foot, which would reduce the swelling, and consequently the pain.

I did not fill the prescription for Vicodin. Instead, I took two ibuprophen tablets after arriving home and elevated my foot on a pillow. Those two ibuprophen tables

I took on the first night of my injury were all the pain relief medication I needed throughout the course of my healing. If I felt pain, I simply elevated my foot and the pain would slowly ebb away. I was fortunate in learning what I needed to know to reduce my pain and facilitate healing without unnecessary pharmaceutical intervention. My son coached me in procedures for returning to a normal life, including negotiating the two flights of stairs that led to my third-story apartment.

Later, when I served as primary caregiver for my brother as he underwent treatment at the UCLA Medical Center for oral cancer, I learned another important lesson in medical anthropology. My brother served as consultant in his own healing experience. The medical staff at UCLA kept him fully informed about his condition. They did not give him false hope. Instead, they kept him apprised of all the potentials of his condition, and they respected his own decisions as to therapeutic options. Ed agreed with the options that were presented to him. As his condition progressed, he made the decision to be readmitted to the UCLA Medical Center for terminal care. He was never treated like a patient; he was a full partner in his medical treatment.

It is not reasonable to expect a physician to wager his or her training and livelihood on the goals of a patient who expects the physician to overcome all the negative lifestyle choices the patient has made. Many of these choices are not reversible. On the other hand, we all make bad lifestyle choices. The health-care professional delivers his or her understanding of health-giving or health-restoring treatments.

It does not serve medicine to assign physicians and other health-care professionals to the status of factory workers. Both medical professionals and factory workers require precision and both have specialized knowledge. The specialized knowledge of factory workers requires repetition. Each bolt or particular model of car must be identical. The specialized knowledge of medical professionals requires them to make rapid-fire decisions to save lives or improve the quality of lives. It is tempting, in an industrialized society, to require standardized exactness in producing goods and services; however, humans—unlike laboratory animals and the products of technology— are highly variable in their genetic, biological, social, and cultural potentials. What works in the laboratory does not necessarily work in the clinic.

I have only one complaint in the treatment I received for my skin condition: I was deprived of my right to informed consent. The physician decided that he knew what was best for me, and he did not provide me with the information that I needed to comply with his instructions. Had I known that he had prescribed beta-blockers, I would never have taken them. By not fully informing me, he endangered my life. A beta-blocker is not a "mild tranquilizer" as he described it. All medications, whether biomedical or complementary, have side effects. We need to know what they are so we can make responsible health choices. As I stated earlier in this book, the physician prescribes, and the patient decides.

IV

CONTEMPORARY ISSUES IN HEALTH AND HEALING

Medicine, to produce health, has to examine disease; and music, to create harmony, must investigate discord.

—Plutarch, *Demetrius*

According to Jared Diamond (1987) and others, epidemics became prevalent when humans settled down into intensive agriculture. In fact, Diamond calls this shift in subsistence patterns, "the worst mistake in the history of the human race." As humans domesticated plants and animals, they reduced the diversity of plants and animals available for human use. Humans are omnivores, which means they require a varied diet. In addition, the food surplus produced by this shift to extensive agriculture gave rise to large populations, cities, and stratification. These three factors, among others, increased human exposure to disease organisms. Large populations provide an environment within which viruses and bacteria can adapt and multiply. Cities increase the exposure of humans to each other, as well as to the bacterial and viral colonies that flourish in human wastes and byproducts. Stratification produces large numbers of people who are inadequately fed and housed. These conditions give rise to epidemics. The following chapters discuss the factors relating to health and disease in contemporary human populations, including the role of medications and herbs in controlling disease.

Chapter 12, "The Social Context of Epidemics," explains why epidemics occur in populations that are crowded together. It also explains why globalization produces conditions that promote the spread of these diseases.

Chapter 13, "Medicines, Herbs, and Dietary Supplements," explores the role of plant materials in human existence, both historically and in contemporary context.

Chapter 14, "Public Policy and Health-Care Delivery Systems," examines the relationship of medical systems—both traditional and contemporary—to the ability of human populations to resist disease and restore health. It also considers without judgment the relationship between biological predispositions to certain forms of illness and the ability of specialists to address conditions that give rise to medical conditions.

13

The Social Context of Epidemics

CASE STUDY
Epidemiology and Gender

An Australian government patrol officer passing through the New Guinea highlands in 1953 provided the first official description of *kuru*, a fatal neurological disorder very common among the Fore and less common among neighboring groups. The Australian government official wrote: "Nearing one of the dwellings I observed a small girl sitting down beside a fire. She was shivering violently and her head was jerking spasmodically from side to side. I was told that she was a victim of sorcery and would continue thus, shivering and unable to eat, until death claimed her within a few weeks."[1] The strange etiology of the disease, known as *kuru*, the Fore word for "trembling" or "fear," made it difficult to treat. The disease primarily afflicted women and children. Fore considered it to be due to sorcery; Western observers thought it to be a psychosomatic disorder caused by the fear of sorcery. Anthropologists Shirley Lindenbaum and Robert Glasse eventually traced the disease to cannibalism. The disease primarily afflicted women because they prepared the bodies of dead kuru victims for consumption and burial: "They first removed hands and feet, then cut open the arms and legs to strip out the muscles. . . . After severing the head, they fractured the skull to remove the brain. Meat, viscera, and brain were all eaten" (1979:20). Fore did not eat all those who died, and not all Fore were cannibals. Men ate pigs, the more desirable protein, so they were not as likely to succumb to kuru (Lindenbaum 1979). For women, kuru victims were the most desired source of protein: "the layer of fat on those who died rapidly [heightened] the resemblance of human flesh to pork, the most favored protein" (1979:20). Women ate the less desirable sources of protein: small game, insects, frogs, and dead humans. They also fed these sources of protein to their children: "Both cannibalism and kuru were thus largely limited to adult women, to children of both sexes, and to a few old men, matching again the epidemiology of kuru in the early 1960s" (1979:20).

The diagnosis of kuru was a significant event in epidemiology and in the development of medical anthropology. It reminded both anthropologists and medical care professionals that epidemics are social as well as biological.

The Biology of Kuru

Kuru has since been classified as a transmissible spongiform encephalopathy disease (TSE), also known as a prion disease. According to the U.S. National Institute of Neurological Disorders and Stroke, "The hallmark of a TSE disease is misshapen protein molecules that clump together and accumulate in brain issue. Scientists believe that misshapen prion proteins have the ability to change their shape and cause other proteins of the same type to also change shape."[2]

Prion diseases are a class of neurological disorders that include Creutzfeldt-Jakob disease and bovine spongiform encephalopathy (mad cow disease). These diseases are transmissible and have no cure. Writing of Creutzfeldt-Jakob disease, the U. S. National Institute of Neurological Disorders and Stroke states: "There is no treatment that can cure or control CJD. Current treatment is aimed at alleviating symptoms and making the patient as comfortable as possible."[3] About 90 percent of CJD patients die within a year. The onset and progression of symptoms occur rapidly: "In the early stages of disease, patients may have failing memory, behavioral changes, lack of coordination and visual disturbances. As the illness progresses, mental deterioration becomes pronounced and involuntary movements, blindness, weakness of extremities, and coma may occur."[4]

The Social Context of Kuru

The incidence of kuru among the Fore reflected the social relationships between men and women. Marriage created alliances between kin groups in different villages. This promoted solidarity within the kin group, but residence patterns favored male solidarity. Upon marriage, women left their own village and moved to the village of their husbands. Males could rely on multiple sources of power: They remained among their biological relatives in their natal village and they also controlled **sorcery**, a means of causing one's enemy harm through control over allies in the spirit world. The rates of disease among Fore reflected power relationships within the group, so that men could control distribution of more desirable sources of protein (pigs) and were also more likely to use sorcery. Because of this power imbalance, women attributed their higher rates of disease to male sorcery, thus exacerbating tensions between the sexes.

The kuru episode among Fore is classified as an **epidemic**, which affects many individuals within a single population. Many infectious diseases in the world today are described by the term **pandemic**, which means they occur over a wide geographic area and affect an exceptionally high proportion of the population. According to the U.S. Surgeon General, "Epidemiology is the study of patterns of disease in the population. Among the key terms of this discipline . . . are *incidence*, which refers to new cases of a condition which occur during a specified period of time, and *prevalence*, which refers to cases (i.e., new and existing) of a condition observed at a point in time or during a period in time."[5]

Disorders described as psychological and those considered to be biological have reached epidemic proportions in different parts of the world. For example, such "psychological" disorders as autism and attention deficit hyperactivity disorder (ADHD) have reached epidemic proportions in parts of the United States, whereas malaria and HIV/AIDS have reached pandemic proportions in other parts of the world, as well as the United States in the case of HIV/AIDS. Two major biological pandemics confronting humans today are malaria and HIV/AIDS.

THE MALARIA PANDEMIC

Many diseases that affect humans require a **vector**, an intermediary organism that carries the disease-causing pathogen from one person to another. In many cases, the vector hosts the pathogen during a crucial stage of its life cycle. For example, the *Anopheles* mosquito hosts the parasite *Plasmodium falciparum*, which causes one form of malaria, during the early stages of its developmental cycle. The mosquito bites a person infected with malaria and ingests blood carrying an embryonic form of *Plasmodium falciparum* into its own body. The protozoan spends most of its developmental stages inside the body of the mosquito. When the mosquito sucks the blood of another person, the more fully developed pathogen is transmitted to that individual's blood.

Symptoms of malaria vary greatly, as does the severity of the disease. In extreme cases, malaria can cause death. According to the U.S. Centers for Disease Control, malaria is curable if it is diagnosed and treated promptly and correctly.[6] The onset of symptoms after a bite by the Anopheles mosquito can also vary from seven to thirty days, depending in part on the species of the malaria-causing organism. In general, the onset of symptoms is more rapid if the infective agent is *P. falciparum*. Slower onset of symptoms is more likely if the infective agent is *P. malariae*.

The onset of malaria can be delayed by weeks or months if travelers take anti-malarial drugs for prophylactic purposes. Malarial symptoms may appear long after the traveler has left the malaria-endemic area. The Centers for Disease Control notes that this is particularly likely with the species *P. vivax* and *P. ovale*. These species "can produce dormant liver stage parasites; the liver stages may reactivate and cause disease months after the infective mosquito bite":[7] "Such long delays between exposure and development of symptoms can result in misdiagnosis or delayed diagnosis because of reduced clinical suspicion by the health-care provider. Returned travelers should always remind their health-care providers of any travel in malaria-risk areas during the past 12 months."[8]

The U.S. Centers for Disease Control and Prevention distinguish between "uncomplicated malaria" and "severe malaria." A classical malaria attack lasts six to ten hours and consists of a cold stage involving sensations of cold and shivering; a hot stage involving fever, headaches, and vomiting, as well as seizures in young children; and a sweating stage involving sweats, a return to normal body temperature, and a feeling of tiredness. In general, a malaria patient experiences a combination of a number of symptoms, including fever, chills, sweats, headaches, nausea and vomiting, body aches, and general malaise. Residents of countries where malaria is common may recognize the symptoms and treat the symptoms themselves. In countries where malaria is uncommon, symptoms of the disease may be misdiagnosed as influenza, a cold, or some other common infection.

Severe malaria involves serious organ failures or abnormalities in the patient's blood or metabolism. These may manifest as cerebral malaria, with abnormal behavior, impairment of consciousness, seizures, coma, or other neurological abnormalities; severe anemia due to destruction of red blood cells; hemoglobin (red blood cells) in the urine due to destruction of red blood cells; fluid buildup in the lungs or acute respiratory problems; abnormalities in blood coagulation and a decrease in blood platelets; and cardiovascular collapse and shock.

Other problems associated with severe malaria include acute kidney failure; hyperparasitemia, in which more than 5 percent of red blood cells are infected by malaria parasites; excessive acidity in the blood and tissue fluids; and **hypoglycemia** (low blood sugar). Symptoms of hypoglycemia include nervousness, sweating, intense hunger, trembling, weakness, palpitations, and difficulty in speaking.

Forty-one percent of the world's population lives in malaria-prone areas. This includes parts of Africa (especially sub-Saharan Africa), Asia, the Middle East, Central and South America, the Caribbean, and the South Pacific, including Australia. Worldwide, 350 million to 500 million cases of malaria occur each year. Malaria causes between 1 million and 3 million deaths annually, mostly among children in sub-Saharan Africa.

Preventing Malaria

The most effective way to prevent malaria is to eliminate standing pools of water required by Anopheles mosquitoes during crucial stages in their development. Singapore is an island country between two countries plagued by malaria: Malaysia and Indonesia. Despite its proximity to these two countries, Singapore is free of the disease. The country has accomplished this miracle by fining residents who fail to empty standing pools of water. The only exceptions to this law are swimming pools and fish ponds. Swimming pools contain chlorine, which kill mosquito larvae, and fish are natural predators on mosquito larvae.

In Africa, two important preventatives of malaria are DDT and mosquito nets. DDT kills the mosquitoes that carry malaria. Mosquito nets prevent the Anopheles mosquito, which carries the malaria parasite, from attacking potential victims who have gone to sleep or are preparing to go to sleep, the time when the Anopheles mosquito is most active. Internationally, DDT has been banned in a number of countries, including the United States.

Malaria is closely associated with agriculture, because agriculture and horticulture produce the standing pools of water needed for Anopheles mosquitoes to breed. The first effective treatment for malaria was the bark of the cinchona tree, which contains quinine, and was introduced to Europe by Catholic Jesuit missionaries in the seventeenth century.[9] Quinine was used to treat both malaria and syphilis. Chloroquine was the most effective treatment for malaria until recent years, when *Plasmodium falciparum* became resistant to the drug.

DDT was developed to control malaria by killing mosquitoes during World War II, but it was eventually used to control insects that fed on agricultural crops. The use of DDT for agribusiness (agricultural and business) purposes led to its ban by many countries in the 1970s. The World Health Organization still advises the use of DDT to combat malaria in areas where the disease is common. The preferred use is spraying down walls of living spaces, where mosquitoes land. The public health use of small amounts of DDT is permitted under the Stockholm Convention on persistent organic pollutants (POPs), but is prohibited for large-scale industrial or agricultural use.

The debate is complex. Early in this century, several African countries proposed re-introducing DDT as a means of controlling malaria among their populations; however, this posed marketing problems. Africa is an important agricultural continent, with agricultural products providing a key source of income. Using DDT to control malaria among its populace would reduce the viability of African agricultural products on the international market.

One alternative is to use insecticide-treated mosquito nets, which are twice as effective against Anopheles mosquitoes as nontreated nets and 70 percent more effective than no nets at all. The most commonly used net costs around $2.50 U.S., but they should be retreated with insecticide every six months. A new type of net, called Olyset, releases insecticide for about five years and costs about $5.50 U.S. This net both protects the individual using the net and kills the mosquitoes attempting to penetrate the net, a double benefit.[10]

Cultural Barriers in Preventing Epidemics

An ongoing argument against health programs is that indigenous people do not understand the concept and, therefore, do not take advantage of projects introduced from outside. A report by *The New York Times* suggests otherwise. An offer to provide mosquito nets to Ponyamayiri, Ghana, a "poor, dusty village of 550 people,"[11] drew a line of takers. Four babies had died of malaria in the previous October. When the families lined up for mosquito nets, the children were given polio vaccine, measles vaccine, vitamin A, and deworming medicine. Neither the children, nor their caretakers, were asked whether they wanted these additional treatments. The assumption was that they were not competent to make these decisions on their own.

Yet, they were competent enough to ask for mosquito nets.

This assumption of incompetence regarding medical care is an example of neo-colonialism; however, this assumption of incompetence also occurs in industrialized countries. Physicians prescribe; patients accept the prescriptions with much the same compliance and misinformation that often happens in reactions to religious intonations. People yield to the supposed wisdom of the experts.

The problem in providing medical care to third world countries is in coordinating the efforts of the various aid campaigns involved, all of whom are competing for available funds. Though these public health programs have been described as "spectacularly successful," they are difficult to fund. Mark Grabowsky, a public health doctor with the U.S. Centers for Disease Control and Prevention, says he had an epiphany on a visit to a mission hospital in Gula, Uganda, when a doctor there told him. "If you get rid of measles, we can close the measles ward. If you get rid of malaria, we can close the hospital."

HIV/AIDS

According to the World Health Organization,[12] which monitors infection and treatment of diseases internationally, an estimated 38.6 million people are living with HIV worldwide. Approximately 4.1 million people became infected with HIV in 2005, and 2.8 million people died of the disease during that time. Leading the world in adopting "more progressive" approaches to reducing HIV among injection drug users in 2005 were Iran, Malaysia, and the Kyrgyz government.

The Genetic Basis of HIV/AIDS

A study published in 2007 in the *Proceedings of the National Academy of Sciences* used genetic analysis to trace the spread of HIV/AIDS from Africa to the United States. The research team, headed by Michael Worobey, an evolutionary biologist at the University of Arizona, analyzed five blood samples collected in 1982 and 1983 from Haitian AIDS patients in Miami. The samples had been preserved in frozen storage by the U.S. Centers for Disease Control and Prevention. Worobey and his colleagues compared the sequences of two viral genes with human immunodeficiency viruses from around the world. The study used as a baseline virus samples from Central Africa, considered some of the earliest forms of HIV.

Based on estimated rates of mutation in the HIV, researchers were able to estimate that the preserved viruses were genetically closest to the earliest viruses in Africa. The researchers found, with 99.7 percent probability, the HIV subtype B originated in Haiti, rather than in the United States. HIV subtype B is the most prevalent form in most countries outside Africa. The findings suggest that the subtype B virus was transmitted from Africa through Haiti to the United States.

Worobey, lead author of the published findings, hypothesized that the virus spread to Haiti by workers who had gone to the Democratic Republic of Congo (formerly Zaire) after that country achieved independence in 1960. The mutation timeline suggests that the virus was carried to the United States by Haitian immigrants between 1966 and 1972. The virus was first detected in Los Angeles in 1981. Findings of the 2007 study challenge earlier speculation that the virus had been exported from the United States to Haiti by means of a tourist sex trade during the 1970s and early 1980s.

HIV Susceptibility

Studies have indicated that people of African descent are more susceptible to HIV infection than people from other descent groups. In the United States, African Americans comprise 13 percent of the population, but account for nearly half of all newly diagnosed infections.[13] This had previously been attributed to high-risk behavior among African Americans, an attribution that could contribute to ethnic stereotyping. As is the case with most health issues, the basis for the disparity between African Americans and other U.S. ethnic groups is influenced by both biology and culture.

In a paper published in the journal *Cell Host & Microbe,* Sunil K. Ahuja of the South Texas Veterans Health Care System reported that a genetic mutation among Africans renders them 40 percent more susceptible to HIV infection than people in other descent groups. The mutation occurs in a single base of DNA in the gene for a receptor on the surface of red blood cells, the Duffy antigen. The antigen is absent in 90 percent of Africans and 40 to 50 percent of African Americans, but present in almost all Americans of non-African descent.[14] An **antigen** is a protein or carbohydrate capable of stimulating an immune response. The capacity to trigger an immune response can alert the body to activate its defenses against an invading organism, such as HIV. African Americans are more likely than Africans to have the antigen because there has historically been gene flow between African Americans and other descent groups in the United States.

The genetics researcher Ahuja suggests that the genetic mutation was **selected for** in Africa because it provided protection against a virulent form of malaria; however, it could be **selected against** in the United States because it renders people of African descent 40 percent more susceptible to HIV infections.[15] The mutation also has benefits for individual patients in that it slows the progression of HIV, the virus that causes AIDS. This extends the period of time AIDS patients are likely to survive. The mutation also has a selective advantage for the microbe in that it is likely to be transmitted to the next generation.

This human-HIV relationship illustrates why medical issues cannot be subjected to simplistic moral models. In a particular environmental context, humans and HIV have adapted to each other. Both are struggling to survive. The mutation that makes humans susceptible to HIV promotes the survival of humans where malaria is present, such as in Africa. The survival of humans promotes the survival of HIV. In the United States, malaria is as yet not a health issue. Therefore, the beneficial aspects of the mutation that blocks production of the Duffy antigen for protection against malaria does not provide a selective advantage in the United States.

Trends in the HIV/AIDS Pandemic

In November 2006, the United Nations and the World Health Organization reported mixed results in efforts to prevent the spread of AIDS internationally. The AIDS pandemic continued to grow in all regions of the world during 2006 and resurged in some areas where successes in containing the disease had proved effective. Though the rate of growth has slowed since the pattern of HIV infection was first detected, the international organizations estimated that the AIDS toll for 2006 would be 2.9 million people dead and 4.3 million infected with HIV. At the time of this writing, United Nations Secretary-General Kofi Annan said, "In a short quarter of a century, AIDS has drastically changed our world." At the time of the report, 39.5 million people were living with HIV, slightly more than .06 percent of the world's population.

The 2006 AIDS and HIV report revealed dramatic regional differences in infection rates, demography, and causes of infection. During the 1990s, rates of HIV infection declined in Uganda due to international efforts to educate high-risk populations and promote condom use. The 2006 report indicated that the significant decline in infection rates was leveling off and that the demographic had shifted. At the time of the report, infection rates appeared to be rising in rural areas and among pregnant women. Dr. Paul De Lay, director of evaluations for UNAIDS, noted that data indicated the increased infection rate was due to behavioral changes, including increasingly erratic condom use and rising numbers of men who had sex with more than one partner during the previous year. He attributed the increase in risky behavior to complacency among the public and to a decline in the intensity of prevention programs, funding, and political commitment.

In Thailand, the number of new infections continued to drop at the time of this writing; however, married women at this time accounted for one-third of new infections. Health officials were discouraged by this change in the epidemic's demography because married women were previously thought to be low-risk.

HIV/AIDS Infection and Injected Drug Use

Though most people living with HIV reside in sub-Saharan Africa, the "most striking" increases in new infection occurred in Eastern Europe and Central Asia, where 270,000 new infections were expected by the end of 2008. That was a 70 percent increase from two years before, and one-third of the new cases occurred among 15- to 24-year-olds, almost all of them in Russia and Ukraine. Kevin De Cock, director of the HIV/AIDS department at the World Health Organization (WHO), attributed increased rates of HIV infection in Eastern Europe, Central Asia, and East Asia to an increase in intravenous drug use.

On the other hand, infection rates sharply declined among 15- to 24-year-olds in Kenya. A more than 25 percent drop among this demographic in both rural and urban areas resulted in a national decline in HIV infection rates. A similar trend occurred in urban areas of Zimbabwe, Ivory Coast, and Malawi, as well as in rural areas of Botswana.

Infection rates in Latin America, the Caribbean, and North America were stabilizing at the time of this writing, but Karen Stanecki, UNAIDS senior adviser on demographics, did not consider the stabilization of infection rates in the United States to be good news. She recommended more focused prevention programs in the United States. De Cock recommended prevention programs targeting intravenous drug users, since these programs have been effective in reducing infection rates elsewhere. In Portugal, prevention programs aimed at intravenous drug users led to a 31 percent decline in new diagnoses between 2001 and 2005.[16]

AIDS figures mean more than numbers. Human lives and well-being are at stake, and some segments of the population bear a disproportionate share of the burden. Among these are migrant workers and sex-industry workers. In both Africa and India, HIV/AIDS rates soared as migrant wage labor replaced locally based economies. Men leaving their homes and families encounter prostitutes, any of whom may be infected with HIV. When they return home, these men infect their wives, and subsequently, their children. The same is true among migrant workers in the United States. Research has yet to show whether migrant workers traveling together as families suffer equal rates of HIV/AIDS infection; however, existing profiles of migrant workers suggest they would not.

EPIDEMICS, ANIMALS, AND SOCIAL STATUS

Epidemics became a significant part of the human lifestyle when agriculture produced the food surplus that gave rise to cities and made ongoing human contact with domesticated animals possible. With the rise of agriculture, most human diseases have resulted from contact with domesticated animals. Bird flu, chicken pox, and mad cow disease are modern examples of diseases that have evolved in domesticated animals and become adapted to survival in the human body.

The food surplus made possible by agriculture that gave rise to cities also produced a high degree of stratification (unequal access to power and resources). Cities promote the development and spread of infectious diseases because people live in close contact with each other. The social complexity characteristic of stratified societies means that a small elite has access to food resources and medical care, whereas a large and impoverished social class does not.

Infectious diseases can also develop through close contact with undomesticated animals in the environment. AIDS is an example of a disease that has spread from wild animals to humans. The suspected origin of HIV (human immunodeficiency virus) is a mutation from SIV (simian immunodeficiency virus) acquired in the process of hunting and butchering nonhuman primates. The most common assumption is that HIV was transmitted to humans from the Central Common Chimpanzee (*Pan troglodytes*) through prolonged contact from humans hunting the chimpanzees as "bush meat." SIV was apparently not fatal to apes because it had a long history within which to adapt to its host. A disease-causing organism that kills its host is an imperfectly adapted species because it must quickly find a new host in order to survive.

The first HIV cases were seen in Kinshasa, the Democratic Republic of Congo, in 1930. In 2006, an international team of researchers from the universities of Nottingham, Montpelier, and Alabama, as well as the Project Prevention du Sida au Cameroun (PRESICA) in Cameroon, determined that HIV adapted to humans by means of chimpanzees. SIV does not cause AIDS-like symptoms in chimps, whereas the genetically similar HIV does cause such symptoms in humans. This indicates that HIV is imperfectly adapted to the human body's biological environment, whereas SIV is adapted to chimpanzees. SIV and chimpanzees have adapted to each other, whereas HIV and humans have not had time to do so.

Rats, Bubonic Plague, Poverty, and Social Status

The crowding and unhygienic conditions characteristic of medieval cities promoted the spread of bubonic plague, which has a complex form of transmission. It is transmitted either through the bite of a rat or the bite of a flea that has fed on an infected rat. In all cases—flea, rat, and human—the infected organism dies. The bacteria multiply quickly inside a flea, blocking its stomach so that it cannot absorb nutrients. The flea begins to feed voraciously, trying to satisfy its hunger, but the ingested blood cannot enter its blocked stomach, so it vomits the tainted blood back into the bite wound. When the flea feeds on another host, it spreads the bacteria to another victim.

Social policy relating to epidemiology is often guided by classification of groups on the basis of ethnicity or social status. A particular group may become stigmatized by outsiders as being especially susceptible to disease because of some presumed defect in the victim. In his book *Blaming the Victim* (1976), William E. Ryan notes that poor people are often blamed for their poverty as a means of diverting responsibility for poverty from the rigid stratification of social status to the behaviors and cultural patterns of the poor. Thus, blaming the victim permits more affluent members of society to justify their own position and avoid taking responsibility for people in impoverished circumstances. Blaming the victim has implications for health maintenance and health care policy because the malnutrition and crowded conditions typically associated with poverty provide a fertile ground for producing new diseases and limiting the ability of the poor to gain access to medical care.

Affluent members of society may think they are insulated from diseases transmitted by people who are malnourished and lacking in medical care, but they are not. Poor people pick lettuce, scrub the floors, and tend the children of people more affluent than themselves. The affluent may refer to their workers as "unclean," but they typically rely on services provided by the "unclean" members of society. It is in the best interests of elite members of society to protect the health of those who provide their food, clean their homes, and tend their children.

The nineteenth century cholera epidemic in India provides this lesson. British colonials considered cholera to be a problem confined to the streets. They ignored the fact that people from the streets made their own privileged lives possible.

HIV AND TUBERCULOSIS:
AN EPIDEMIOLOGICAL TIME BOMB

Under normal circumstances, a healthy human body can fight off the bacteria that cause the disease of tuberculosis. Tuberculosis (TB) can remain dormant for years before manifesting symptoms. It becomes dangerous in cases of poor nutrition and hygiene, as was the case in European cities. Once the tuberculosis bacterium was isolated, vaccines and medications could target the ravages of the bacteria on the human body. Tuberculosis is a life-threatening disease that primarily affects the lungs and annually kills nearly 2 million people worldwide. Signs of tuberculosis have been found in Egyptian mummies and in bones dating back at least 5,000 years. "Today, despite advances in treatment, TB is a global pandemic, fueled by the spread of HIV/AIDS, poverty, a lack of health services and the emergence of drug-resistant strains of the bacterium that causes the disease."[17]

In general, our immune system is well-adapted to dealing with the tuberculosis bacterium. This is our first and most effective line of defense. In fact, the most effective line of defense against any form of disease is our own immune system. We become vulnerable to infectious diseases when we neglect our own health.

Tuberculosis can target almost any part of our bodies, including the joints, bones, urinary tract, central nervous system, muscles, bone marrow, and lymphatic system."[18] In general, tuberculosis is not easy to catch. It preys on individuals whose immune system is compromised through diet or other conditions. Tuberculosis is an especially infectious disease because it can be transmitted from one human to another through sneezing, coughing, or even breathing. The bacterium travels on the minute drops of moisture emitted during exhalation. It does not require the vectors of fleas, rats, or mosquitoes to transmit the disease from one human to another.

In recent years, more virulent forms of tuberculosis have emerged, due to several factors. The worldwide spread of HIV has reduced humans' ability to resist the invasion of tuberculosis bacteria. In addition, the antibiotic treatment for tuberculosis is almost as disruptive to a human's life as the disease itself. Thus, people afflicted with tuberculosis may stop treatment before their disease is fully cured. When this happens, only the weaker tuberculosis bacteria are killed, whereas the more hardy tuberculosis bacteria survive. This is why an individual taking antibiotics for a bacterial disease must complete the entire regimen. Those bacteria that survive are more likely to transmit their resistance to antibiotics to their offspring, thus perpetuating a more virulent form of the disease.

Infectious diseases transmitted by nonhuman vectors can be controlled or eradicated by eliminating the vector or the breeding grounds of the vector. For example, though Singapore is surrounded by countries that have high rates of malaria, Singapore is itself is malaria-free. Singapore has eradicated malaria by enacting laws that levy stiff fines against those who allow standing water on their premises. The only exceptions are swimming pools, which are chlorinated, and aquariums or pools that contain fish. In both cases, larvae of the malaria vector cannot survive. The chlorine is toxic to the larvae, and the fish eat the larvae.

But what happens when the vector is a human being?

The Human Disease Vector

Diseases transmitted from one human to another are the most difficult to eradicate because prevention and eradication measures must be enacted directly upon the diseased human, rather than upon the nonhuman vector that transmitted the disease. Human vectors are protected by laws; nonhuman vectors are not.

By the year 2007, people in the United States thought they were insulated against transmission of tuberculosis; however, TB had begun to reemerge as a health threat due to a number of factors. The overuse and misuse of antibiotics in the United States produced new strains of TB that were resistant to treatment. International migration and immigration brought new cases of TB to the United States. Treatment for TB includes strong and unpleasant side effects, so patients diagnosed with TB were not following through on their treatment regimens.[19] This led to development of new and more drug-resistant strains of the disease.

The year 2007 marked a turning point in public awareness and the actual threat of TB in the United States. During May of that year, a lawyer from Atlanta, Georgia, was diagnosed with a drug-resistant form of TB and was cautioned by the U.S. Centers for Disease Control and Prevention against traveling on public air transportation. Guidelines issued the previous year by the World Health Organization state that patients with multidrug-resistant TB "must not travel by public air transportation" until they prove to be noninfectious.

One day before the CDC sent the lawyer a letter notifying him that he had a particularly resistant form of the disease, the lawyer had flown from Atlanta, Georgia, in the United States, to Paris aboard a commercial jetliner holding more than 300 passengers and flight crew, two days earlier than planned. The purpose for his trip was his wedding and honeymoon, two days after his meeting with county health officials.

County health officials notified the Georgia Division of Public Health, which in turn, notified the U.S. Centers for Disease Control and Prevention. The CDC did not learn that the infected individual had left the country until May 17, more than two weeks after he had been told of his condition. The CDC learned on May 22 that the individual had XDR-TB. XDR is the abbreviation for "extensively drug-resistant tuberculosis." According to the World Health Organization, XDR is resistant to first- and second-line treatments. It can develop when first- and second-line treatments are misused or mismanaged and therefore become ineffective: "Because XDR-TB is resistant to first- and second-line drugs, treatment options are seriously limited. It is therefore vital that TB control is managed properly."[20]

The man and his wife had traveled to Greece and Italy before the man was contacted by the CDC at his hotel in Italy and advised not to return to the United States on public air transportation. The man, his bride, and her eight-year-old daughter responded by cutting the honeymoon short and returning to the United States via a roundabout way, taking short flights in Europe and then arriving in Montreal, Canada, on May 24. He drove across the U.S. border at Champlain, New York.

In running the man's passport through a computer, the U.S. border inspector received a warning with instructions that he should hold the traveler, don a protective mask in dealing with him, and telephone health authorities. The infected individual was instead cleared for entry into the United States and was contacted by the CDC by phone in New York. The individual diagnosed with XDR-TB was cleared to enter the United States; the border inspector who cleared him to enter was relieved of duty.

The infected man later told reporters he tried to sneak into the United States by way of Canada because he was afraid he would die if he didn't reach the United States. He did not seem concerned about the many people who may die as a result of being in contact with him.

The CDC did not notify the Italian Health Ministry of the man's condition, as required by international treaties. Instead, a day after they learned the seriousness of the man's condition, CDC officials contacted a doctor working in Italy who had worked for the organization in the past. That doctor contacted the Italian Health Ministry to let them know about an unidentified tuberculosis case and said the CDC would be in touch. A day later, on May 24, the Italian Health Ministry still had not heard from the CDC. Dr. Maria Grazia Pompa, head of Italy's tuberculosis surveillance program, contacted the CDC and said, "Weren't you supposed to contact us?"

On May 25, a day after the man had entered the United States, the CDC sent an e-mail to Dr. Pompa advising her of the details of the TB case. They did not advise Canadian authorities that a man diagnosed with XDR-TB was in their country until after he had left. The case indicates the role of class and connections in addressing health-care issues. The man's new father-in-law was a microbiologist working for the U.S. government, whose specialty at the CDC was TB and other bacteria. He said he had given the patient "fatherly advice" about traveling with the illness. The man's father was a lawyer who tape-recorded their meeting with CDC officials, during which an exchange in which legal issues about the advisability of the man's taking the trip were raised. After returning to the United States, the man was flown by a CDC plane to avoid contact with passengers traveling on air transportation in the United States.

Epidemics are often associated with impoverished urban conditions because of overcrowding and lack of adequate nutrition. Malnutrition is associated with both the development of new diseases, or new resistant strains, and their spread because malnutrition reduces the effectiveness of the immune system for fighting off disease. The case of TB Andrew illustrates the point that epidemics are not only about controlling disease vectors. They are about the difference in treatment accorded the rich and connected as opposed to that accorded the poor and disenfranchised. Because of his powerful contacts, TB Andrew was allowed to expose thousands of people in several nations to a disease for which no effective treatment had yet been found.

DEVELOPMENTAL DISORDERS

The human lifestyle has changed dramatically in the last few hundred years, especially with respect to industrialization. Industrialization produces a regimented lifestyle in which people spend most of their lives indoors. It also produces an environment in which toxic substances are continually emitted. No organism with a life cycle as long as that of the human species could possibly adapt so quickly to these changed conditions. In the following pages, we will discuss two developmental "disorders" diagnosed since the rise of industrialization. These "disorders" might have been adaptive during the several million years in which the hominid[21] line subsisted as foragers.

Biology and Behavior: Autism

The mind-body dichotomy characteristic of the Western philosophical tradition typically attempts to determine whether a particular health condition is caused by biology or behavior. A more recent formulation of this dichotomy is to determine whether the health condition is genetic or environmental. Recent studies cast new light on the relationship of genetics and environmental factors in reference to **autism**.

Autism is a behavioral disorder that afflicts one in 150 children in the United States. It manifests as a range of developmental problems in three crucial areas of development: social skills, language, and behavior. There is variability in the symptoms and degree of autism: "The most severe autism is marked by a complete inability to communicate or interact with other people."[22] Autistic children develop normally for the first few months, or years, of life and then become less responsive to other people. In the area of social skills, autistic children tend to display the following symptoms:

- Fails to respond to his or her name
- Has poor eye contact
- Appears not to hear others at times
- Resists cuddling and holding
- Appears unaware of others' feelings
- Seems to prefer playing alone—retreats into his or her "own world"[23]

Of these, the three most significant are the failure to respond to his or her name, the inability to maintain culturally appropriate eye contact, and the tendency to be unaware of others' feelings. Our name marks our social identity. Consistent failure to respond to one's name indicates resistance to social interactions with others. Failing to maintain eye contact is more ambiguous, since it may be a mark of shyness, rather than autism. This characteristic alone does not define autism.

The most serious of these indicators is unawareness of others' feelings because humans are social animals. We rely on each other for survival. Being aware of other people's feelings allows us to function successfully in social groups. The inability to recognize and interpret the emotions of others is not unique to autism. It is also characteristic of **antisocial personality disorder**, a more severe form of the inability to relate to others that expresses itself in "chronic behavior that manipulates, exploits, or violates the rights of others. This behavior is often criminal."[24] The difference between the two is that an individual suffering from autism detaches or disassociates from social interaction. An individual suffering from antisocial personality disorder, previously called psychopathology or sociopathology, actively seeks to harm others.

Autism is also expressed in the inability to use language. An individual suffering from autism typically exhibits the following symptoms:

- Starts talking later than other children
- Loses previously acquired ability to say words or sentences
- Does not make eye contact when making requests
- Speaks with an abnormal tone or rhythm—may use a singsong voice or robot-like speech
- Can't start a conversation or keep one going
- May repeat words or phrases verbatim, but doesn't understand how to use them[25]

Autism also manifests in behavior that is apparently related to an attempt to simplify and routinize the environment. Based on its manifestations, the routinization appears to be an attempt to screen out unfamiliar or distressing aspects of the environment. Behavioral aspects of autism include the following:

- Performs repetitive movements, such as rocking, spinning, or handflapping
- Develops specific routines or rituals
- Becomes disturbed at the slightest change in routines or rituals
- Moves constantly
- May be fascinated by parts of an object, such as the spinning wheels of a toy car, rather than to the object overall.
- May be unusually sensitive to light, sound, and touch

Autistic children tend to reject social aspects of the environment in favor of the more mechanistic (and therefore controllable) aspects of the environment. For example, one of my students, a child psychiatrist, noted that children without autism tend to note the social aspects of a photo, drawing, or painting of a human, such as that individual's expression, whereas autistic children focus on a nonsocial component, such as a hat. Analysts at the Mayo Clinic note: "Young children with autism . . . have a hard time sharing experiences with others. When someone reads to them, for example, they're unlikely to point at pictures in the book. This early-developing social skill is crucial to later language and social development."[26]

Autism and Biological Development

There is wide variability in the way autistic children develop as they mature. Some children who manifest symptoms of autism as children may "become more engaged with others and show less marked disturbances in behavior."[27] The symptoms of other autistic individuals may become more severe with adolescence, a time when biological and social changes occur rapidly.

The majority of children with autism are slow to acquire new knowledge or skills, a factor that is not related to intelligence: "An extremely small number of children with autism are 'autistic savants' and have exceptional skills in a specific area, such as art or math."[28] The issue with these autistic individuals is not one of intelligence but the ability to communicate their esoteric knowledge to others. This aspect of individual personality has been observed during hundreds of years, but has only recently been attributed to autism. Individuals with this syndrome become focused on a single attribute of a phenomenon, rather than the relevance of the entire phenomenon.

The manifestation of autism has never been reduced to a single "cause." It appears to have both genetic and cultural/environmental origins. French researchers in 2006 sequenced a gene called SHANK3 in more than 200 people with autism spectrum disorder. They found mutations in the gene in members of three families in the studies.[29] Autism spectrum disorders were described almost simultaneously in the United States and Germany. Based on his studies of eleven children, Dr. Leo Kanner of the Johns Hopkins Hospital in the United States developed the term "early infantile autism" to describe symptoms of abnormal development behavior. At the same time, the German scientist Hans Asperger described a milder form of the disorder. Because of Asperger's description, autism is now often referred to as Asperger's disorder.

Autism spectrum disorders are typically detected by the age of three years, and in some cases, as early as 18 months. These symptoms are typically noticed first by the parents: "When an engaging, babbling toddler suddenly becomes silent, withdrawn, self-abusive, or indifferent to social overtures, something is wrong."[30] All children with ASD (autism spectrum disorder), whether the extreme or milder form, exhibit deficits in social interaction, verbal and nonverbal communication, and repetitive behaviors or interests. They may also have unusual responses to sensory experiences, such as sounds and visual stimulation, ranging from mild to severe.[31]

The SHANK3 gene sequence has been linked to neurological functioning, which makes it a prime suspect in the development of autism. The French study, though provocative, is not conclusive because it focused on autistic children, and did not compare the rate of gene mutations among families in which autism occurs with populations considered normal. Thus, the relative influence of biology and socialization cannot be definitively determined.

Two studies performed in the United States share with the French study the focus on genetic factors, and to a lesser extent, the lack of comparison with nonautistic populations. One of these studies identified a genetic mutation that causes autism in about 1 percent of cases. This study does not link incidence of autism to environmental factors, such as the social context. This study, headed by geneticist Mark J. Daly of Massachusetts General Hospital, was conducted by a multidisciplinary team called the Autism Consortium and reported early in 2008 in the *New England Journal of Medicine*. This study noted that deletions or duplications of a segment of chromosome **locus**, called 16p11.2, occurred in children with autism, but not in their parents, an indication that the altered coding resulted from a spontaneous **mutation** occurring either after fertilization or in the process of producing sex cells, sperm and egg. This particular locus is considered a genetic "hot spot," since it is particularly susceptible to mutation.

Not all mutations are negative. They are among the factors that provide diversity in the gene pool of a population. Diversity in the gene pool of a population is desirable because it allows some members of a population to survive in the event of an environmental catastrophe. As the human population has grown, from 1.9 billion people in 1900 to 7 billion early in the third millennium, diversity in the gene pool may contribute to the survival of the species. Though humans value the ability to interact socially, the ability of some individuals with autism to focus on solving a particular problem may enhance the survival of the human species as a whole. Other characteristics of autism, associated with some cases, include increased aggression, which seems less likely to ensure the survival of the human species.

The study reported above, by the Autism Consortium, indicated a correlation between the mutation and autism, but not a definitive causal factor. The deletions or repetitions in the locus 16p11.2 were found in twenty-four of 2,252 people in families with at least one autistic family member, but in only two out of 18,834 people without the disorder. Thus, the mutation can be a predictor of autism, but does not determine autism, since not everyone with the mutation develops autism.

Early in 2008, three other groups of researchers independently reported in the *American Journal of Human Genetics* that a gene CNTNAP2 could be implicated in autism. These studies included much larger groups of subjects than those in the Autism Consortium. The gene CNTNAP2 produces a protein that allows brain cells to communicate with each other. Geneticist Aravinda Chakravarti of the Johns Hopkins University School of Medicine, who led one of the studies, suggests that the genetic factor may be a necessary but not sufficient cause for the disorder.

Child development specialists who work with autistic children suggest that autism results from the interaction of a genetic predisposition with the social environment within which the child develops. Based on my own (unsystematic) observations of children with autism and other behavioral disorders, I would suggest that environmental factors may include overstimulation or overly controlled social environments. The ability of humans and other primates to survive depends on **plasticity**, the ability to evaluate a social or other environmental context and behave appropriately. Autistic individuals appear to lack—or have a reduced capacity for—the characteristic of plasticity, a capacity that allows humans to quickly evaluate and function in a variety of social and physical environments.

Biology and Behavior: ADHD

The complex relationship among psychology, biology, and behavior is illustrated by a longstanding debate in the United States concerning such childhood behavioral disorders as attention deficit hyperactivity disorder. In the 1960s, a time of intense interest in and research on psychological processes, it was assumed that extreme act-ing-out behavior was due to socialization. Parents, especially the mother, were blamed for the child's inappropriate responses in social situations. By the 1980s, the ability of scientists to measure brain wave patterns led to a biochemical theory of childhood mental disorders as being caused by genetics. Thus, such conditions as what came to be known as attention deficit hyperactivity disorders were treated with psychiatric drugs.

It is difficult, however, to isolate whether a particular behavior is due to biology or to the culture that produces a particular form of socialization, because both genes and culture are transmitted in families. It becomes even more complicated when one considers that, just as alterations in brain wave patterns produce changes in behavior, changes in behavior produce alterations in brain wave patterns.

ADHD is characterized by "a persistent pattern of abnormally high levels of activ-ity, impulsivity, and/or inattention that is more frequently displayed and more severe than is typically observed in individuals with comparable levels of develop-ment.[32] Approximately 3 to 7 percent of school-age children have been diagnosed with ADHD.[33] ADHD is typically diagnosed in children between the ages of three and five, based on patterns of "excessive locomotor activity, poor attention, and/or impulsive behavior."[34]

Medications used to treat ADHD contain stimulants, of which the most common are methylphenidate and amphetamine. Methylphenidate, the active ingredient in Ritalin, the most often prescribed ADHD medication, "has effects similar to, but more potent than, caffeine and less potent than amphetamines. It has a notably calming and 'focusing' effect on those with ADHD, particularly children."[35] It has been long observed that medications that stimulate activity in adults are calming to children. The reverse is also true. Medications that are calming for adults produce hyperactivity in children.

Researchers at Brookhaven National Laboratory administered normal therapeutic doses of methylphenidate to healthy, adult males. Using positron emission tomogra-phy (PET), researchers confirmed that the drug increased subjects' dopamine levels. Dopamine is a neurotransmitter that affects neurons involved in voluntary movement, learning, memory, and emotion, including the ability to experience pleasure and pain. The researchers at Brookhaven National Laboratory speculate that methylphenidate amplifies the release of dopamine, thereby improving attention and focus in individ-uals who have dopamine signals that are weak (Volkow, et al. 2002).

Researchers at the University of Texas at Austin have studied the chemical processes that underlie addiction and therapeutic processes involving dopamine. They note, "Cocaine and other drugs of abuse can alter dopamine function. Such drugs may have very different actions. The specific action depends on which dopamine receptors [in the brain] the drugs stimulate or block, and how well they mimic dopamine."[36]

Methylphenidate, like cocaine, increases the level of dopamine in the synapse, the process that transmits information from one neuron to another, by preventing dopamine reuptake. After a synapse, the reuptake system returns the dopamine to the sending neuron, where it is an enzyme called monoamine oxidase (MAO). This enzyme usually breaks down dopamine. Amphetamine increases the level of dopamine in the synapse by helping to release more dopamine. "It's interesting that amphetamine and cocaine produce affect [the conscious subjective aspect of an emotion considered apart from bodily changes] behavior and heart function in similar ways."[37] However, they accomplish this through different chemical processes.

Based on the available research, the National Institute on Drug Abuse supports the use of stimulants as well as psychotherapy to treat ADHD because these treatments "improve the abnormal behaviors of ADHD, as well as the self-esteem, cognition, and social and family function of the patient" (Konrad, et al. 2004).

NIDA acknowledges reports that methylphenidate has been used for recreational purposes by people for whom it is not prescribed, but distinguishes the effects of medical use of stimulants from those of recreational use. Those who become addicted to stimulants for recreational use ingest large amounts of the substances very quickly, which "induces rapid increases of dopamine in the brain"[38] "In contrast, the therapeutic effect is achieved by slow and steady increases of dopamine, which are similar to the natural production by the brain. The doses prescribed by physicians start low and increase slowly until a therapeutic effect is reached. That way, the risk of addiction is very small."[39]

As noted repeatedly in this book, all ingested, injected, inhaled, and absorbed substances have side effects. Among side effects of stimulants are reduced appetite, especially in very young children; rebound effect, which involves increased irritability or depression that can be worse than before the medication regime began; headache; jittery feeling, which can be accentuated if combined with caffeine or other medications containing stimulants; gastrointestinal upset; anxiety; increased blood sugar levels; increased blood pressure; tics and stereotyped (repetitive) responses; psychosis or paranoia, especially in individuals who are predisposed to psychiatric disorders; and seizures, especially in patients predisposed to epilepsy. Other side effects include difficulty in sleeping, irritability, and depression, all of which could be due either to the ADHD or another psychiatric disorder.[40] There have also been cases of sudden deaths among those taking these stimulants; however, these appear not to exceed the rate of sudden deaths among the overall population.[41]

Physicians prescribing medications take into account whether the side effects outweigh the benefits of treatment for a particular condition. Patients seeking treatment for their condition should do the same.

EVOLUTION AND EPIDEMIOLOGY

It is a commonly held misperception that science and biomedicine can ultimately eliminate disease and other forms of human suffering. Anthropological studies of evolution do not bear this out. Just as humans have adapted to the environment in which our ancestors have evolved, disease organisms also have adapted to the environments in which they survive and thrive, which is often in the bodies of living organisms. The biological anthropologist Michael Alan Park writes:

> We tend to think of diseases as abnormalities—and for individuals suffering from them,
> they are. But diseases are as much a part of life as any other aspect of our biological
> world. Since many diseases are caused by other living organisms—viruses, bacteria, and

protozoa—and are carried by other species, they are really perfectly natural. Disease-causing species have adapted to the biology of their hosts, and the hosts at least attempt to adapt to the disease-causing species. Diseases are thus excellent examples of evolutionary processes. (2008:373–374)

Just as humans have evolved many mechanisms to promote their survival—including the immune system and processes that promote stasis—organisms that cause disease in human populations have also evolved mechanisms that promote their survival. Some of these mechanisms promote survival in particular environments. For example, the genetic code that produces sickling of hemoglobin cells in humans also provides protection against malaria in areas of the world where the malaria protozoan is found. Hemoglobin (red blood cells) carries oxygen to all parts of the body. Thus, it is essential for survival. However, normal round hemoglobin can also carry the malaria protozoa. Sickled hemoglobin cannot carry malaria protozoa, but it also cannot carry sufficient oxygen to promote survival. Thus, an individual with genetic coding for both normal and sickled hemoglobin is most likely to survive in regions where malaria is common.

The process of adaptation to a particular environment is similar for the bacteria, viruses, and protozoa that cause many diseases in humans. These disease-causing organisms, however, have an important advantage over humans: They have a short life cycle, and therefore, can adapt very quickly to a less than ideal environment. In comparison, humans mature slowly and live a long time. Therefore, we cannot evolve new disease-resistant mechanisms within a single lifetime, nor even within several lifetimes. We must rely on the mechanisms evolved in our ancestors over many generations of adapting to the diverse ecologies of our planet.

In general, these human adaptations have been effective; however, there are conditions that can overwhelm our adaptive mechanisms. These include an impaired immune system due to diet, lifestyle, and exposure to disease organisms for which we have no immunity, as well as exposure to disease organisms that have evolved resistance to our immune defenses. Our bodies exert a selective pressure on disease organisms. In turn, viruses, bacteria, and protozoa exert a selective pressure on our bodies.

An important advantage that humans have over disease-producing organisms is **culture**, which is knowledge, beliefs, and customs that we learn from others and transmit from one generation to the next. We have evidence of cultural adaptations in **hominid** populations in Ethiopia in the form of stone tools dating back to at least 2.6 million years ago. Cultural adaptations in the form of wooden and other types of tools no doubt date back even further; however, these types of biodegradable cultural products do not survive in the fossil record.

For at least the last 100,000 years, **cultural evolution** has been an important part of human adaptation to particular environments. Since humans evolve very slowly in biological terms, but very rapidly in terms of culture, both biology and culture have played important roles in the ability of humans to maintain health and resist disease. During the earliest stages of hominid evolution, our ancestors were foragers. They lived by hunting and gathering. At some point, fishing would also have become part of hominid **subsistence practices**, converting environmental resources to human use.

Since humans are large **mammals** with long life spans, our subsistence needs exert strong pressures on the environment. Foraging, a subsistence pattern typical of our ancestors and surviving into modern times, involves moving from place to place to avoid overexploiting any one locale. Foragers traditionally live in small groups spread out over a relatively large territory. Because they lived in small, dispersed populations, they were typically not subject to epidemics, since organisms that cause epidemics require large, dense populations.

The geographer Jared Diamond notes: "Epidemics couldn't take hold when populations were scattered in small bands that constantly shifted camp. Tuberculosis and diarrhea disease had to await the rise of farming, measles and bubonic plague the appearance of large cities" (1991:74[1987]). However, foragers were subject to infections and would have been exposed to new forms of diseases as they migrated into new foraging territories.[42]

Evolutionary Trends in Epidemiology

The anthropologist George Armelagos identifies three trends in the relationship between humans and diseases. He calls these "epidemiological transitions." The first epidemiological transition took place about 10,000 years ago, when people began to settle down and produce food rather than pursuing it from place to place. The two main forms of subsistence during this period were agriculture and pastoralism.

Agriculture produced a large food surplus that permitted a high degree of task specialization, since a small percentage of the population could produce food for all the rest. Task specialization led to a high degree of stratification, differences in social status. Agriculture also led to the rise of cities—large, dense, sedentary populations—which facilitated the transmission of epidemic diseases through greater exposure to human contact and increased populations of disease vectors, such as rats and their fleas.

Domestication of plants also reduced the diversity of the human diet. Humans are omnivores. Through the process of millions of years of natural selection, humans became adapted to a highly varied diet, consisting of both plants and animals, based on what was available seasonally and locally. The more limited the diet, the more limited the nutritional possibilities available to humans. A diet consisting of limited nutritional possibilities reduces the human capacity to resist disease.

The domestication of animals produced other disease possibilities. Due to long contact between humans and domesticated animals, organisms that produced diseases in domesticated animals became adapted to humans. Some examples of diseases introduced to humans in this way include smallpox, chicken pox, and more recently, mad cow disease. Disease organisms adapted to wild animals are less likely to be transmitted to humans because the degree of exposure is less extensive, thus typically this does not allow for the evolution of the disease organisms to become adapted to humans. An exception to this rule is HIV, which evolved from the simian immunodeficiency virus.

In a more exceptional case, a wildlife biologist at Grand Canyon National Park in Arizona died of pneumonic plague in 2007 after performing a **necropsy** on a mountain lion that had tested positive for the disease. A necropsy is a postmortem examination or autopsy. According to the U.S. Centers for Disease Control and Prevention, plague is caused by the bacterium *Yersinia pestis*. The disease is found in rodents and their fleas and occurs in many areas of the world, including the United States.[43]

Pneumonic plague is one of several forms of plague identified by the CDC, all of which are caused by *Y. pestis*. Pneumonic plague occurs when *Y. pestis* infects the lungs. Unlike other plagues, pneumonic plague can be spread from person to person on moisture droplets expelled by coughing, sneezing, or breathing. Bubonic plague is spread by the bites of infected fleas. Antibiotics are the prescribed treatment for plague. Though the National Park Service does not state this, the infected biologist evidently inhaled *Y. pestis* while conducting the necropsy.

Armelagos notes that, during the last years of the nineteenth century, modern medical science provided immunizations and antibiotics, along with other public health measures. Thus, many infectious diseases were brought under control, though diseases in general were not eliminated from the human condition. As a result of humans living longer and of changes in lifestyle, there was a shift from infectious diseases to chronic degenerative diseases, such as cancers and cardiac, circulatory, and pulmonary diseases. These are characteristic of developed, industrialized countries. They also reflect differences in class, which includes a more sedentary and less healthy lifestyle, less physical activity, more stress, environmental pollution, and less healthy diets. Among the factors involved in less healthy diets are less reliance on homegrown foods, which are more diverse and contain more nutrients, and a move to a mass-produced diet that relies on processing. Processing reduces the variability of available nutrients and includes additives that promote long shelf-life rather than longer human life.

The third epidemiological transition involves the development of new diseases and the return of old diseases. The emergence of new and more antibiotic-resistant forms of bacteria has been blamed on the overuse and inappropriate use of antibiotics. Michael Alan Park attributes one cause of the emergence of antibiotic-resistant bacteria to selective pressures linked to the overuse of antibiotics, which gives "microorganisms a greater chance to evolve resistance by exposing them to a constant barrage of selective challenges. . . . Some bacteria reproduce *hourly*, and the processes of mutation and natural selection are speeded up in these species" (2008:378). Park adds that another factor in the development of new diseases is change in human activity that brings more people into contact with more diseases: "As people and their products become more mobile, and as our populations spread into previously little-inhabited areas, cutting down forests and otherwise altering ecological conditions, we contact other species that may carry diseases to which they are immune but that prove deadly to us" (2008:378).

Human exposure to diseases for which they had not evolved an immune response has accelerated with global warming, a process that changed the earth's ecology during the twentieth and twenty-first century.

GLOBAL WARMING AND EPIDEMIOLOGY

In 2007, people in the village of Castiglione di Cervia in Italy suffered from weeks of high fever, exhaustion, and excruciating bone pain, a condition they had not previously experienced. We become accustomed to illnesses that regularly afflict us, our relatives, and our neighbors, even if those diseases can be life-threatening. When symptoms that have not previously been experienced begin to afflict people, especially if they occur in clusters, it is natural for humans to seek some way of assigning blame. As noted in chapter 4, being able to name something is the psychological equivalent to being able to control it.

The people of Castiglione di Cervia began to ask the age-old question: "Who or what has caused this affliction to come upon us?" In times past, the question might have been addressed by burning a "witch" or looking for some other **preternatural** cause, an extraordinary phenomenon that exceeds what is ordinary or regular. In the Age of Science, the people of Castiglione di Cervia looked for a human or natural cause. Among the culprits named were pollution in the river, the government, and recent immigrants from Africa.[44] These are all influences that people may feel powerless to resist because, under situations of crisis, they become defined as the threatening "Other" (Womack 2001).

The ominous "Other" that proved to be afflicting the residents of Castiglione di Cervia was both more ordinary and more diffuse, therefore more difficult to control. The name of the disease was chikungunya fever, a viral illness spread by the bite of infected mosquitoes. The disease follows a cyclical pattern with an inter-epidemic period of seven to eight years. Chikungunya is not a life-threatening infection; the treatment recommended by the World Health Organization is rest and convalescence.[45] The pain involved can be treated with an **analgesic** (pain medication) and long-term anti-inflammatory therapy. The condition has been reported from a number of tropical regions ranging from East Asia to Africa, as well as from countries around the Indian Ocean.

Symptoms of chikungunya fever are similar to those of dengue fever, which is a hemorrhagic disease, also spread by a mosquito. It is found in tropical regions of Asia, Africa, and North America. Whereas chikungunya has previously had a limited distribution and is typically not fatal, dengue fever is found around the world in tropical regions. It is a frequent cause of hospitalization and death, especially among children.[46]

The most ominous factor in the case of the chikungunya outbreak in Italy is not the Tiger mosquito that is the disease vector, but that this vector was found in southern Europe, a nontropical region where it has not previously occurred. Its occurrence in southern Italy at this time is a product of global warming. Humans can draw on technology to abate some of the effects of global warming. We can fan ourselves or run air conditioners as long as adequate fuel supplies are available. We can draw on culture. We can wear sunshades or parasols when we go outdoors. Nothing humans can do, however, can abate the effects of global warming on our ecosystem.

Climate on earth is a product of the sun's energy and the temperature of the ocean. Changing ocean temperatures reshape the global temperature. Some temperate zones will become tropical. Other temperate zones will be covered with ice. Islands and beaches will disappear. Many species of large mammals, which are most demanding on the earth's resources, may no longer survive in their natural habitat. Humans are large, resource-hungry mammals. The change in world temperatures poses a wholly new challenge for epidemiology and for the practice of medicine in general.

With global warming, as measured by the rise in the world's ocean temperatures, the earth's climate is shifting. The climate on land is largely shaped by the ocean's tides. As these shift, some areas on earth will grow warmer, others will grow colder. Thus, the pattern of infectious diseases will also shift. The true danger of global warming for humans is not directly due to the change in temperatures. Humans survive primarily by culture. We can build shelters and heat or cool our domiciles. The true danger will come from changes in the ecosystem. Some plant and animal species on which humans depend will become extinct, while others will evolve into new species. These new species may not be compatible with human life. **Microbes**, microscopic organisms, evolve faster than humans because their lives are shorter. New diseases are likely to emerge more quickly than the human body can develop immunity to them.

14

Medicines, Herbs, and Dietary Supplements

CASE STUDY
A Brief History of Herbs and Healing

For more than four million years, our hominid ancestors relied primarily on plants for survival, supplemented by meat from the hunt.[1] Such extreme reliance on plants would have required sophisticated knowledge of the nutritional and medicinal properties of plants. These early ancestors would also have known to avoid plants toxic to humans. Contemporary Lacandon Maya of southern Mexico classify ailments on the basis of symptoms and cultivate herbs demonstrated to be effective in treating those symptoms. For example, diarrhea or an upset stomach may be treated by one of three plant species. *Bursera simaruba* is a species of tree occurring from southern Florida to South America. *Ficus obtusifolia* is a species of fig. Wild clove (*Eugenia caryophyllata*) has anesthetic and antiseptic properties. "Most of the treatments involve chewing the leaves or bark, or boiling a plant's leaves or bark, and drinking the resulting liquid" (McGee 2002:160). Some medicines are administered externally, as in the case of a woman who produced "bone medicine" by boiling the leaves of an unidentified plant (possibly wild clove) in water and applying the liquid to the aching muscle. Wounds are treated by collecting leaves from the Bäbah tree (*Sapindus saponaria*), drying the leaves, and sprinkling the resulting powder on the wound. Many modern medicines have been developed by extracting the active ingredient from herbs or other substances and testing these extracts for their effectiveness in treating specific disorders. An example from China is the use of extracts from *Artemisia annua*, a plant that has been used an anti-malarial in Asia for 2000 years. In 1972, Tu Youyou discovered artemisinin in the plant's leaves, a drug named *qinghaosu* by the Chinese. Artemisinin is still widely used in China and Southeast Asia for treating symptoms of malaria. For about a decade, the Western world was skeptical about the use of artemisinin as a medicine, partly because artemisinin is volatile. More recently, trials have shown that artemisinin combined with other substances, such as lumefantrine, is more than 90 percent effective in treating malarial symptoms, especially for the chloroquine-resistant *Plasmodium falciparum.*

Most healing systems involve some form of ingesting, infusing, injecting, or topically applying concoctions made from plants and animal materials. Throughout known history, shamans and other healers have used medications to supplement or provide the central ingredient for other forms of healing. Terms to designate substances associated with healing fall into three categories. Substances that have been tested according to scientific procedures are "medications." The term "drugs" has a dual meaning. It can refer to scientifically tested medication, but it can also be used to describe self-administered substances such as cocaine, heroin, crystal methamphetamine, and other mood-altering chemicals.

Traditional healers and other individuals involved in "natural" healing typically rely on herbal concoctions to relieve symptoms. In some cases, these herbs provide the basis for scientific medications, which are extractions or synthesized versions of herbs occurring naturally. Dietary supplements fit into an entirely different category. The use of dietary supplements presumes that the ordinary human diet does not meet our nutritional needs, a provocative issue.

TRADITIONAL PHARMACOLOGY:
HEALING AND DREAMING

In the United States, we owe much of what we understand about psychological aspects of traditional pharmacology to the work of Richard Evans Schultes, whose academic training was based at Harvard. Schultes became a hero in the 1960s for his studies of hallucinogenic plant species in South America. Perhaps his greatest gifts to botany (and, more generally, to science) were his willingness to travel to remote regions to discover new plant species, his willingness to offer himself as a research subject, and his ability to dramatically convey his knowledge in the classroom.

Schultes called the vast continent of South America "the land where the gods reigned" (Davis 2004:15). He based this description on the preparation *ayahuasca*, known indigenously as *yagé*, described variously as "the vision vine, the vine of the soul, the most celebrated hallucinogen of the Amazon" (Davis 2004:16).

Largely as a result of Schultes' explorations, the hallucinogen became a recreational drug in the United States in the 1960s. In South America, the drug was used by *curanderos* (shamans) to guide them in their healing journeys into the spirit world. Among anthropologists and psychologists, this journey is described as a journey into the unconscious. Wade Davis writes: "Sacred to all the tribes of the upper Amazon, [*yagé*] is the embodiment of the jaguar, a magical intoxicant capable of freeing the soul, allowing it to wander into mystical encounters with ancestors and animal spirits" (2004:16).

Yagé is made by scraping off the bark of the liana plant and heating it in water. The water is then drunk by healers. The shamans studied by Schultes attributed their healing powers to the plant itself, which allowed them to see which herb or herbs a sick person needed: "The plant made the diagnosis. It was a living being, and the Ingano [an indigenous group of Colombia] acknowledged its magical resonance as reflexively as Schultes accepted the axioms of his own science" (Davis 2004:17).

The shamans who taught Schultes about the experiential properties of the psychotropic plants in their environment were primarily interested in their healing effects. The philosophy underlying the use of psychotropics in traditional shamanic healing traditions differs from that underlying the use of medications in Western biomedicine. Pharmaceuticals used in Western biomedicine are evaluated on the basis of how they operate directly on the medical condition being treated. Psychotropics used by traditional healers are aimed at transforming the cognitive patterns of the healer so that he or she can "see" the underlying condition—whether social, biological, spiritual, or psychological—that produced the illness.

These psychotropic drugs should by no means be considered recreational. Using them requires a period of training under the tutelage of a shaman who has demonstrated the ability to heal. The psychotropics are designed to displace the ordinary perceptions of the healer that may obscure the "true" cause of a disorder. The "true" cause may lie in the unconscious conflicts of the suffering person. It may be "caused" by living in a hostile social environment, or it may be "caused" by factors that can never be determined scientifically. Doctors do not practice medicine without a license. Shamans do not practice healing without a long period of training.

Use of hallucinogens without training can lead to psychosis, rather than the ability to heal. A young man of my acquaintance felt himself become a bird after ingesting LSD in a Honolulu hotel room. The hallucinogenic experience feels so authentic, no doubt he could feel the growth of his feathers and the alteration of his body form. Unfortunately for him, the man's psychological state defied the physical limitations of his biology. He crashed after "flying" out the window of his hotel room, and became paraplegic as a result.

One explanation of hallucinogens is that they disrupt the neural pathways (synapses) that are formed in the first years of our lives. The human brain requires order, so it reforms neural pathways appropriate to the context. The individual who "flew" out the window probably had an unacknowledged death wish. He had a desire to "leave the earth." This explanation was supported by his later choice of suicide. He drank liquid Drano, a caustic substance used for cleaning out drains.

The ability to experience altered states of consciousness develops as part of the sophisticated neural pathways characteristic of humans. We all enter an altered state of consciousness when we dream. Dreams address our unconscious conflicts. This is what gives rise to the term "dream work," which is essential for maintaining psychological equilibrium. People who are not allowed to enter into dream states begin to exhibit psychotic symptoms. Unlike the use of hallucinogens, dreaming is protected by our body's survival mechanisms. When we dream, our bodies enter a temporary state of paralysis. Thus, we can have many psychological adventures without physical danger. We also have the waking response. If a dream becomes too frightening, we wake up, thus avoiding an extreme physical response, such as a heart attack or stroke.

People who sleepwalk have a faulty paralysis mechanism, a flaw that allows them to act out their dreams. People who ingest hallucinogens override their bodies' protective mechanisms. They act out their unconscious impulses. If they have cleared the "demons" out of their unconscious, or if they have learned to negotiate with them through the shamanic career, they can survive the horrors of a waking nightmare, a "bad trip." If, however, they have not undergone this "education," a "bad trip" can be fatal. Repeated "bad trips" can lead to psychosis.

None of us really understands the content of our unconscious thoughts. That is why it is called the "unconscious." It contains material (experiences and thoughts) that can be too frightening to be made available to our conscious awareness. Hallucinogens bypass the conscious pathways that prevent us from delving too deeply into unconscious material. Shamans undergo a long period of training that allows them to face and understand the "demons" in their unconscious. The shamanic journey and shamanic training are, in fact, a prolonged period of psychoanalysis. Those who skip the "journey" and go straight to the experience are courting psychosis.

SCIENCE AND CONTROLLED EXPERIMENTS

In recent medical history, the "wisdom" of the body has been superseded by the specialized training of medical professionals. Emeran Mayer and Clifford B. Saper suggest that early healing systems were based on the body's ability to self-regulate and overcome invading organisms through both psychological and physiological processes:

> It is striking to realize that only a handful of the drugs that were prescribed at the turn of the last century by Western physicians are still in clinical use (opiates, digitalis, aspirin, and quinine). Presumably, most of the rest of what physicians were doing at that time, and what they did for millennia before that, relied upon the healing effects of endogenous physiological systems, activated by state of mind. (Mayer and Saper 2000:3)

Predominantly in the United States and Europe, medical interventions take the form of surgery and the administration of medications tested under scientific procedures. Scientific medicine is based on controlled experiments to determine whether a particular substance is more effective than a placebo. The scientific approach has proved remarkably effective in isolating ingredients that target a particular condition.

The Physiology of Medication

Medications react differently depending on whether they are inhaled, ingested, injected, or absorbed through the skin. These are all chemical processes, and the same substance, administered differently, can produce different reactions. For example, a study reported in the December 14, 2006, *New England Journal of Medicine* found that flu shots administered in the arm were 67 to 77 percent effective in preventing the flu in adults, whereas the FluMist nasal spray was 30 to 57 percent effective.

Many variables are involved, including what is added to deliver the vaccine in an inhalable form. Others involve the processes through which the body absorbs the medication. Substances administered orally undergo the gastric processes of the alimentary system. Inhalants are absorbed into the blood stream through the sensitive nasal passages. Injections pass almost immediately into the blood stream, and thus, are less altered by the chemistry of ingesting and inhaling.

Genetics, Medicine, and the Struggle to Survive

Researchers made a huge breakthrough in cracking the human genetic code when they completed the sequencing of the human genome in spring of 2003. The genome is the entire genetic code of an organism, and the process of sequencing its coding provides a basis for determining where particular traits are located on a DNA molecule. Knowing the sequence of coding is significant for medicine because it allows us to address and perhaps treat disorders that are genetically based. The anthropologist Michael Alan Park explains the importance of **evolution** and **genetics** in our lives:

> We benefit from this knowledge every day of our lives. We eat foods from species of plants and animals bred according to the principles of genetics and selection. We know the causes of many of the illnesses that beset us because we understand the genetic operations of our cells, and we have insight into how some organisms (such as viruses and bacteria) are adapted to other organisms (like us), and vice versa. Many of the antibiotics and other medicines that help us treat those illnesses work only because of the interrelatedness of all life. (2008:105)

Like us, disease organisms are struggling to survive. It is not personal. It is a battle between our immune system and the disease organisms that pit their survival against our immune system. We and our disease organisms are evolving together. Our weapons in this ongoing battle are our immune system, our lifestyle, and our avoidance of organisms that cause disease. When these weapons fail to protect us, we must rely on drugs that are more effective than our immune system in destroying invading organisms.

There is a downside to taking drugs to treat disease, in that all drugs have side effects. In fact, all ingested substances—including foods—have side effects. While studying the interrelationship of behaviors, cognition, and performance among professional and high-level athletes, I learned that food—and the context in which it is ingested—was linked to performance in the minds of the athletes and their trainers. At the time of my study, one motto was, "Proteins for power; carbohydrates for speed."

Athletes linked consuming certain kinds of foods with their performance in competition (Womack 1982). Linking food with performance makes sense in a practical and nutritional sense. Food and drink fuel the human body, just as gasoline is fuel for many machines. We would never think of driving a car without gasoline, but we often operate our bodies without considering what kind of fuel our bodies might require for the demands we make on them.

In recent years, the Mediterranean diet has been touted as the "ideal" diet for the human species. This is a vast over-simplification. It is the "ideal" diet for people whose ancestors evolved genetic coding for the Mediterranean climate, lifestyle, and resources available to them. It is not "ideal" for people who ancestors evolved above the Arctic Circle. Humans are the most biologically varied species on earth. Our ancestors adapted biologically and culturally to the environments that provided them with their resources. Sherpas who live in the high mountains of the Himalaya would be selected against if they tried to survive on a Mediterranean diet. They could not possibly acquire enough Mediterranean resources to keep them alive. You can't grow olive trees in snow. And you can't acquire fish from rocky soil.

My ancestors evolved in the British Isles and along the western coast of Europe. Fish were plentiful; olives were not. As a part of research for this book, I went on a vegetarian diet. It was a sensory delight to anticipate what vegetables I would select at the market, how I would prepare them, and how delicious they would taste as I ate them. After all, I grew up on a farm in Missouri, where edible species of both plants and animals are abundant. My ancestors, and my own body, had adapted to an environment that supported variability in plant and animal species. But tuna, an ocean fish, had to be shipped to us in aluminum cans. On the other hand, my mother's homemade cottage cheese, produced by milk from our own cows, spoiled me forever for mass-produced cottage cheese. I keep buying mass-produced cottage cheese, taking a bite or two motivated by a sense of duty, and then storing it in the refrigerator for the little organisms that find the mass-produced cottage cheese a wonderfully nurturing environment. After three months of an exclusively vegetarian diet, both my body and brain shut down. Ravi Wadhwani, my Ayurveda consultant, had advised me against such an extreme regime. And he was right. But I don't regret the experiment.

My "experiment" in an extreme dietary regime caused me to lose a significant amount of weight, which I much appreciated, but it also taught me that maintaining health and resisting disease is a holistic process. Lifestyle provides the most important model for maintaining health and resisting disease. However, when disease-causing organisms overwhelm our body's natural defense mechanisms, humans have historically and prehistorically called upon the pharmacopoeia of their particular environment and culture to combat disease. With the advent of science, use of drugs to combat disease and sustain health changed in terms of paradigm and practice. Contemporary biomedicine draws on the efficacy of science to diagnose and treat illness. This requires statistical measures of efficacy.

DRUG TRIALS

Whether over the counter (OTC) or prescription, medications must undergo a series of controlled trials before they can be marketed for the public. The trials begin with long-term development and testing by pharmaceutical companies, involving years of experiments in animal and human cells. The tests are aimed at determining whether the medications submitted for testing are effective against the conditions for which they are tested, as well as identifying any negative or potentially dangerous side effects. If this phase of testing is successful, the pharmaceutical company that has developed a medication can submit the data to the U. S. Food and Drug Administration requesting approval to begin testing the drug in humans.

Clinical trials, testing of an experimental drug in humans, typically take place in three phases. Phase I focuses on assessing the drug's safety and involves testing the substance on a small number of healthy volunteers (20 to 100), who are usually paid for participating in the study:

> The study is designed to determine what happens to the drug in the human body—how it is absorbed, metabolized, and excreted. A phase I study will investigate side effects that occur as dosage levels are increased. This initial phase of testing typically takes several months. About 70 percent of experimental drugs pass this initial phase of testing.[2]

The second phase of clinical trials focuses on assessing the drug's efficacy. This phase involves up to several hundred patients and lasts from several months to two years: "Most phase II studies are randomized trials. One group of patients will receive the experimental drug, while a second "control" group will receive a standard treatment. . . . Only about one-third of experimental drugs successfully complete both phase I and phase II studies."[3]

Phase III studies involve larger numbers of subjects, from several hundred to several thousand patients, and last for several years: "This large-scale testing provides the pharmaceutical company and the FDA with a more thorough understanding of the drug's effectiveness, benefits, and the range of possible adverse effects. . . . Seventy to 90 percent of drugs that enter phase III studies successfully complete this phase of testing."[4]

Both Phase II and Phase III studies are typically double-blind, meaning that neither the patient nor the researchers know who is getting the experimental drug. This aims at avoiding the psychological side effects of patients' expectations. A patient who thinks she or he is getting an experimental drug is likely to show improvement simply due to optimism. A patient who thinks she or he is getting a placebo is likely to experience deterioration in the condition being tested due to negative expectations. The experimenter can subtly convey information about the experiment through body language and facial expressions. Double-blind experiments are aimed at avoiding psychological factors that may skew results of the experiment.

The Economics of Clinical Trials

If a Phase III study is successfully completed, a pharmaceutical company can request FDA approval for marketing the drug:

> In late phase III/phase IV studies, pharmaceutical companies have several objectives: (1) studies often compare a drug with other drugs already in the market; (2) studies are often designed to monitor a drug's long-term effectiveness and impact on a patient's quality of life; and (3) many studies are designed to determine the cost-effectiveness of a drug therapy relative to other traditional and new therapies.[5]

Both preliminary experiments in developing new drugs and clinical trials are expensive to conduct, and there is no certainty of profit by the pharmaceutical company. If the company can get FDA approval to conduct clinical trials, the cost is shared by the pharmaceutical company and the U.S. National Institutes of Health. This shared arrangement is based on the idea that pharmaceutical companies have a chance to benefit economically and the American public has a chance to benefit by improved health care.

FDA approval of a drug for marketing typically requires a follow-up study by the pharmaceutical company to determine if problems arise when a medication is in widespread distribution. The FDA, however, does not have a strong record of insisting on these follow-ups.

Physicians who participate in clinical trials are typically paid on a per-patient basis, a practice that could lead them to prescribe drugs for patients whose conditions do not warrant that course of treatment. Some precautions are built into the system. Any physician awarded a research grant by a pharmaceutical company or the National Institutes of Health must obtain approval from an Institutional Review Board to conduct the study. Institutional Review Boards are established by institutions, such as universities or research organizations, to review biomedical and behavioral research involving humans. In the United States, these are regulated by the FDA and by the Department of Health and Human Services. This aims to prevent unethical or harmful experiments from being conducted on humans.

The purpose of Institutional Review Boards is to examine protocols of a research project to ensure that the research does not harm human subjects and to assess the scientific merit of the project. The National Institutes of Health requires subjects to sign an "informed consent" form, which describes the study, including the risks involved and what might happen to a patient in the study. It also advises patients that they have the right to leave the study at any time.

The Public's Right to Know

Perhaps the greatest danger in clinical trials is not for the participants, but for the general public. Problems that do not show up in a clinical trial conducted on only a few hundred or a few thousand patients may become significant when the medication is used by millions of people in varied states of health, in various circumstances, of different ages, and with varied lifestyles. Also, patients in clinical trials are carefully monitored by physicians observing research protocols. CenterWatch, a clinical trials listing website maintained by Thomson Corporation, notes that [patients in clinical trials] "typically will get excellent care from the physicians during the course of the study."[6] Such "excellent care" is ordinarily not available to the broad spectrum of patients who will be taking the medication.

A number of drugs that have stood up to the scrutiny of clinical trials have proved to have harmful side effects. As a result of publicity about the possibility of these side effects, the U.S. Congress, scientists, and advocacy groups have requested that the results of clinical trials be released to the public. This would allow patients to make informed decisions about whether to take high-risk drugs for what may be low-risk conditions.

Physicians and medical researchers control the testing of drugs and medical healing techniques. Ultimately, however, they cannot control the lifestyles of individuals, and lifestyles may be a key factor in the outcome of medical conditions.

Drugs and Aging

Our bodies change as we grow older. That may sound like a truism, and it is, but the ways in which our bodies change can sometimes be unexpected. Yu-Xiao Yang of the

University of Pennsylvania School of Medicine led a study of the relationship of medicines prescribed for heartburn to the risk of hip fractures among older Americans. The study was funded by the National Institutes of Health, the American Gastroenterological Assn/GlaxoSmithKline Institute for Digestive Health, and several drug manufacturers.

The drugs studied—which included Nexium, Prilosec, Prevacid, and Protoniz—block production of acid in the stomach and are among the most widely used in the United States. Together, they account for annual sales of more than $10 billion. The University of Pennsylvania researchers concluded that the drugs, which block stomach acid, also block absorption of calcium. Yang notes, "The perception is that the drugs are completely safe, and doctors dispense them without thinking too much about the risks and the benefits."[7]

According to the National Institutes of Health, an estimated 300,000 Americans older than sixty-five suffer hip fractures. About 20 percent die of complications and an additional 20 percent are consigned to nursing homes.[8]

Yang and his colleagues conducted their research on a database of British hip fracture patients older than fifty matched with a group of 135,386 individuals who had not suffered hip fractures. They found that using the drugs for one year increased the risk of hip fractures by 44 percent. Long-term users of the drugs who also ingested high dosages incurred as much as 260 percent of the normal risk. Men were twice as likely as women to suffer hip fractures. Patients taking a different class of acid inhibitors—including Tagamet, Zantac, Pepcid, and Axid—had a 21 percent increase of fractures after one year.[9] The University of Pennsylvania findings are similar to those of a smaller Danish study published earlier; however, the Danish study did not indicate a higher risk associated with long-term usage of the drugs or with higher dosages.[10]

A team of researchers at McGill University in Montreal, headed by David Golzman, found similar results among individuals over fifty who took antidepressants daily. About 10 percent of those using antidepressants fractured a bone over a five-year period, compared to a 2 percent fracture rate for those who did not take daily does of antidepressants. The study focused on a class of antidepressants known as selective serotonin reuptake inhibitors (SSRIs), including Prozac and Zoloft.[11]

A "PILL-POPPING SOCIETY"

The United States has been called a "pill-popping society" because many members of the public believe that any problem—whether biological or psychological—can be solved by taking a pill. As noted earlier, all substances—whether ingested, injected, inhaled, or absorbed through the skin—have side effects. Some side effects are known as a result of stringent testing procedures. In these cases, the decision to prescribe or take a pill is based on which is worse, the medical condition or the side effects. Some side effects can be unpredictable due to patients' differing physiology, psychology, and lifestyle. In other cases, side effects may show up years after the medical regime was undertaken.

In the 1960s, a New York gynecologist named Robert A. Wilson wrote a book called *Feminine Forever*, which promoted the use of the hormones estrogen and progestin (a synthetic form of progesterone) as a way of combating the "tragedy of menopause." He asserted that estrogen could keep women energetic, young-looking, and straight-backed into old age.

Defining menopause as a "tragedy" reinforces prevailing American views that growing old is something to be avoided. Aging was considered especially "tragic" for women because it meant they would lose their reproductive powers, and with it, their appeal for men. As noted in chapter 7, this is not a universal belief. Among the French, for example, women between thirty-five and fifty-five have proverbially been considered at their peak. Mireille Guiliano, president and CEO of Clicquot Inc. writes of the ages between fifty-five and seventy-seven:

> The French rightly acknowledge there is a particular mystique to *"une femme d'un certain âge"* [a woman of a certain age], an expression with layers of meaning, including respect but also worldliness and hints of seduction. Our media have no trouble projecting the sexiness of Catherine Deneuve and Charlotte Rampling. Here the difference between France and America is amazing. In Europe, men naturally find women of this age group desirable, even sexy, and are often caught turning around to look at one entering a restaurant. If she is eating alone, they are more likely to flirt with her than to pity her. It's inconceivable in New York, where eye contact seems to have gone the way of smoking. (2005:247)

With typically French pragmatism, Guiliano adds: "With increased life expectancies, this stage, dismissed as old age just a few decades ago, is for many one of the most vital times of life." (2005:245). She suggests that reaching and enjoying *"un certain âge"* might require some investment in oneself: "Well-being, while not rare, is more fragile in these years, when health problems that might roll off a younger woman's back can have much more serious effects. For this reason, pampering oneself is important" (2005:245).

In the United States, physicians other than Wilson jumped on the hormone replacement bandwagon for what they described as health reasons. It was expected that the hormones estrogen and progesterone would protect women against heart disease and stroke; however, clinical results of prescribing hormone replacement therapy gave cause for concern. In 1993, the U.S. government funded a study called the Women's Health Initiative. The study tracked 17,000 women and, contrary to expectations, found a slight but significant increase in breast cancer, heart attacks, blood clots, and strokes. Following guidelines aimed at protecting research subjects, the study was halted three years before scheduled.

After the practice of prescribing estrogen and progesterone for women began to be discouraged in 2003, breast cancer rates in the United States dropped by 7.2 percent, a dramatic decline. About 200,000 cases of breast cancer had been expected in 2003, but about 14,000 fewer women actually were diagnosed with the disease. Breast cancers that seem to be fueled by estrogen dropped 8 percent in 2003, twice the rate of breast cancers that do not feed on the hormone. New cases of breast cancer that feed on estrogen fell 12 percent in women between fifty and sixty-nine. A seemingly logical connection between the "female" hormones, estrogen and progesterone, was not supported by the actual practice of prescribing the drugs. This is a good example of why it is important to fund clinical trials of drugs before they are released to the general public. We all would like a panacea to solve all our problems but presumed panaceas, like all drugs, have side effects.

Misuse of Over-the-Counter Drugs

According to an annual study by the National Institute on Drug Abuse, released in December 2006, the profile of drug abuse by American teenagers has shifted. Fewer teens reported drinking alcohol, smoking cigarettes, or using illegal drugs such as marijuana during 2006, but more were abusing legal drugs, such as cold medicine. The ingredient dextromethorphan appears to hold the secret to the appeal of cold medicines for "getting high."

Dextromethorphan (DXM), a semisynthetic narcotic, is a cough-suppressing ingredient in about seventy OTC (over the counter) cold and cough medicines. Cold medicines with "DM" or "Tuss" in the title or name contain DXM.[12] Effects of DXM include euphoria, enhanced awareness, impaired judgment, loss of coordination, dizziness, nausea, seizures, panic attacks, psychosis, brain damage, and addiction. Overdosing can result in coma and death.

"Getting high" may require large doses of cold and cough medicine, especially since tolerance may develop with prolonged use. Internet sites advise young users to drink cough syrup expeditiously to absorb enough DXM prior to vomiting, which will occur as a result of the large amount of cough syrup required for intoxication. "Teens have been reported to drink three or four bottles of cough syrup in one day and take up to 20–30 tablets of Coricidin at once."[13]

Coricidin, prescribed for high blood pressure, contains the cough suppressant dextromethorphan and chlorphenamine maleate (an antihistamine). Some varieties of Coricidin may also contain acetaminophen (an analgesic/fever reducer) and guaifenesin (an expectorant). "Cold turkey" withdrawal from an addiction to DXM includes symptoms such as restlessness, muscle or bone aches, insomnia, diarrhea, vomiting, and cold flashes with goose bumps.[14]

According to a study conducted at the University of Michigan, over-the-counter cold medicine was used "fairly recently" to "get high" by as many as one in fourteen high school seniors. It is difficult to track the rates of OTC use of cough and cold medicine, since 2006 was the first year the annual study, now in its thirty-second year, has tracked the use of cough and cold medicine by teens. The study also reported an increase in the use of prescription drugs, such as the painkillers OxyContin and Vicodin and the stimulant Ritalin.

The study conducted by the University of Michigan, surveyed 50,000 students in the eighth, tenth and twelfth grades at more than 400 schools nationwide. Nearly 10 percent of high school seniors admitted to using excessive dosages of Vicodin, a slight increase over the previous year. Nine percent of eighth-graders sniffed glue, spray paints, cleaning fluids, or other inhalants, a slight decrease.

Misuse of Prescription Drugs: Viruses

It is common practice in the United States to prescribe antibiotics for such ailments as influenza and colds, both of which are caused by viruses. Antibiotics are not effective against viruses, though they have long been effective in treating bacterial infections. A number of scientists and physicians in the United States have cautioned against the risks of prescribing antibiotics to treat illnesses for which they are ineffective.

At the time of this writing, physicians cautioned against the use of antibiotics to treat sinusitis, an ailment usually caused by a virus that runs its course in twelve weeks, with or without treatment. Dr. Don Leopold, chair of the University of Nebraska Medical Center's Department of Otolaryngology, stated that there are no approved drugs to treat sinus infections and no recommended course of treatment.[15] Dr. David Spiro, a pediatrician and professor at Oregon Health and Science University, said the number of cases treated by antibiotics is "extremely high for a condition that, for the most part, self-resolves."[16] Guidelines released by the American Academy of Pediatrics and the American Academy of Family Physicians recommended that medications should only be prescribed for children and antibiotics used if the condition persists or doesn't improve.

Saline flushing is recommended for most cases of sinus infections, but patients are typically not receptive to them because they expect to be given prescriptions for antibiotics. Irresponsible prescription of antibiotics, and their misuse, increases the likelihood that new infectious diseases will emerge as strains of bacteria develop resistance to existing antibiotics. This is already evident in the development of resistant forms of staphylococcus microbes.

Resistance to Prescription Drugs: Bacteria

Gonorrhea, a sexually transmitted disease caused by the bacterium *Neisseria gonorrhoeae*, has long been effectively treated in the United States using antibiotics. In the 1930s and 1940s, antibiotics from a class of medications known as sulfonamides were used effectively. After the *N. gonorrhoeae* bacterium became resistant to sulfa drugs, penicillin was effectively used to treat gonorrhea until late in the twentieth century.

Since 1986, the U.S. Centers for Disease Control has monitored the development of resistance of *N. gonorrhoeae* to antimicrobials in the United States through the Gonococcal Isolate Surveillance Project (GISP). Data collected by GISP in 2003 indicated that 16.4 percent of isolates were resistant to penicillin, tetracycline, or both.[17]

As *N. gonorrhoeae* resistance to penicillin and tetracycline increased, a class of antibiotics known as fluoroquinolones became the most effective treatment of gonorrhea. Some degree of resistance to fluoroquinolones had been noted since 1991; however, the degree of resistance was not sufficient to argue against use of this class of medications. Since 2001, an increasing number of bacterial strains that cause gonorrhea have become resistant to the fluoroquinolones, leading the CDC in 2007 to recommend that doctors stop prescribing these antibiotics for treatment of gonorrhea and to begin using a different class of antibiotics, known as cephalosporins.

The CDC's recommendations were based on GISP monitoring of resistance rates among heterosexual males in twenty-six American cities. The highest rates of resistance, nearly 27 percent of gonorrhea cases, was detected among heterosexual males in Philadelphia, with rates nearly that high in similar populations in San Francisco. Dr. John Douglas, director of the CDC's Division of Sexually Transmitted Diseases Prevention, has stated, "We are running out of options to treat this disease, [and there are] no new drugs for gonorrhea in the drug development pipeline."[18]

Responses to the "Pill-Popping Society"

Since the 1960s, when youths in the United States sought an escape from a society based on "plastics,"[19] Americans have sought a way out of the mainstream. In many cases, this "escape" has been achieved through alternative forms of medical treatments, "natural" foods or health-related products, and/or psychotropic substances. This trend was reversed in some segments of the population leading up to and immediately after the beginning of the third millennium. At this time, science became a popular health metaphor, and large segments of the population sought the "salvation" of longevity through pharmaceuticals, surgeries, and other medical applications. All extremes produce a backlash, and this began to become apparent in medicine when **autism** became a popular diagnosis for variability in childhood development.

Among some segments of the population, the increase in autism diagnoses was attributed to vaccinations of children required for admission to public schools. Twenty states, including California, allow medical exemptions from these vaccinations. These exemptions have been traditionally based on a belief in some form of formal religious practice. More recently, parents are basing their requests for exemptions on their belief that the vaccines are linked to autism and other disorders.

According to Saad B. Omer, an assistant scientist at the Johns Hopkins Bloomberg School of Public Health, the rate of personal belief exemptions is increasing, from less than 1 percent in 1991 to 2.54 percent in 2004.[20] In previous decades, those who did not vaccinate their children were believed to be poor and uneducated; however, the picture has changed. Those who refuse vaccinations for their children are likely to be well-educated and financially stable. The percentage varies according to region and appears to be based in personal beliefs about medical practices and lifestyle in general.

In San Diego, California, a controversy arose in 2008 concerning vaccinating children for measles, after an outbreak in which twelve children developed the disease. This was considered unusual, even in a city having a population of more than 3 million people. Concern was expressed that unvaccinated children were exposing vaccinated children to the risk of measles, since the MMR (measles, mumps, and rubella) vaccine is only 95 percent effective against measles.

The underlying issue is a contest between parental rights and the rights of government organizations to enact and enforce laws relating to what is considered the common good. Measles was considered a common childhood disease in previous decades in the United States. Treatments were conservative, primarily involving bedrest and isolation.

An online publication by the U.S. Centers for Disease Control[21] assesses the risks of being vaccinated with the MMR vaccine, noting, "A vaccine, like any medicine, is capable of causing serious problems, such as severe allergic reactions. The risk of MMR vaccine causing serious harm, or death, is extremely small."[22] It adds, "Getting MMR vaccine is much safer than getting any of these three diseases. Most people who get MMR vaccine do not have any problems with it."[23]

Mild problems identified by the CDC include fever (up to 1 person out of 6); mild rash (about 1 person out of 20); swelling glands in the cheeks or neck (rare). Moderate problems include seizure caused by fever (about 1 out of 3,000 doses);

temporary pain and stiffness in the joints, mostly in teenage or adult women (up to 1 out of 4); temporary low platelet count, which can cause a bleeding disorder (about 1 out of 30,000 doses). Severe problems include a serious allergic reaction (less than 1 out of a million doses). Other problems that have not been linked directly to the vaccine are deafness; long-term seizures, coma or lowered consciousness; and permanent brain damage.

It is not the purpose of this analysis to advocate either for or against MMR vaccination. During my childhood, measles, mumps, and rubella were considered common childhood diseases. We were usually isolated to prevent spreading these diseases to others, but long-term health issues concerning them were believed to minimal. Other diseases, such as polio, were viewed as debilitating and were, therefore, addressed through vaccinations.

Polio Vaccination: A Historical Success

Vaccines administered in childhood have historically been effective in eliminating or reducing the incidence of such illnesses as polio. According to information provided by the Global Polio Eradication Initiative, supported by the World Health Organization, the U.S. Centers for Disease Control, and UNICEF, "Poliomyelitis (polio) is a highly infectious disease caused by a virus. It invades the nervous system, and can cause total paralysis in a matter of hours."[24]

More than 50 percent of polio cases affect children under three, but the disease can occur at any age. The virus is transmitted from person to person through the mouth and then multiplies in the intestine. It is spread primarily through contamination by feces of drinking water. Most people infected with poliovirus display no symptoms and can thus inadvertently spread the disease for several weeks before symptoms become manifest. One in 200 infections can cause irreversible paralysis, usually in the legs.[25] Five to ten percent of people who become paralyzed by the polio virus die when their breathing apparatus becomes paralyzed.

Polio has been virtually eliminated in industrialized nations through vaccines administered to children and by treatment of drinking water; however, vaccinated individuals who display no symptoms can spread the disease to unvaccinated people by being host to the virus: "Until the 1950s, polio crippled thousands of children every year in industrialized countries. Soon after the introduction of effective vaccines in the late 1950s . . . and early 1960s, . . . polio was brought under control, and practically eliminated as a public health problem in industrialized countries."[26]

Studies conducted in developing countries during the 1970s indicated that thousands of children were crippled every year by the disease, so that immunization programs were introduced worldwide, "helping to control the disease in many developing countries":

> Today, the disease has been eliminated from most of the world, and only seven countries world-wide remain polioendemic. This represents the lowest number of countries with circulating wild poliovirus. At the same time, the areas of transmission are more concentrated than ever—98 percent of all global cases are found in India, Nigeria and Pakistan.[27]

The success of vaccination programs in controlling diseases such as polio has led to the belief that vaccination programs can address and control all infectious diseases, but questions remain: Should all currently nonfatal infectious diseases be controlled through vaccination programs? Might control of these diseases by vaccination lead to even more dangerous diseases or more fatal variations of contemporary diseases if/when the disease-causing organisms become resistant to vaccination? The history of medicine suggests that the short life span of disease-causing organisms allows them to adapt more readily to changing conditions than humans are able to do.

THE NATURAL HISTORY OF HERBS

Our early hominid ancestors were foragers who moved from place to place, gathering plants and, less often, hunting for animals. As these hominid species foraged, it is likely they discovered plants that would ease the pain of injuries and help them heal from illnesses. These may have been our first herbalists.

As of at least 10,000 years ago, humans have based much of their survival needs on domesticated plants and animals. Deni Bown, author of *Encyclopedia of Herbs* (2001), suggests that the horticulture of herbs has historically been spread through trade, warfare, and migration. The earliest written and visual records of planted herb gardens are from Egypt, dating to around 4,000 years ago. Chamomile (Chamaemelum nobile) was identified by pollen analysis as the main herbal ingredient in the embalming oil use to mummify Rameses II, who died in 1224 BC. Bown notes:

> The lives of people and plants are more entwined than is often realized. Our passion for aromatics and flavorings inspired exploration and was a significant factor in colonial expansion. Some herbs have such power to change our physiological functioning that they have assumed social and religious importance, and in some cases revolutionized medicine, creating fortunes for those who harvest, process, and trade them. (2001:16)

Though it is prevalent in the Western world to distinguish between "good" and "bad" substances, herbs and other medications have the potential for both "good" and "evil." The Swiss physician and alchemist Paracelsus[28] (1493–1541) wrote that "All substances are poisons; there is none which is not a poison. The right dose differentiates between a poison and a remedy."[29]

What Is an Herb?

The official botanical definition of an herb is "a small, seed-bearing plant with fleshy, rather than woody parts" (Bown 2001:18). A broader definition includes trees, shrubs, annuals, algae, lichens, and fungi, which are valued for their flavor, fragrance, medicinal, and healthful qualities, as well as for economic and industrial uses. Economic and industrial uses include pesticides and dyes. In this book, we will focus on the nutritional and medical properties of herbs.

Bown notes that herbs work differently from medicines, in that medicines deliver only the known, tested active ingredients. Bown describes the philosophy underlying herbal medicine: "The whole plant (and extracts derived from it) contains many ingredients that work together, and which may produce a quite different effect (known as a synergistic effect) from that of a constituent if given on its own" (2001:19).

This is an important difference. Medicines are typically based on a single active ingredient plus a binder that facilitates administration of that ingredient. Any possible mediating ingredients in herbs will have been eliminated in the process of conducting clinical trials and preparing the medicine for market.

Well-trained herbalists recognize that all herbs—as well as all ingredients ingested or inserted into the human body—have side effects. One difference between herbs and medically prescribed medications is that the dosage of herbs is typically diluted, whereas the dosage of medicines is standardized. This has negative results on both sides. Individuals dosing themselves with herbs may imbibe overdoses in the belief that there is a difference between "good" and "bad" herbs. Medically prescribed dosages are based on statistical averages that may not hold true for individuals taking a particular drug.

Are Herbs Better than Science-Based Medicine?

Popular opinion in the United States suggests that herbs are more effective and less dangerous than medicines produced by pharmaceutical companies. This is not borne out by research. As an example, the herb black cohosh is believed by women and herbalists in the United States to relieve symptoms of menopause, such as hot flashes. Since a 2002 federal study showed that women who undertook estrogen replacement therapy ran an increased risk of breast cancer and heart disease, black cohosh became a leading alternative to hormone therapy. About 2 million American women turn fifty each year, and about 80 percent of them show some symptoms of menopause.[30]

The 2002 study was led by epidemiologist Katherine M. Newton of Group Health, a health system based in Seattle. It was sponsored by the National Institute on Aging and the National Center for Complementary and Alternative Medicine, both components of the National Institutes of Health, and published in the *Annals of Internal Medicine*. Controlled clinical trials demonstrated that the herb was no more effective than a placebo. Only estrogen significantly reduced hot flashes. Newton said, "In the doses we used, and the way we used it, it did not work."

The study involved 351 women, aged forty-five to fifty-five, averaging about six symptoms a day. Half were in the midst of menopause and half were post-menopausal. The women were divided into five groups: (1) One group was given 160 milligrams of black cohosh per day. (2) A second group was given a mixture of nine herbs, plus 200 milligrams of black cohosh per day. (3) The third group was given the herb mixture and women were encouraged to eat more soy foods. (4) The fourth group was given estrogen with or without progestin. (5) The fifth group was given a placebo. "Women receiving either black cohosh or the herb mixture had an average reduction of 0.5 symptoms per day compared with those in the placebo group, a statistically insignificant finding. Women receiving estrogen . . . had a reduction of four symptoms per day. Those consuming soy . . . had more symptoms . . . for reasons that are not clear."[31]

The results of this study alone do not suggest that women should stop using black cohosh to relieve menopausal symptoms. It is a cost-benefit decision. Reducing menopausal symptoms by using prescribed hormone replacement medications run a risk of potentially fatal illnesses, such as breast cancer and heart disease. Women who use black cohosh have reduction of symptoms similar to those of placebos, which have been shown to reduce symptoms in some cases and for certain types of disorders.

Many websites promote the use of black cohosh for relieving menopausal symptoms, but few list potential side effects. One website, for example, describes black cohosh as a phytoestrogen and affirms that it can restore "your hormone imbalance and relieve the discomfort of PMS & menopause symptoms." In American popular culture, soy has been promoted as a solution to many kinds of health problems. In the study mentioned above, women who consumed soy products had more, not fewer, menopause symptoms. I use this example to cite the divergence between American popular culture and a disinterested evaluation of health care procedures.

Lack of Regulations

Herbal medicines and dietary supplements are not regulated by the FDA because this organization does not have authority over these forms of medications. The American public assumes it is protected by the FDA from overstated claims by manufacturers of herbal medicines, dietary supplements, and cosmetics; however, the FDA has been stripped of this oversight by members of the U.S. Congress, who are protecting their own constituencies, those who manufacture these products.

Deni Bown, author of *Encyclopedia of Herbs* (2001) writes, "A number of herbs discussed in this book are potentially dangerous. They are subject to legal restrictions regarding formulation, use, and sale." (2001:19). These restrictions are based on three main categories: (1) poisonous herbs sold for therapeutic use; (2) herbs that may be hazardous as garden plants; (3) herbs that have become pernicious weeds outside their country of origin.

A popular view that medicines produced through scientific methods are "unnatural" and "bad," whereas herbal medicines are "good" and "safe," is a binary opposition that does not hold up in practice. All medications—whether produced according to scientific methods, based in traditional herbal remedies, or marketed as herbal dietary supplements—must be evaluated according to a cost-benefit analysis: "Is the relief of symptoms I'm getting worth the side effects I'm suffering." That question can only be answered through the interaction of the patient and the health-care provider.

Health-care providers can make recommendations, but the patient has the power to make the final decision. The United States is a litigious society, which permits people to avoid responsibility for their decisions. This erodes the ability of health-care providers to make the efficacious recommendations they would make for members of their own families. Our litigious society requires health-care providers to consider their patients as potential enemies who could cost them their livelihoods and invalidate their professional training. This is a lose-lose situation for both patients and health-care providers.

SCIENTIFIC METAPHORS

In spite of its emphasis on science, Western medicine is still bounded about with metaphor. The debate over medical marijuana use, which dominated media at the beginning of this century, illustrates the juxtaposition of symbols and scientific discourse. Marijuana is the common name for the hemp plant *Cannabis sativa*. It is viewed by many to be an effective treatment for pain and nausea, including when these symptoms are caused by diseases such as cancer and the side effects of chemotherapy. Marijuana also stimulates the appetite, which can be useful in treating appetite loss attending certain types of illness, such as AIDS. Marijuana also appears to be effective in treating such organic disorders as glaucoma, a condition that can lead to blindness because of pressure within the eye. Officially, however, marijuana is viewed as a dangerous drug, especially in the United States. Marijuana is illegal in most states for medicinal purposes and illegal in all states for recreational purposes.

Opponents of legalizing marijuana for medical purposes fear that recognizing the plant's medical value would open the door to legalizing it for recreational use. Those who take this position suggest that THC (tetrahydrocannabinol), the ingredient presumed to be therapeutic in marijuana, should be extracted and administered in pill form. As medical anthropologists could predict, a THC pill is unlikely to be as effective in treating symptoms as use of the marijuana plant in its native form, even if researchers have correctly identified the active ingredient, because a pill is not processed by the body as easily as the same chemical administered in a more diffuse form. This is partly because a pill releases its active ingredients more rapidly, and its effectiveness may be altered by digestive processes. In addition, as noted earlier, anthropologists have long observed that herbs consumed in their native form according to traditional practices do not produce the addictive or extreme reactions characteristic of recreational use of extracts.

Diplomacy, Efficacy, and Medical Research

Officials and a pharmaceutical researcher in Britain took a diplomatic approach to adapting cannabis (marijuana) for medicinal use. Highly publicized arrests of multiple sclerosis patients who had been medicating themselves with marijuana in 1997 led to officially fostered research into developing a more "medicinal" marijuana. Alan Macfarlane, the British Home Office's chief drug inspector, described its parameters: "We insisted that they develop a proper medicine. It had to be textured like a medicine, look like a medicine, behave like a medicine and be delivered like a medicine."

In other words, the job of converting cannabis into medicine involved repackaging. This was not an entirely cynical public relations campaign. A tenet of Western medicine is that dosages be controlled rather than randomly administered. Based on their studies of Moroccan hashish, British researchers discovered that the marijuana ingredient CBD (cannabidiol) had greater therapeutic properties and fewer psychoactive properties than the more widely publicized THC. As a result of government-sponsored research, a British pharmaceutical company, GW Pharmaceuticals, began marketing a spray consisting of about 425 chemicals found in marijuana leaves. Unlike the native plant, the spray provides more consistent quality and gives physicians the ability to regulate dosages.

Based on a small sample of twenty-four patients, Oxford researchers determined that plant-derived cannabis medicinal extracts (CME) can alleviate neurogenic symptoms unresponsive to standard treatment. The patients suffered from such neurological disorders as multiple sclerosis and spinal cord injury, as well as brachial plexus damage in which the nerves that conduct signals from the spine to the shoulder, arm, and hand are damaged. One subject experienced phantom pain after a limb amputation due to neurofibromatosis, a genetic disorder that causes tumors to form on nerves and causes abnormalities in the skin and bone deformities.

The cannabis extract CBD (cannabidiol) significantly reduced pain. THC (delta-9-tetrahydrocannabinol) significantly reduced pain, muscle spasm, and spasticity, while improving subjects' appetites. The combination of THC and CBD significantly reduced muscle spasm and improved sleep. All three CMEs produced relief in other parameters measured, including bladder control, coordination, alertness, happiness, relaxation, optimism, energy, sense of well-being, and feelings of being refreshed. Derick T. Wade et al. write, "Individual patients also reported benefits with other symptoms such as co-ordination, bladder and bowel control, and visual acuity but these were not studied systematically" (2003:22). Authors of the study note that CBD had analgesic and antispasticity properties without psychoactive side effects:

> Early experience with rapid initial dosing with THC:CBD indicated the need for more gradual introduction to CME. When over-dosing did take place supportive measures were all that were required. Patients disliked intoxication and wished to avoid it, in contrast to recreational users. During self-titration this was the dose-limiting effect in several patients, and was the primary reason for withdrawal in three cases. However, with careful self-titration, most patients were able to achieve useful symptom relief at a subintoxication dose. Soreness from the alcohol solvent was noted in a few patients and caused one to withdraw. (Wade et al. 2003:24)

The researchers add, "No patients were suspected of abusing CME, and most used doses that were much less than the maximum permitted" (Wade et al. 2003:24–25).

The Oxford study confirms earlier research revealing that patients self-titrating after surgery administer to themselves lower dosages of pain medication than would have been administered by their caretakers. This could be due in part to the fact that patients administer lower doses as needed rather than according to a set formula and schedule. The ability to control one's pain also has powerful psychological benefits, including reduction of feelings of fear and helplessness.

Because the Oxford study used whole-plant cannabis medicinal extracts, it also supports what anthropologists have long proposed, that indigenous use of substances do not have the negative side effects associated with recreational extracts, such as cocaine or medicines that extract only the active ingredient in the herb. The researchers write:

> Recently, standardized whole-plant cannabis medicinal extracts (CME) have become available for clinical research. This is important because many components of the plant other than THC may have therapeutic potential or synergistic activity. These include nonpsychoactive cannabinoids such as cannabidiol (CBD), as well as various terpenoids and flavonoids. (Wade et al. 2003:19)

Terpenoids are an abundant and volatile plant compound that form the basis for a variety of phenomena, including flavorings, perfumes, and pharmaceuticals, as well as those having antimicrobial and antifungal properties.[32] Flavonoids have antioxidant properties that have been shown to have antibacterial, anti-inflammatory, antiallergic, antimutagenic, antiviral, antineoplastic, antithrombotic, and vasodilatory activity.[33] In other words, they can perhaps guard against the mutations that lead to such diseases as cancer, heart disease, and stroke. Much of the research on terpenoids and flavonoids is still in its infancy, and therefore is controversial. Maintaining health is the result of the interaction of many factors other than dietary intake, including activity, attitude, and stress levels, as well as social and physical environment.

In 1985, the U.S. Food and Drug Administration approved an oral cannabis-derived medicine called Marinol. In 2006, the U.S. Food and Drug Administration approved advanced clinical trials for the marijuana-derived drug Sativex, developed by GW Pharmaceuticals. Lester Grinspoon, an emeritus professor of psychiatry at Harvard Medical School and author of *Marijuana, the Forbidden Medicine* (Yale University Press, 1997), describes the actions of the U.S. Food and Drug Administration as "contradicting itself" because the agency reiterated its position that cannabis has no medical utility.[34] Grinspoon adds:

> There is very little evidence that smoking marijuana as a means of taking it represents a significant health risk. Although cannabis has been smoked widely in Western countries for more than four decades, there have been no reported cases of lung cancer or emphysema attributed to marijuana. I suspect that a day's breathing in any city with poor air quality poses more of a threat than inhaling a day's dose—which for many ailments is just a portion of a joint—of marijuana.[35]

Grinspoon notes that orally administered Marinol requires one and a half hours to take effect. Sativex, which is administered by holding a few drops of the liquid under the tongue acts more quickly, but not so quickly as inhaling marijuana. Grinspoon writes, "One of the most important characteristics of cannabis is how fast it acts when it is inhaled, which allows patients to easily determine the right dose for symptom relief."[36] Because Sativex and Marinol are slow-acting, "self-titration," or self-dosage is difficult. Research in hospitals involving other painkillers has determined that patients typically do not overmedicate themselves using "self-titration." In fact, they typically administer less of a painkiller than would be administered according to prescription.

Much of the debate over medical marijuana is cultural, rather than chemical. Puritanical values continue to dominate the discourse in the United States. A puritanical value in the United States is that anything that feels good or tastes good must be harmful, or even sinful. We have forgotten the lessons of the Prohibition era early in the twentieth century. Prohibition of buying or imbibing alcoholic substances did not prevent people from doing this. It just made them criminals.

15

Public Policy and Health-Care Delivery Systems

CASE STUDY
Atomic Bomb Testing and Marshall Islanders

After World War II, the United Nations transferred administration of the Marshall Islands in the Pacific, among other islands in the Trust Territory of the Pacific—Islands (TTPI), to the United States with the stipulation that the United States promote the health and well-being of the citizens of the trust territory and "protect the inhabitants [of the Trusteeship] against the loss of their lands and resources" (UN Trusteeship Council 1958). Anthropologist Holly M. Barker writes, "From 1946 to 1958, the U.S. government used its territory to detonate 67 atomic and thermonuclear weapons in the air, on the land, and in the seas surrounding the Marshall Islands" (2004:20). Marshallese told Barker their experiences both during the unannounced blasts and the pattern of birth defects that occurred afterward. "I cannot describe what it was like. It felt like the air was alive. . . . Everything was crazy . . . That afternoon, I found my hair was covered with a white power-like substance. It had no smell and no taste when I tried tasting it. Nearly all the people on Rongelap [atoll] became violently ill" (2004:51). A mother described the birth defects of her two sons born after the blasts. Both quickly died: "My second son, born in 1960, was delivered live but missing the whole back of his skull—as if it had been sawed off. So the back part of the brain and the spinal cord was fully exposed. . . . You knew, it was heartbreaking having to nurse my son, all the while taking care his brain didn't fall into my lap" (2004:54). A number of the babies born in the decades after the nuclear tests were described as "looking like grapes," which has been described as disrupted cell division. Barker conducted a linguistic analysis to assess how the nuclear testing experience affected both the quality of Marshall Islanders' lives and their ability to gain compensation from the U.S. government. She writes, "Anthropologists are uniquely qualified to understand and articulate problems facing communities and to take actionable steps to assist communities, particularly communities where we work. . . . If our research is going to help the people, it must be owned by them. It is essential to include the people we work for

289

in every phase of our work, from designing a research approach, to gathering and analyzing data (2004:158).

By using methods of linguistic analysis, Barker emphasizes the insider perspective in evaluating the experiences of Marshall Islanders as a result of U.S. nuclear testing. Statistics may provide an abstract vision of the enormity of such an event. The language used by those who experienced the event illustrates its personal cost.

Medical anthropologists have studied health and disease in many contexts. Their contribution has focused on the social consequences of disease ratios and demographic circumstances. A number of these studies have been described in previous chapters of this book. This chapter will focus on social conflicts, malnutrition, population, and access to medical care.

THE GENEVA CONVENTIONS

After the horrors of World War II, during which millions of Jews, gypsies, Russians, and others died, an international committee of Allies convened in Geneva, Switzerland, to prevent such a horror from ever happening again. But humans are fragile. They forget quickly, and in many cases, they have never learned of the horrors that humans have inflicted on other humans. The Geneva Conventions, rules for conduct during war, were aimed at preventing large-scale torture of the human species. The conventions specified what conditions were permissible in treatment of prisoners and other personnel involved in conflicts.

The Geneva Conventions were not adopted for entirely humane reasons. Participants in the coalition were concerned about protecting themselves and their own people. They understood that disregard of humane standards was a threat to the survival of the human species as a whole. The detonation of two atomic bombs by the United States in Japan at the end of World War II may have provided a stimulus for such an undertaking. It became clear that new forms of technology could mean the extinction of the human species. In a 1961 address to the United Nations, U.S. President John F. Kennedy stated:

> Unconditional war can no longer lead to unconditional victory. It can no longer serve to settle disputes. It can no longer be of concern to great powers alone. For a nuclear disaster, spread by words and waters and fear, could well engulf the great and the small, the rich and the poor, the committed and the uncommitted alike. Mankind must put an end to war or war will put an end to mankind.[1]

In the introduction to his book *Philosophy of History* (1832), Georg Wilhelm Friedrich Hegel wrote, "What experience and history teach is this—that people and governments have never learned anything from history, or acted on principles deduced from it." We daily find this to be true. What we failed to learn from World War II is that any one of us can be detained and tortured at any time. What we should have learned from subsequent events is that any powerful government can set aside the Geneva Conventions at any time.

A group of Harvard Medical School researchers led by J. Wesley Boyd found that American medical students receive inadequate instruction about military medical ethics and the ethics required of physicians under the Geneva Conventions. The survey of students at eight U.S. medical schools found that 94 percent had received less than one hour of instruction about military medical ethics. They also found that only 37 percent of medical students were aware that the Geneva Conventions apply whether or not war had been declared. Of the students, 33.8 percent did not know that the Geneva Conventions state that physicians should "treat the sickest first, regardless of nationality," 37 percent didn't know that the Geneva Conventions prohibit threatening or demeaning prisoners, as well as depriving them of food or water for any length of time, and 33.9 percent could not state under what circumstances they would be required to disobey an unethical order from a superior. The study was published in the *International Journal of Health Services*.

The American Medical Association defines torture as "the deliberate, systematic, or wanton administration of cruel, inhumane, and degrading treatments or punishments during imprisonment or detainment."[2] The AMA policy adds: "Physicians must oppose and must not participate in torture for any reason. Participation in torture includes, but is not limited to, providing or withholding any services, substances, or knowledge to facilitate the practice of torture. Physicians must not be present when torture is used or threatened."[3] AMA policy also specifies the conditions under which physicians may examine or treat prisoners:

> Physicians may treat prisoners or detainees if doing so is in their best interest, but physicians should not treat individuals to verify their health so that torture can begin or continue. Physicians who treat torture victims should not be persecuted. Physicians should help provide support for victims of torture and, whenever possible, strive to change situations in which torture is practiced or the potential for torture is great.[4]

The AMA policy statement, issued in December 1999, does not state what sanctions, if any, would be applied to a physician who did not comply with the organization's policy on torture.

SOCIAL INEQUALITY AND AVAILABILITY OF MEDICAL CARE

The 2006 World Health Report, compiled by the World Health Organization, reveals a great disparity between the need for medical care and the availability of medical care worldwide. The report estimates a worldwide shortage of almost 4.3 million doctors, midwives, nurses, and support workers. The most severe shortage was in sub-Saharan Africa, where there was need for a 139 percent increase in medical personnel. Critical shortages were identified in 36 countries of the African continent. The next most critical area was South and East Asia, with shortages concentrated in six of the eleven countries.

The 2007 World Health Organization Report acknowledged the continued looming threat of an influenza pandemic, outbreaks of Ebola, Marburg disease (hemorrhagic fever), and other infectious diseases, natural disasters, and high rates of women who die in pregnancy and childbirth in developing countries; however, the report also cited positive developments in international health care. Among these positive effects were that "public and private partners came together to improve global health with notable results."[5] Specifically, the WHO Report noted that progress had been made to halt resurging yellow fever in Africa.

Yellow fever is caused by a virus transmitted by a mosquito. It can be particularly injurious because it is spread by the lymphatic system, and therefore attacks internal organs, including the heart, kidneys, adrenal glands, and the liver. Symptoms include fever, muscle pain (including a severe backache), headache, shivers, and loss of appetite, as well as nausea or vomiting. Among 15 percent of patients, a toxic phase develops within twenty-four hours that includes bleeding from the mouth, nose, eyes, and stomach. Half the patients who develop this complication die within two weeks. The other half recover without significant organ damage. Vaccines are available to protect against yellow fever, and a single dose confers protection for ten years or more.[6] The disease is largely confined to tropical regions, including South America and Africa. In Africa, the disease is primarily located in the moist savanna zones of West and Central Africa during the rainy season, though outbreaks can occur in urban areas and villages. To a lesser extent, the disease can also occur in tropical forests.[7]

Infectious Diseases and Charitable Organizations

Among the organizations involved in promoting health care internationally is the Bill and Melinda Gates Foundation, established by the founder of Microsoft and his wife. The policy statement of the organization reports that "The foundation is guided by the belief that all lives, no matter where they are lived, have equal value. The mission of our Global Health Program is to encourage the development of life-saving medical advances and to help ensure they reach the people who are disproportionately affected."[8]

The organization focuses its funding in two main areas: extending access to existing vaccines, drugs, and other medical tools to fighting diseases common in developing countries; and promoting research to develop health solutions that are effective, affordable, and practical.[9] The foundation's priorities for diseases and conditions are as follows: (1) acute diarrheal illness, which "contributes to the deaths of 2 million to 3 million young children each year";[10] (2) acute lower respiratory infections, including pneumonia, "which kill about 2 million young children every year";[11] (3) child health; (4) HIV/AIDS; (5) malaria; (6) poor nutrition; (7) reproductive and maternal health; (8) vaccine-preventable diseases; and (10) other infectious diseases, including "sexually transmitted infections, infections involving multicellular organisms such as worms, and those caused by parasites transmitted through insects."[12]

The Bill and Melinda Gates Foundation was criticized in an article in the *Los Angeles Times* for not addressing all the ills afflicting international populations. In fact, the article suggested that addressing only a few of these ills led to an increase in other health problems.[13] The article ignores several important issues involved in addressing international health problems. Charitable organizations, such as the Bill and Melinda Gates Foundation, are obliged to define and specify their goals so they can be held accountable for their contributions.

In the past, some "charitable" organizations have obtained U.S. income tax advantages by making contributions that could not be traced or accounted for. In addition, it is an unfortunate fact of human existence, as well as that of other animals, that survival of one life-threatening event does not guarantee that one will survive a later life-threatening event. If more people stay alive, there will be more people who encounter other hazards that challenge the human condition. If, for example, I am successfully treated for cancer, this does not guarantee that I will not be killed in an accident on the way home from the treatment, or that I will not develop an untreatable illness later on. The more people there are on earth, the more potential there is for diseases to develop and for accidents to happen. This does not negate the attempt to deal with what Shakespeare called "the slings and arrows of outrageous fortune."[14]

Health Care and Population Disparities

The disparity in available medical may be exacerbated by increases in world population and shifts in the population distribution. According to the 2004 Revision of the United Nations Population Estimates and Projections, the world's population is expected to reach 9.1 billion by the year 2050, and 34 million people will still be added annually by mid-century, even if fertility levels decline. Further, there will be a major shift in the world population demographics between now and 2050 from the developed regions of the world to less-developed regions of the world:

> Today, 95 percent of all population growth is absorbed by the developing world, and 5 percent by the developed world. By 2050, according to the medium variant,[15] the population of the more developed countries as a whole would be declining by about 1 million persons a year and that of the developing world would be adding 35 million annually, 22 million of which would be absorbed by the least developed countries. (2004:xviii)

Between 2005 and 2050, the population is expected to at least triple in a number of developing countries. Among them are Afghanistan, Burkina Faso, Burundi, Chad, Congo, the Democratic Republic of Congo, the Democratic Republic of Timor-Leste, Guinea-Bissau, Liberia, Mali, Niger, and Uganda. This demographic shift has profound implications for public policy, since increases in poverty and malnutrition are likely to make major demands on health care delivery systems. The 2006 projections do not include warfare conditions, such as have occurred in Iraq, Afghanistan, Africa, and Eastern Europe.

The U.S. Census Bureau notes that between 1804 and 1922, a period of 118 years, the world population increased from 1 billion to 2 billion. Between 1987 and 1999, a period of only 12 years, the world population increased from 5 billion to 6 billion. The world population is expected to reach 9 billion by 2050. The U.S. Census Bureau predicts that the population grown rate will slow due to two factors: increased use of contraception and the AIDS pandemic.[16]

MEDICINE AND PUBLIC POLICY

It is not a secret that the richest and most powerful people in the world have access to the most expensive medical care. It is not necessarily clear that this is the "best" medicine in terms of quality of life. Just because an individual can be kept alive by extreme interventions does not mean that these are the best interventions for a particular patient. For all of us at the time of death, our fear of death may trump our fear of life. Ultimately, however, death may relieve us of burdensome lifestyle obligations. Heirs waiting at the bedside may be torn between anticipation of an inheritance and grief over loss of a significant elder, accompanied by anxiety over the assumption of adult responsibilities.

A philosophy in Western Europe and the United States is that there should be equal access to health care for all people regardless of their life circumstances; however, social circumstances often mediate against this. Rishi Manchanda, a senior resident in UCLA's combined internal medicine/pediatrics residency program, describes the difficulties in providing medical care to poor and uninsured individuals in the United States.[17] Health-care professionals are required to spend part of their training caring for indigent patients; however, their training does not extend to fully understanding health-care funding or management of health care for indigents or those not covered by insurance.

Manchanda notes that indigents and uninsured patients are not assured that they will be treated by the same medical personnel. He quotes a male patient who arrived at a free clinic as saying, "Every time I come here, I meet a new doctor. Don't make me tell you everything about me all over again."[18]

Further, the medical care specialists treating him had little knowledge of procedures required for filling medical prescriptions and instructions. Patients may be given prescriptions for which there was no systematized means of filling them. Patients may be marked as "noncompliant," diagnosed as a conscious choice, when their noncompliance may be mandated by prevailing prescription or treatment guidelines.

POPULATION AND PUBLIC POLICY

Probably the most serious epidemic challenging medicine today is the vast number of humans on the planet. Though the dramatic increase in population, a fourfold increase between 1900 and the present, had been long predicted, and anthropologists as well as others had ignored the predictions, ugly specters—including overpopulation and new forms of disease—began to appear. In his 1976 book, *Anthropology and Contemporary Problems*, John Bodley wrote of a rapidly changing world in which small-scale societies were being obliterated by the emergence of an industrial civilization, which Bodley calls a "brilliant short-term success": "We have eliminated the earlier primitive cultures, which were proven long-run successes, and there are now clear indications that civilization has accumulated enough internal problems to be self-terminating. We seem about to become victims of our own evolutionary progress" (1976:vii).

Bodley viewed what he called "primitive cultures" to be well-adapted to their environments, whereas "civilized" cultures threaten to overrun the same earth that has supported human life for more than 100,000 years and our hominid ancestors for more than 4 million years.[19] To avoid self-termination, Bodley advises, we must consider all that we know about human groups, obtained through ethnographic research, in an attempt to "compare their solutions to basic human problems with our own solutions" (1976:vii). Bodley adds, "Perhaps this is anthropology's most critical purpose" (1976:vii).

We no longer classify human societies as either "primitive" or "civilized," but anthropologists today are dealing with the drastic changes Bodley predicted would take place. About the only problem Bodley did not address in his book was the spread of infectious diseases, such as AIDS and the resurgence of tuberculosis, which have begun to afflict large numbers of people around the world and seem to have made the survival of the human species more tenuous. Bodley, however, did anticipate medical anthropology by calling for more engagement on the part of anthropologists:

> [*Anthropology and Contemporary Human Problems*] is a treatment of and a call for more anthropological research into the problems of overconsumption, adaptation to environment, resource depletion, hunger and starvation, overpopulation, violence, and war. Anthropologists have dealt with these issues in many different ways, in many different times, and in many different cultures. This book attempts to relate these anthropological insights to the contemporary world. (1976:v)

Bodley bases his work on that of anthropologists, as well as that of authors in other disciplines, who have cautioned the American public about the dangers of overexploiting the world's resources. In his 1968 book, *The Population Bomb*, biologist Paul Ehrlich warned that the "population explosion" would lead to famines in which millions of people would starve to death. Ehrlich was echoing what others had said before. Notably, the British economist Thomas Malthus had warned of such a probability more than 160 years earlier: "[The] power of obtaining an additional quantity of food from the earth by proper management and in a certain time, has the most relation imaginable to the power of keeping pace with an unrestricted increase of population" (cited in Bodley 1976:139). In 1972, Ehrlich and Ehrlich compared the rapid growth of the human population to devastation by natural forces:

> The explosive growth of the human population is the most significant terrestrial event of the past million millennia. . . . No geological event in a billion years—not the emergence of mighty mountain ranges, not the submergences of entire subcontinents, nor the occurrence of periodic glacial ages—has posed a threat to terrestrial life comparable to that of human overpopulation. (1972:1)

As the total population increases, the health of individuals almost inevitably decreases. More people are competing for decreasing sources of food and other resources. As Malthus noted, a population increases beyond the capacity of the earth (environment) to support it. As the human population increases, we turn more areas of the earth's surfaces into uninhabitable environments or overtax the environments we have previously exploited. As we save a life, we condemn other humans, and other forms of life, to extinction. This is an inevitable product of the competition for survival. Even knowing these inevitable consequences, it is difficult

to condemn other members of our species to extinction without attempting to provide them with adequate medical care. Statistics mean nothing when we are face to
face with the eyes of a hungry child.

Who Benefits from Hunger?

The inequities of social status become even more troubling when we compare the
resources available to one population but not to another. The pets of humans in
affluent populations eat better than humans in the poorer regions of the world. This
is not a competition of humans against other species. It is a competition of humans
against other members of their own species. Those who have great wealth exploit
those who have less wealth.

As the geographer Jared Diamond (1991) has pointed out, exploitation of the
poor by the rich has been the case in human history since the agricultural revolu-
tion. Specifically, the food surplus generated by intensive agriculture—which began
to displace foraging about 10,000 years ago—leads to a high degree of task specialization and resulting status inequalities among settled populations. The increase in
status differentiation requires the development of policing organizations to protect
the rich from the predations of the poor. The wealth generated by producing agricultural surpluses also gives rise to the need for standing armies to protect against
invaders seeking to acquire the stored wealth of sedentary populations.

Even as some observers were warning against the effects of a dramatically increasing world population, others were lauding its effects on the world economy. Colin
Clark, a British economist and statistician, linked population growth to "progress":
"[Population growth] brings economic hardship to communities living by traditional methods of agriculture; but it is the only force powerful enough to make such
communities change their methods, and in the long run transforms them into much
more advanced and productive societies" (quoted in Bodley, 1976:140–141).

Clark suggested that the earth's resources are "immense" and that "the beneficial
economic effects of large and expanding markets are abundantly clear" (quoted in
Bodley, 1976:141). Clark is correct in stating that "large and expanding markets"
convey economic benefits, but it is evident from his argument that these benefits do
not extend equally to all members of society. People who exploit a large consumer
market base obtain more economic benefits than those who buy from them. And
those who buy are limited by their incomes in what they can buy.

An abundance of labor typically pushes wages down as people compete for jobs,
so that population growth enriches those at the higher rungs of the economic lad-
der, but impoverishes those on the lower levels. Even the poorest of us benefit the
economy by providing labor and a market, however limited. Both the super-rich and
the super-poor contribute to what Bodley calls a "culture of consumption"
(1975:4–5). Bodley considers "the level of consumption" to be a more critical variable than overpopulation: "Quality of life, or standard of living, must be considered
in any attempt to assess the carrying capacity for given environments. Population
pressure is always relative to particular cultural conditions" (1976:141).

A major difference in the economic disparity is that affluent humans have medical means to control their own fertility and conserve their own wealth, but they
have the ability to deny it to people who do not have the same access to fertility

restricting procedures. Thus, fecundity among the impoverished people of the world contributes to the prosperity of those who have the means to restrict their own reproductive capacity and to deny it to the people they exploit.

What Disparity in Wealth Means for Health and Healing

The sickest people on earth are generally the poorest because they do not have access to the most nutritious food resources or to adequate medical care. The people I am calling "poor" are those who do not have access to adequate resources in general. Poverty is relative. Farmers who live in rich environments can always provide for their needs, even if they don't have much money in the bank. And the farm, if paid for, can provide collateral for a loan in times of crisis. Even farmers or horticulturalists in inhospitable areas can eke out a few small plants or forage for wild plants and animals.

Those who suffer most in terms of deprivation are the urban poor. Though they may have better access to health care than the rural poor, they cannot produce or gather enough food to meet their nutritional needs. Further, they are subject to crowding and pollution. These three factors alone—pollution, crowding, and poor nutrition—can produce tremendous health problems. Pollution provides a medium in which bacteria and viruses can thrive. Disease-causing organisms are disseminated through contact, so crowding facilitates their spread. Humans are vectors for transmitting certain types of diseases. Poor nutrition impairs the immune system, so malnourished individuals cannot defend themselves against infection. An undernourished, untreated, and overworked population subject to pollution can become a gigantic petri dish for breeding new diseases and new strains of existing diseases. Ultimately, these diseases spread to the rich, as India's cholera epidemic of the nineteenth century illustrates.

"The best laid schemes . . ."

"The best laid schemes o' mice and men Gang aft a-gley." Robert Burns' words from his poem "To a Mouse" illustrate the difficulty in designing health-care delivery programs that consider such factors as local social and cultural contexts, evaluation of need priorities, and coordination of funding agencies. Sub-Saharan Africa is the region most often identified as in urgent need of crisis intervention. In recent decades it has been afflicted by high rates of HIV/AIDS infection, famine, malnutrition, political instability, lack of educational facilities, and rates of population growth that exceed the resource base. These problems have been added to the longstanding problem of malaria and other infectious illnesses indigenous to the region.

Relief agencies, such as the World Health Organization, agree that many of the problems could be resolved using inexpensive solutions, such as distributing vitamins and mosquito nets. According to a December 2006 report in *The New York Times*, Africans in the village of Ponyamayira, Ghana, were eager to accept mosquito nets to protect their children from malaria. When they arrived to pick up the mosquito nets, aid workers also administered polio vaccine, vitamin A, deworming medicine, and measles vaccine to their children. On the surface, this sounds like an effective approach, but it failed on two sides: It was not coordinated with local cultures, and it did not coordinate the aid efforts of the many agencies involved.

The policy was described as "a winning strategy" by a World Health Organization official and as "spectacularly successful" by the head of the Global Fund to Fight AIDS, Tuberculosis and Malaria. But funding for the program was canceled after its introduction. Dr. Arata Kochi, who leads the global malaria program for the World Health Organization, explains the problems with the program: "There were too many cooks."[20]

Anthropologists might explain it differently: The program did not take culture and social organization into account. There were at least two cultures involved here, often with competing goals. Aid workers wanted to solve the problems of the region and announce success in doing that. Indigenous people just wanted to keep their children healthy. Further, they wanted to be involved in the decisions about what keeps their children healthy. They understood the importance of mosquito nets in protecting their children and themselves from malaria-causing mosquitoes. They were not consulted or informed about the other medical interventions they were forced to undergo.

Informed parents can be valuable partners in the prevention and treatment of disease. Arrogant and undertrained health care workers can subvert the most ambitious programs aimed at preventing and treating infectious diseases.

THE HUMAN COST OF MALNUTRITION

Nancy Scheper-Hughes was drawn into the field of medical anthropology in 1965 as a Peace Corps volunteer and community development/health-care worker. In the months following a military coup in Brazil, Scheper-Hughes took up her work in a shantytown in Northeast Brazil called the Alto Do Cruzeiro (Crucifix Hill). The nine states that make up the area are the poorest in the country. In 1982, Scheper-Hughes returned to Alto Do Cruzeiro as an anthropologist.

During her initial stay in the shantytown, Scheper-Hughes was introduced to the high cost of poverty and its effect on infant mortality. Largely because of the high rate of infant and child mortality, life expectancy in the Northeast is only forty years:

> Approximately one million children in Brazil under the age of five die each year. The children of the Northeast, especially those born in shantytowns on the periphery of urban life, are at a very high risk of death. In these areas, children are born without the traditional protection of breast-feeding, subsistence gardens, stable marriages, and multiple adult caretakers that exists in the interior [of Brazil]. (Scheper-Hughes 2003:219[1989])

Rapid and large-scale industrialization was displacing many sharecroppers, who were being replaced by farm machinery. Women in the shantytowns found work as domestics in the homes of the rich or as "scabs" on sugar plantations. Child care was an ongoing problem:

> The women of the Alto may not bring their babies with them into the homes of the wealthy, where the often-sick infants are considered sources of contamination, and they cannot carry the little ones to the riverbanks where they wash clothes because the river is

heavily infested with schistosomes and other deadly parasites. Nor can they carry their young children to the plantations, which are often several miles away. (2003:219 [1989])

According to Scheper-Hughes, "the average woman of the Alto experiences 9.5 pregnancies, 3.5 child deaths, and 1.5 still births. Seventy percent of all child deaths in the Alto occur in the first six months of life, and 82 percent by the end of the first year. Of all deaths in the community each year, about 45 percent are of children under the age of five" (2003:221[1989]). Scheper-Hughes asserts that mothers cope with the high rate of child loss by postponing investment in a child until it has displayed a "knack" or "taste" for life.

Scheper-Hughes observes that the postponement of parental investment by mothers is likely to contribute to the high rate of infant mortality; however, she notes that what she calls "selective neglect" and "passive infanticide" has been historically and cross-culturally widespread in areas where resources are scarce. She adds that these "active survival strategies" could contribute to overall survival, since resources not directed toward infants who "want" to die can be invested in promoting the survival of healthier siblings. Mothers in Scheper-Hughes' study who did not expect their infants to survive withheld nutrition as well as other forms of nurturance.

Scheper-Hughes does not precisely state what criteria mothers look for when evaluating an infant's "knack" or "taste" for life; however, birth spacing and subjective evaluations of an infant's health, as measured by its vitality, could be factors in postponing parental investment. Where resources are scarce, such subjective evaluations of an infant's chances for survival could promote the survival of more vigorous infants.

According to UNICEF, 11 million children each year—about 30,000 a day—die before reaching their fifth birthday, mostly from preventable or treatable causes."[21] The highest child mortality rates are in sub-Saharan Africa, an average of 173 deaths per 1,000 live births, more than twenty-four times the rate of child death in industrialized countries. South Asia ranks second, with ninety-eight deaths per 1,000 live births, fourteen times the rate of child deaths in industrialized countries. In sub-Saharan Africa, HIV/AIDS is contributing to an increase in child death rates, but "the cause of most deaths in developing countries remains the same as in the past: easily treated or prevented killers such as pneumonia, diarrheal diseases and malnutrition for which affordable solutions exist."[22]

Malnutrition can contribute to high death rates among both children and adults by eroding the immune system. UNICEF attributes many of the problems afflicting children to the "poor nutrition and health of mothers throughout their life and before, during and after pregnancy."[23] This bears on the health of children in a number of ways. The health and nutrition of the mother shape the development of the child before birth. In addition, a mother's poor health and nutrition may cause her to die during pregnancy and childbirth. If she survives pregnancy and childbirth, her ability to care for her children may be negatively affected by poor nutrition and health. UNICEF defines early childhood as "the period up to when a child begins school, with special attention given between birth and three years of age. It includes the prenatal months, since a woman's health before and during pregnancy has a major impact on the survival, growth and development of her child."[24] UNICEF recommends saving the child by empowering the mother, economically and nutritionally.

Even if children survive the effects of malnutrition, they may suffer from life-long disability that could prevent them from participating fully in their society. They may not reach their full growth potential or may be susceptible to disease. According to UNICEF, at least 10 percent "of all children—over 200 million in all—suffer some form of physical and/or mental disability or learning impairment. An even larger number suffer from diminished learning capabilities and other disadvantages that compromise their prospects for a productive and capable life."[25]

Malnutrition and Intelligence

Malnutrition can lead to significant drops in intelligence quotient (IQ). The American Association on Mental Retardation (AAMR) identifies nutrition, along with genetics, as a biomedical factor that could cause retardation. Other causes are social factors related to social and family interaction, "such as child stimulation and adult responsiveness," behavioral factors that can include maternal substance abuse, and "educational factors . . . related to the availability of family and educational supports that promote mental development and increases in adaptive skills."[26] The AAMR adds that "factors present during one generation can influence the outcomes of the next generation. By understanding inter-generational causes, appropriate supports can be used to prevent and reverse the effects of risk factors."[27]

An important factor in retardation is malnutrition. The advocacy organization Bread for the World lists effects of severe malnutrition as:

1. Studies have shown that malnutrition during the first two years of life causes a child's brain to shrink or atrophy, impairing both mental and physical development.
2. Malnutrition affects behavioral development by reducing IQ, slowing motor skills, and increasing learning disabilities.
3. Malnutrition early in life also stunts growth. Those who grow up without an adequate diet are commonly short for their age and height.
4. Malnutrition often causes hair to grow in a reddish color and fall out easily.
5. Vitamin deficiencies caused by malnutrition lead to vision problems, such as blindness in children and night blindness in adult women.
6. Malnutrition and infection often come together. Malnutrition weakens the immune system and throws off the body's hormone balances, making it easier for infections to set in.
7. Malnourished children often have bacterial overgrowth in the small bowel, which can lead to infection and diarrhea.
8. Infections related to a weakened immune system reduce appetite, cause withdrawal from solid foods, decrease absorption of nitrogen and other nutrients because of diarrhea, increase metabolic losses of potassium, magnesium, zinc, vitamins A, B2, C and so on through urine.
9. Hormone balances are thrown off. Insulin levels go down. Thyroid hormone levels change.[28]

The affluent cannot afford to ignore malnutrition among the poor because the affluent and the poor interact with each other in various ways. Malnourished individuals may not be able to resist infectious diseases or may serve as breeding grounds for new infectious diseases. The most effective approach for preventing the development and spread of new diseases is preventing malnutrition.

The organization Bread for the World notes that the highest concentrations of malnutrition are in Nepal, Bangladesh, and sub-Saharan Africa. The organization recommends a treatment regimen combining antibiotics, a specifically designed amount of calories each day for weight recovery, and a nutritious protein- and vitamin-rich diet.[29]

As global warming progresses, the poorest regions of the world are being hardest hit. Low-lying regions of Bangladesh are being inundated, forcing an ever-increasing population to abandon their homes and move to higher ground. Thus, the twin forces of increasing population and decreasing land area can increase rates of malnutrition.

Malnutrition and Behavior

Helping the poor is often viewed as a form of charity that helps only the poor. In social animals, such as humans, providing food resources for the poor may also help the affluent. A team of scientists at the University of Southern California has conducted a long-term study of the effects of malnutrition since 1972. Longitudinal studies of this type provide the best evidence of the costs malnutrition exacts on individuals and on populations. The study was initially funded by the World Health Organization and the Mauritian government, but as of this writing, it was also funded by the U.S. National Institute of Mental Health. The study was originally designed by Sarnoff Mednick, director of USC's Social Science Research Center. The initial study involved having physicians assess the nutritional levels of approximately 2,000 three-year-olds from two towns on the island of Mauritius. Follow-up studies indicated that malnutrition could lead to antisocial and behavioral problems at ages eight, eleven, and seventeen. The study determined that giving children vitamin supplements and increasing the level of protein in their diets reduced antisocial and aggressive behavior. Children in the original study are now thirty-five years old, on average.

The current study, led by USC fellow Jianghong Liu, focuses on the children of the original participants. The longitudinal study has revealed that malnutrition results in poor brain development, reducing IQ levels. Low IQ levels have been linked by the research team to higher levels of aggression.[30]

What Is Malnutrition?

According to the International Food Policy Research Institute (IFPRI), insufficient food consumption, along with infection and poor health, is the primary cause of malnutrition. According to reports of the United Nations Administrative Committee on Coordination/Sub-Committee on Nutrition (UN ACC/SCN), protein-energy malnutrition (PEM), measured by low body weight, affects 34 percent of all preschool age children in the Third World. Insufficient food consumption can lead to deficiencies in key nutrients that can lead to anemia (iron deficiency) and blindness (vitamin A).

As of 1990, more than half the children suffering from protein-energy malnutrition were in South Asia, a region composed of India, Pakistan, Bangladesh, Nepal,

Sri Lanka, and Bhutan. The next largest number of underweight children was in sub-Saharan Africa, followed by China and Southeast Asia.[31] These figures can be misleading, since India and China make up about 36 percent of the world's population. Also, the pattern of childhood malnutrition may have changed, since both India and China have undergone great economic growth since this study was conducted.

Two studies on children of India indicated a mixed picture related to disparities in wealth and education, as well as with regional variation. Though India has implemented a number of programs aimed at combating malnutrition, not every child in a region may have access to them. In some cases, low-caste or Muslim children may be excluded. The Indian government released data for twenty-two of India's twenty-nine states compiled by the National Family Health Survey. In the northern state of Uttar Pradesh, 47 percent of children under three were found to be clinically underweight. In Madhya Pradesh, in central India, the proportion of clinically underweight children was 60 percent. In southern Tamil Nadu, the proportion of underweight children has dropped to 33 percent. As noted below, the IFPRI notes that programs targeting PEM in Tamil Nadu have been successfully implemented.

At the other end of the scale, a study conducted by the Delhi Diabetes Research Center during the same period found that nearly one in five children in the Delhi metropolis in northern India aged ten to sixteen was either overweight or clinically obese. Delhi is one of the most prosperous regions of India, and its economy has been greatly boosted in recent years by industrialization and outsourcing of jobs from the United States. Obesity can bring health problems of its own. At the same time, the proportion of underweight fell very little from 35 percent to 33 percent, suggesting a disparity in access to food resources. Overall, India has long produced a surplus of food grains, indicating that distribution, rather than production, is the source of the problem.

It is well known that rates of underweight and obesity are related to social status. What is not so well known is the exact dynamic of nutrition and underweight or obesity. In India, childhood obesity is most likely to occur in high-status or wealthy families, who have access to an abundance of all kinds of food. In the United States, childhood obesity is linked to low-income families who base their subsistence on high-calorie, high-carbohydrate diets. Researchers at the University of Wisconsin-Madison noted that more than a third of three-year-olds in low-income households in major U.S. cities are overweight or obese. Latino children were most likely to be overweight or obese, with 45 percent at risk, compared to 32 percent among white and African American children. The researchers identified two factors that protect children from obesity: breast-feeding for at least six months and not allowing children to take a bottle to bed.

The study is controversial, however, because developmental rates differ in children. At the time of this writing, the U.S. Centers for Disease Control and Prevention did not label anyone younger than twenty as obese, since rapid growth early in life makes it difficult to compare desirable weights for children and adults. Whereas the international measure for optimal childhood weight is based on standardized weights, the U.S. Centers for Disease Control uses the body mass index, or BMI, which gauges the relationship of weight to height. None of these measures is exact, since heights and weights vary from one group to another due to genetics. In addition, a rate of malnutrition that makes a child underweight may also stunt his or her growth. Despite differences in measurement, both the U.S. Centers for Disease

Control and Prevention and the American Obesity Association agree that American children are becoming increasingly overweight. The percentage of American children in the 95th percentile for BMI has more than doubled over the last two decades, to nearly 19 percent in 2004.

Though they are important in evaluating at-risk populations, standardized measures do not tell the full story about childhood health. Behavioral measures, such as vitality and willingness to join in childhood activities, are perhaps a more reliable measure, but they are more difficult to evaluate and impossible to quantify. Therefore, they are difficult to evaluate and impossible to submit to agencies that grant research funds.

Cross-Cultural Measures of Malnutrition

According to the IFPRI projection, virtually all regions in the world "will experience a reduction in the absolute numbers of underweight children, with the notable exception of Sub-Saharan Africa. . . . Even an optimistic scenario puts the number of malnourished [preschool children] at about 34 million in the year 2020."[32] The pessimistic scenario places the number of malnourished children in sub-Saharan Africa at around 60 million. The predictions for sub-Saharan Africa are based on a population growth rate of 3 percent per year, the highest in the world.[33] High population growth rates are linked to higher rates of poverty, and therefore, to higher rates of malnutrition in regions where economic growth does not keep pace with population growth.

The IFPRI report predicts that the most dramatic reduction in malnutrition rates among preschool aged children would occur in China and Southeast Asia, including Indonesia, Thailand, the Philippines, Vietnam, Malaysia, Myanmar (Burma), Laos, and Kampuchea.[34] The report noted that systematic programs aimed at reducing malnutrition have been successfully implemented in Thailand, Zimbabwe, Indonesia, Costa Rica, Chile, and in Tamil Nadu in India. The report concludes:

> In Thailand, the prevalence of underweight children was reduced from 36 percent to 13 percent over a period of eight years, through a national program and policy that both attacked poverty and promoted explicit nutrition programs. Increases in incomes and reduction in poverty are important, but experiences in several countries indicate that even where there are no rapid improvement in incomes, malnutrition can be reduced by explicit programs and policies that aim at improving household access to food and health services and improving child care practices such as breastfeed and proper weaning of infants.[35]

Malnutrition and the Prosperity of Nations

Malnutrition is not only a problem for individuals. It is also a problem for nations. Ethiopia has recovered from famines that plagued the nation, but malnutrition continues to prevent Ethiopia's economic growth. According to a report in *The New York Times*, at least 10,000 children under the age of five died in 2005 in the northern region of Wag Hamra alone.[36] The cost of supplying nutrients is cheap, when figured on a per-child basis, but the magnitude of the problems overwhelms even the most dedicated agencies.

Medical anthropologist Sonia Patten describes an interdisciplinary program aimed at addressing malnutrition in Malawi, in southeastern Africa. The original impetus of the program was a USAID grant aimed at promoting exchange between universities in developing nations and U.S. universities. The goal of the program, University Development Linkages Program (UDLP) was to strengthen developing nation colleges and universities by giving them access to U.S. facilities and other university resources (Patten 2003:407). The program in which Patten participated involved two American universities and an agricultural college associated with the University of Malawi system in Africa. The U.S. team quickly identified malnutrition among children as a problem that needed to be immediately addressed:

> We recognized that three out of five children in the country were undernourished. Worse, the mortality rate for children under five was 24 percent, or nearly one in four. The problem was caused by the fact that children received insufficient protein and calories, which left them vulnerable to a host of infectious diseases, potential mental impairment, serious deficiency diseases such as kwashiorkor and marasmus, and premature death. (Patten 2003:407)

Kwashiorkor is a form of malnutrition caused by inadequate protein. Early symptoms of malnutrition, including kwashiorkor, are fatigue, irritability, and lethargy. If protein deficiency continues, symptoms include failure to grow, loss of muscle mass, edema (swelling), and decreased immunity. As the condition progresses, symptoms include a large and protuberant belly, skin conditions including dermatitis, changes in pigmentation, and thinning of the hair. Though these conditions occur primarily in impoverished countries, as many as 50 percent of elderly persons in U.S. nursing homes may suffer from inadequate protein-calorie intake.[37]

Marasmus is a form of serious protein-energy malnutrition. This typically occurs in developing countries at the time a child is weaned, and therefore deprived of the proteins available in breast milk. According to the World Health Organization, 49 percent of the 10.4 million deaths occurring in children under five years of age are associated with PEM.[38] Marasmus is an adaptation to insufficient energy intake: "Children adapt to an energy deficit with a decrease in physical activity, lethargy, a decrease in basal energy metabolism, slowing of growth, and finally weight loss."[39]

Patten notes that nutritional deficiencies occur when children are weaned:

> We learned from [researchers indigenous to Malawi] and from field research that mothers breastfeed their babies for two or three years. This assured that the children received sufficient protein and calories during their early years. However, that changed when the children were weaned. The indigenous weaning food is a thin gruel of water and corn flour, and babies receive small amounts of it beginning at about four months of age. When mothers wean their toddlers, it is this gruel that the children eat day after day. It is a nutritionally inadequate weaning food and children soon begin to show its effects— swollen bellies, stunted growth, and increased susceptibility to malaria, measles, and other infectious diseases. (Patten 2003:407)

Patten and the team she worked with developed an ingenious solution to the problem of adding protein to the children's diets through the use of goat's milk, but the plan needed cooperation from a variety of sources. The goats in Malawi villages were meat goats sold for revenue, not milk goats. It required the importation of Saanen dairy goats from South Africa, Damascus goats from Cyprus, and Anglo-Nubian goats from the United States. The most successful imports were Saanen goats from South Africa, perhaps because of the geographical closeness of South Africa to Malawi.

The next project was to gain cooperation from village chiefs so that women could control the dairy productivity of goats. The experiment was based on the social organization of each of three villages. In the central region of Malawi, most people belong to the Chewa ethnic group, which is matrilineal and matrilocal. At first, the male chiefs of the two villages selected for the study were skeptical because they did not consider it right for women to own goats. But since the death of a child was a great sorrow, and the men were aware of the problem of malnourished children, they eventually agreed to the arrangement. Researchers discovered that the third village selected was not suitable because of a large number of animal thefts, and the prime suspects were a family living in the village.

The program was closely monitored and supported by the research team. Eventually, it was combined with a program for growing soybeans for the times when milk production was low. The balance of power was sustained because village chiefs oversaw the project, and both men and women provided the labor required for caring for the goats and soybeans. Patten concludes:

> Our project team designed and tested a locally sustainable approach to alleviate infant and child malnourishment in rural Malawi. Data on changes in the participating children's weights, heights, and upper-arm circumferences show that relatively small amounts of goat milk included in the regular diet make a substantial difference in promoting normal growth in children. Results from a rapid appraisal survey that I helped design indicate that the project is highly valued by rural women. This is confirmed by key village women and by the fact that more women sought to join the program than project resources allowed (2003:413–414).

The program has since spread to other Malawi communities and has been adopted by nongovernmental organizations (NGOs) for introducing locally sustainable efforts in other parts of the country. In addition, several district hospitals have established flocks of goats on their grounds to provide rehabilitation for severely malnourished children.[40]

Top-down management programs typically do not work out over the long term unless they are based on an understanding of indigenous social and economic factors. A major contribution of medical anthropology is to ascertain the local conditions that make social improvements possible. An important issue here is that there is no single magic bullet that solves all epidemiological and nutritional problems. Each program must be individually designed for the specific social and environment conditions that a particular medical and health issue poses.

MEDICAL TOURISM

The practice of Western biomedicine has gone global for a variety of reasons. One of them is cost. A report in *UDaily*, a publication of the University of Delaware, notes:

> The cost of surgery in India, Thailand or South Africa can be one-tenth of what it is in the United States or Western Europe, and sometimes even less. A heart-valve replacement that

would cost $200,000 or more in the U.S., for example, goes for $10,000 in India—and that includes round-trip airfare and a brief vacation package. Similarly, a metal-free dental bridge worth $5,500 in the U.S. costs $500 in India, a knee replacement in Thailand with six days of physical therapy costs about one-fifth of what it would in the States, and Lasik eye surgery worth $3,700 in the U.S. is available in many other countries for only $750. Cosmetic surgery savings are even greater: A full facelift that would cost $20,000 in the U.S. runs about $1,250 in South Africa.[41]

UDaily summarizes comments on medical tourism by Frederick J. DeMicco, who is chair of the Hotel, Restaurant and Institutional Management Department at the University of Delaware, and Marvin Cetron, founder and president of Forecasting International. These experts explain that other reasons for medical tourism are that state-of-the-art medical facilities are not available in some parts of the world, and in others the health care system is overburdened. For example, in Britain and Canada, "the waiting period for a hip replacement can be a year or more, while in Bangkok or Bangalore, a patient can be in the operating room the morning after getting off a plane."[42]

These researchers note that "the hospitals and clinics that cater to the tourist market often are among the best in the world, and many are staffed by physicians trained at major medical centers in the United States and Europe":[43]

Bangkok's Bumrundgrad hospital has more than 200 surgeons who are board-certified in the United States, and one of Singapore's major hospitals is a branch of the prestigious Johns Hopkins University in Baltimore. In a field where experience is as important as technology, Escorts Heart Institute and Research Center in Delhi and Faridabad, India, performs nearly 15,000 heart operations every year, and the death rate among patients during surgery is only 0.8 percent—less than half that of most major hospitals in the United States.[44]

In some countries, research infrastructures rank ahead of those in most Western countries: "India is among the world's leading countries for biotechnology research, while both India and South Korea are pushing ahead with stem cell research at a level approached only in Britain."[45] The quality of postsurgical care may also be better than that found in Western facilities: "In many foreign clinics . . . the doctors are supported by more registered nurses per patient than in any Western facility, and some clinics provide single-patient rooms that resemble guestrooms in four-star hotels, with a nurse dedicated to each patient 24 hours a day."[46]

The market for medical tourism is rapidly growing. At the time of this writing, Singapore drew more than 250,000 patients per year, nearly half from the Middle East, and nearly a half million patients traveled to India for medical care. Medical tourism has become an important economic sector for some countries. DeMicco and Cetron estimate that medical tourism will contribute as much as $2.2 billion to India's economy by 2012. Other countries breaking into this lucrative economic sector are Argentina, Costa Rica, Cuba, Jamaica, South Africa, Jordan, Malaysia, Hungary, Latvia, and Estonia.

Major centers for medical tourism are Bangkok and Phuket, which draw patients for cosmetic surgery and dental treatments. Eye surgery, kidney dialysis, and organ transplantation are also among the most common procedures sought by medical tourists in Thailand. Six medical facilities in Bangkok have hospital accreditation from the United States. India is also highly sought after for medical treatments: "India has top-notch centers for open-heart surgery, pediatric heart surgery, hip and knee replacement, cosmetic surgery, dentistry, bone marrow transplants and cancer therapy, and virtually all of India's clinics are equipped with the latest electronic and medical diagnostic equipment."

DeMicco and Cetron add that India is a pioneer in some medical practices:

> Unlike many of its competitors in medical tourism, India also has the technological sophistication and infrastructure to maintain its market niche, and Indian pharmaceuticals meet the stringent requirements of the U.S. Food and Drug Administration. Additionally, India's quality of care is up to American standards, and some Indian medical centers even provide services that are uncommon elsewhere. For example, hip surgery patients in India can opt for a hip-resurfacing procedure, in which damaged bone is scraped away and replaced with chrome alloy—an operation that costs less and causes less post-operative trauma than the traditional replacement procedure performed in the U.S.[47]

The Canadian Broadcasting Corporation notes that India is considered the leading country in promoting medical tourism. It adds that India is now leading the field in "medical outsourcing," in which it supplies services to overburdened medical care systems in Western countries.[48]

The CBC observes that medical tourism has been a part of the human experience for thousands of years: "In ancient Greece, pilgrims and patients came from all over the Mediterranean to the sanctuary of the healing god, Asklepios, at Epidaurus. In Roman Britain, patients took the waters at a shrine at Bath, a practice that continued for 2,000 years. From the 18th century wealthy Europeans traveled to spas from Germany to the Nile."[49]

As the CBC notes, medical tourism is mostly available to people who can afford to combine medical treatment with a vacation. Critics have argued that the profitable, private-sector nature of medical tourism is diverting needed resources and personnel away from local populations. In response, the largest of the estimated half-dozen medical corporations in India serving medical tourist, Apollo Hospital Enterprises, has expanded its services to the poor: "It has set aside free beds for those who can't afford care, has set up a trust fund and is pioneering remote, satellite-linked telemedicine across India."[50]

Though Thailand and India are leaders in medical tourism, other countries have expanded their services to accommodate the increasing international demand:

> Cuba . . . first aimed its services at well-off patients from Central and South America and now attracts patients from Canada, Germany and Italy. Malaysia attracts patients from surrounding Southeast Asian countries; Jordan serves patients from the Middle East. Israel caters to both Jewish patients and people from some nearby countries. One Israeli hospital advertises worldwide services, specializing in both male and female infertility, in-vitro fertilization and high-risk pregnancies. South Africa offers package medical holiday deals with stays at either luxury hotels or safaris.[51]

Medical tourism may well change the practice of Western biomedicine. On one level, the West—Europe and the United States—may lose its lead in the practice of biomedicine. On another level, social status may come to play an even greater role in access to biomedical health care.

Notes

INTRODUCTION

1. http://www.medanthro.net/definition.html. Updated January 19, 2007. Since I originally accessed this website in January 2007, it has been redesigned and elaborated. This definition was formulated by medical anthropologists in the American tradition. Another good site defining medical anthropology is the British equivalent, titled "Medical Committee" at http://www.therai.org.uk/committees/medical_anthropology.html (accessed on August 14, 2009).

2. medanthro.net.

3. Or for tenure.

4. UCLA/CURE Neuroenteric Disease Program, Department of Medicine and Physiology, UCLA School of Medicine.

5. Department of Neurology, Beth Israel Hospital, Boston, MA.

CHAPTER 1 MODELS OF THE BODY, THE SELF, AND THE HUMAN EXPERIENCE

1. The 400,000 Dogon speak approximately 120 dialects, many of which are not mutually intelligible. As might be expected, their creation myths vary somewhat, as is the case with all oral traditions. My description is largely taken from Griaule (1965), supplemented with other sources.

2. Since Griaule and others described Dogon culture, expansion of the neighboring Fulani has pushed the Dogon into rocky, arid terrain that is less hospitable for agriculture. As a result, they have constructed dams and wells to grow produce for sale at market. There is some indication that this horticultural shift has produced a related shift in Dogon cosmology, so that Nommo have come to be feared. This is logical in view of the more recent Dogon dependence on water in a region where water is scarce.

3. My interpretation of Good's usage of the word "objective" refers to the Western view of the body as an object independent of the mind. This is reflected in medical practice of distinguishing between physicians, who treat the body, and psychologists, who treat the mind.

4. Symbols are words, images, or behaviors that convey multiple levels of meaning. (Womack 2005)

5. Ian Buruma, *Behind the Mask: On Sexual Demons, Sacred Mothers, Transvestites, Gangsters and Other Japanese Cultural Heroes*. New York: New American Library, 1984.

6. Jane Goodale's research, on which this report is based, was conducted at Snake Bay in Australia.

7. http://www.samoanews.com/friday.01072005/FRothernews/storyl.html. Accessed August 2005. Apparently this site or story has not been maintained.

8. I am indebted for this information to Asian students in my medical anthropology class, taught at El Camino College.

9. http://www.vanishingtattoo.com. Accessed June 2007 and again on August 14, 2009.

10. http://www.nytimes.com/2007/06/17/us/17tattoo.html. Accessed June 2007 at the time article was published. Access is now limited.

11. Divorce is not unique to urban industrialized societies. It is a common characteristic of societies in which the economic system is based on mobility. Among traditional !Kung foragers of Africa, the divorce rate equaled that in contemporary American cities. Anthropologists attribute this to the economic independence of forager women, where women contribute greatly to the economy.

12. *Artilleriiskii Zhurnal*, 1858, No. 2. Trans. Mark Conrad 2002.http://home.comcast.net/~markconrad/USHAKOV.htm. Accessed June 2007.

13. *Artilleriiskii Zhurnal*.

14. The term "White Man's burden" derives from a Rudyard Kipling poem of the same name:

Take up the White Man's burden,
Send forth the best ye greed —
Go, bind your sons to exile
To serve your captives' need . . .

Originally written for Queen Victoria's Diamond Jubilee, "The White Man's Burden," was published in the magazine *McClure's* in 1899, under the title "The White Man's Burden: The United States and the Philippine Islands." It justifies the colonialization of the Philippines by the United States. It was also published under the name "The White Man's Burden" in *The Journal*, Detroit, 1923.

15. See Zunyou Wu, Zhiyuan Liu, and Roger Detels. 1995. "HIV-1 Infection in Commercial Plasma Donors in China." *The Lancet* 346:61–61.

16. See Cindy Sui. "China's Farmers Offer Children for Adoption before AIDS Orphans Them." *Agence France Press*, October 17, 2002.

CHAPTER 2 CONSTRUCTING GENDER:
THE BODY IN SOCIAL CONTEXT

1. This was first pointed out to me by Liz Ryder, based on her fieldwork in New Guinea.

2. Quoted in Chandler Burr, *The Atlantic Online*, http://www.theatlantic.com/doc/print/199706/homosexuality-biology. Accessed December 2007.

3. http://www.coolnurse.com/puberty.htm. Accessed December 2007.

4. Bourdieu echoes, in different terms, George Herbert Mead's analysis in *Mind, Self and Society* (1934) that, as children, we define who we are by taking the role of the "other" in play.

5. Anand Giridharadas, "The Ink Fades on a Profession as India Modernizes," http://www.nytimes.com/2007/12/26/world/asia/26india.html. Accessed December 2007.

6. The traditional wisdom in anthropology is that more male embryos than female embryos are conceived, but that fewer boys are born, possibly as a result of negative selective pressure by the mother's hormones. More recently, evidence suggests the ratio of male-to-female births increases during conditions of environment stress, such as in times of war.

7. Choe Sang-Hun, "Where Boys Were Kings, a Shift Toward Baby Girls," http://www.nytimes.com/2007/12/23/world/asia/23skoera.html. Accessed December 2007.

8. I am indebted to John Duffy, PhD, clinical professor emeritus at the Tulane University School of Medicine and of the Department of History, University of Maryland, for contributing this overview.

9. Portions of the book have been published online at http://blinkytreefrog.livejurnal.com/80660.html. Accessed December 2007.

10. http://www.pe.com/localnews/sanbernardino/stories/PE_News_Local_bauthor13.a2148.html. Accessed December 2007.

11. Pers. comm. 2007.

12. Lévi-Strauss wrote about this concept in a number of contexts, including kinship and mythology. He discusses implications of binary oppositions in his book *The Savage Mind* (*Le pensée sauvage*).

13. Morgan Holmes, "Re-membering a queer body." *Undercurrents*, May 1994:11–13. Published by Faculty of Environmental Studies, York University. Also available at http://www.medhelp.org/www/ais/articles/HOLMES.HTM.

14. Morgan Holmes, "Medical Politics and Cultural Imperaties: Intersexuality Beyond Pathology and Erasure," master's thesis, Interdisciplinary Studies, York University, Ontario, Canada, September 1994.

15. http://living.oneindia.in/kamasutra/facts-about-sex/intersexuals.html. Accessed December 2007.

16. In cases of intersexuality, female genitalia are more likely to be favored over male genitalia in genital surgery aimed at "correcting" intersexuality because female genitalia are easier to construct surgically.

17. Nanda uses the feminine pronoun in describing hijras in conformity to their self-identity as females.

18. It is significant that Tamasha wears a sari, a female garment, which emphasizes her self-identity as feminine. Not all *kothis* wear saris or identify with feminine gender. In their view, they are simply "not-male" (Reddy and Nanda 2005).

19. Gender is socially constructed in all groups.

20. Pedro de Magalhães, "History of the Province of Santa Cruz," ed. John Stetson. *Documents and Narratives Concerning the Discovery and Conquest of Latin America: The Histories of Brazil* 2 (1922):89.

21. http://www.ohsu.edu/news/2004/030504sheep.html. Accessed in 2004.

CHAPTER 3 THE BIOLOGY OF PSYCHOLOGY AND THE PSYCHOLOGY OF BIOLOGY

1. Having grown up in the American Midwest where Calvinistic attitudes are common, I would suggest that carnal desires are less often stifled than engaged in surreptitiously. Medically speaking, research in both Europe and the United States has suggested that the reduction of stress through relaxation and pleasurable activities promotes the maintenance of health.

2. I am indebted to Claude Lévi-Strauss (1963) for this model. He suggested that humans conceptualize the world in binary oppositions, which are then resolved through a third mediating principle. This analysis describes a process of human cognition, rather than a description of the physical properties of the universe.

3. Perry specializes in neurological brain trauma produced by childhood neglect.

4. These refer to the sensory apparatus, hearing, feeling, internal sensations, taste, vision, and smell.

5. The Washington University School of Medicine. "Neuroscience Tutorial. "Basal ganglia and cerebellum." http://thalamus.wustl.edu/course/cerebell.html. Accessed January 2008 and again on August 14, 2009.

6. C. George Boeree. "General Psychology: The Emotional Nervous System." 2002, 2009. http://webspace.ship.edu/cgboer/limbicsystem.html. Accessed January 2008 and August 14, 2009.

7. http://www.willamette.edu/~gorr/classes/cs449/brain.html. Accessed January 2008. The parent website for this research is Willamette University in Oregon.

8. Research on computers is occurring much faster than research on the human brain, so some of these parameters may be obsolete by the time this book goes to press; however, complexity of computers will never equal the complexity of the human brain until computers learn to laugh and cry.

9. http://www.ag.ndsu.edu/pubs/yf/famsci/fs609w.htm. Accessed 2008. The parent website for this research is North Dakota State University.

10. North Dakota State University.

11. North Dakota State University.

12. North Dakota State University.

13. This definition of cognition was provided by medicineterms.com. http://www.medterms.com/script/main/art.asp?articlekey. Accessed 2008.

14. Jeanna Bryner, "Sea Slug Offers Clues to Human Brain Disorders," http://www.livescience.com/animals/061228_brainy_slugs.html. Accessed January 2008.

15. Bryner, "Sea Slug."

16. Bryner, "Sea Slug."

17. http://transcriptome.affymetrix.com/local_index.html. Accessed January 2008. There are several additional respected Internet sources that discuss transcriptome, including the British site bioinformatics.oxfordjournals.org/cgi/content/abstract/21/22/4194 and the American site. www.ncbi.nim.nih.gov/pubmed/14681424.

18. Bryner, "Sea Slug."

19. Bryner, "Sea Slug."

20. Bryner, "Sea Slug."

21. For more information on serotonin, see the Mayo Clinic's "Selective Serotonin Reuptake Inhibitors (SSRIs)" (http://www.mayoclinic.com/health-ssris/MH00066, accessed August 2009) which deals with treatment of depression through SSRIs. It also lists the side effects of SSRIs as follows: nausea; sexual dysfunction, including reduced desire or orgasm difficulties; dry mouth; headache; diarrhea; nervousness; rash; agitation; restlessness; increased sweating; weight gain; drowsiness; insomnia.

22. *Dialogues of Alfred North White as recorded by Lucien Price*, Chapter 17, December 15, 1939. Boston: David R. Godine, 2001.

23. Taken from Richard J. Gerrig and Philip G. Zimbardo, *Psychology and Life*, 15th ed. Boston, MA: Allen and Bacon, 2002.

24. Mark K. Smith, "Howard Gardner, Multiple Intelligences and Education," 2002, 2008, http://www.infed.org/thinkers/gardner.htm. Accessed January 2008 and on August 14, 2009.

25. The University of California, San Francisco, is noted for biomedical research and medical education.

26. Henrietta C. Leiner and Alan L. Leiner began their professional career as mathematicians, then began research in electronic computer systems. They then transferred their interest in the logic of network systems to the organization of the cerebrocerebellar networks in the human brain.

27. Henrietta C Leiner and Alan L. Leiner, "The Treasure at the Bottom of the Brain," 2009, http://www.newhorizons.org/neuro/leiner.htm. Accessed August 13, 2009. This article compares the operation of the cerebellum to the operations of computers. They say, "In computing machines the processing of information is accomplished by both the hardware in

the systerm (the circuitry) and by the software (the messages transmitted between the various parts of the circuitry)."

28. http://www.guardian.co.uk/commentisfree/2006/nov/22/comment.health

29. Ingvard Wilhelmsen, "Hypochondria," http://www.uib.no/med/avd/med_a/gastro/wilhelms/hypochon.html. Accessed January 2008 and August 14, 2009.

30. http://www.psychosomaticmedicine.org/cgi/content/abstract/66/3/435. Accessed January 2008.

31. See www.cas.usf.edu/~jacobsen/FatigueCatastrophizing.pdf (accessed January 2008) and aje.oxfordjournals.org/cgi/content/abstract/156/11/1028, among others.

32. http//wellspanhealth.com/healthnews/healthday/060525HD532907.htm. Accessed January 2008.

33. http//wellspanhealth.com/healthnews/healthday/060525HD532907.htm.

34. See, for example, Arthur Kleinman et al. 1997; Terrence Turner 1993; Robert Desjarlais 1992; Catherine A. Lutz and Geoffrey M. White 1986; M. L. Lyon and J. M. Barbalet 1994; Lila Abu-Lughod and Catherine A. Lutz 1990; and Arjun Appadurai 1990.

CHAPTER 4 METAPHOR, LABELING THEORY, AND THE PLACEBO EFFECT

1. Literally, "horse." Vodou practitioners say that *lwa* "ride" them during possession, much as a human rides a horse.

2. Lisa Stevenson. "The Life of the Name." Paper presented at the UCLA Mind, Medicine and Culture seminar, April 3, 2006, 1.

3. Stevenson, 3.

4. The term "witch-doctor" is no longer used by anthropologists.

5. David L. Rosenhan. "On Being Sane in Insane Places." http://psychrights.org/Articles/Rosenham.htm. This article can be accessed through many websites since it has been much cited and is often used in classes. (The original article is David L. Rosenhan, "On Being Sane in Insane Places," *Science* 179 (1973): 250–258.)

6. Rosenhan, "On Being Sane."

7. Rosenhan, "On Being Sane," 3.

8. Rosenhan, "On Being Sane," 3.

9. Rosenhan, "On Being Sane," 4.

10. Rosenhan, "On Being Sane," 6.

11. Rosenhan, "On Being Sane," 4.

12. Rosenhan, "On Being Sane," 1.

13. These observations about the stigma of naming are my own.

14. This information is from the U.S. Centers for Disease Control and Prevention website, http://www.cdc.gov/ncidod/dbmd/diseaseinfrom/hansens_t.htm. Accessed February 2008.

15. See **peripheral nervous system,** interlinked neurons that convey information from the environment to the central nervous system and instructions from the central nervous system to the peripheral nervous system.

16. U.S. Centers for Disease Control and Prevention website, http://www.cdc.gov/ncidod/dbmd/diseaseinfo/hansens_t.htm. Accessed February 2008.

17. US CDC.

18. US CDC.

19. US CDC.

20. http://kidshealth.org/PageManager.jsp?dn+KidsHealth&lic. Accessed February 2008. This particular Web page is no longer available, although KidsHealth continues to maintain its website.

21. http://kidshealth.org/PageManager.jsp?dn+KidsHealth&lic.

22. The psychological and social skills of shamans will be discussed in chapter 11.

23. Irving Kirsch and Guy Sapirstein, http://www.advance.uconn.edu/1998/981005/10059812.htm. Accessed February 2008; Web page no longer available. A criticism of this research can be found in "Controversial Study Investigates Therapeutic Benefits of Placebo," *Psychiatric Times*, September 1, 1998, 15, 19.

24. Walter A. Brown, "Understanding and Using the Placebo Effect," *Psychiatric Times*, October 1, 2006, 23, 1, http://www.psychiatrictimes.com/print.jhtml;jsessionid+IMWN50HVWHR4AQSNDLOS.

25. Brown, "Understanding."

26. Brown, "Understanding."

27. Brown, "Understanding."

CHAPTER 5 THE HUMAN LIFE CYCLE:
COMING OF AGE

1. See Bolton 1977 and Carter 1977.

2. See Allen 1978, 1988.

3. Molly Hennessy-Fiske, "War Zone Midwives Deliver," *Los Angeles Times*, January 2007. http://www.latimes.com/news/nationworld/world/la-fg-midwife15jan15,06762067.story?coll+la Accessed January 2007.

4. Hennessy-Fiske, "War Zone Midwives Deliver."

5. Hennessy-Fiske, "War Zone Midwives Deliver."

6. "Pre-eclampsia and Eclampsia: Causes and Treatements: Signs and Symptons of Pre-Eclampsia and Eclampsia," http://www.webmd.com/baby/features/pre-eclampsia-eclampsia-causes-treatments. Accessed January 2008 and August 14, 2009.

7. "Pre-eclampsia and Eclampsia."

8. http://www.adhb.govt.nz/newborn/Guidelines/Anomalies/Non-ImmuneHydrops.htm. Accessed January 2008 (this website no longer appears to be active).

9. Note that the United Nations figures report lifetime probability of maternal death, whereas the U.S. statistics refer to each pregnancy and birth. If a woman becomes pregnant seven times in her lifetime, the likelihood that she will die as a result of pregnancy or childbirth increases proportionately.

10. http://www.unicef.org/newsline/mmstat.htm. UNICEF is an international organization that monitors health and disease parameters. Extensive information on these topics is available on the UNICEF website. This particular report was accessed January 2008.

11. UNICEF.

12. UNICEF.

13. Kava (literally meaning "bitter") is an intoxicating and narcotic beverage made from the root of the kava plant. It is an important part of all ceremonial events in Fiji, as well as Samoa.

14. Lafcadio Hearn, *Gleanings in Buddha-Fields*, Rutland, VT: Charles E. Tuttle Co., 1971, 95 (orig. pub. 1897).

15. Hearn, *Gleanings in Buddha-Fields*, 95.

16. Melissa Healy, "On their terms," *Los Angeles Times*, December 18, 2006, F1.

CHAPTER 6 THE HUMAN LIFE CYCLE:
THE REPRODUCTIVE YEARS

1. Erika Hayasaki, "It Wasn't Funny at the Time," *Los Angeles Times*, April 14, 2007, A16.

2. "Puberty," http://www.coolnurse.com/puberty.htm.

3. This observation was contributed by my research assistant Kevin Huynh.

4. http://www.nytimes.com/2006/12/08/health/08kids.html?th=&emc=th&page-wanted=print. Accessed December 8, 2008. This is a report of research on childhood development.

5. *New York Times,* childhood development.

6. *New York Times,* childhood development.

7. *New York Times,* childhood development.

8. http://news.yahoo.com/s/livescience/20061217/sc_livescience/whyteensdostu-pidthings^p. Accessed December 2006.

9. http://www.livescience.com/humangiology/060907_teenage_feelings.html. Accessed September 2006. A more recent article on this topic is S. Burnett, G. Bird, J. Moll, C. Friith, S. J. Blakemore, "Development During Adolescence of the Neural Processing of Social Emotion, *Journal of Neuroscience* 29(6) (2009): 1294–1301.

10. Neural development during adolescence. Accessed December 2006.

11. Neural development during adolescence. Accessed December 2006.

12. Neural development during adolescence. Accessed December 2006.

13. http://www.livescience.com/humanbiology/05017_teen_thought.html. Accessed December 2006.

14. Teen thought. Accessed December 2006

15. Teen thought. Accessed December 2006.

16. Our DNA is unique except for identical twins, who are produced by the splitting of a single ovum fertilized by a single sperm. The DNA coding for identical twins is therefore the same.

17. http://www.ucmp.berkeley.edu/history/malthus.html. Accessed December 2006.

18. http://health.yahoo.com/topic/men/symptoms/article/mayoclinic/914D4A8F-460F-4F5F-A. Accessed December 2006.

19. Men's health. Accessed December 2006.

20. Men's health. Accessed December 2006.

21. Men's health. Accessed December 2006.

22. Men's Health. Accessed December 2006.

23. Nicholas Bakalar, "Childhood: Fathers Influence a Child's Language Development," *The New York Times,* November 14, 2006, http://travel.nytimes.com/w006/11/14/health/14child.html?partner=rssnyt&emo=rss&adxnnl. Accessed August 17, 2009.

24. Robert Roy Britt, "Kids Are Depressing, Study of Parents Finds," *Live Science,* February 2006. The research on parental depression was published in the American Sociological Association's *Journal of Health and Social Behavior.* This article notes "Any parent will tell you kids can be depressing at times. A new study shows that raising them is a lifelong challenge to your mental health. Not only do parents have significantly higher levels of depression than adults who do not have children, the problem gets worse when the kids move out" (http://www.livescience.com/humanbiology/060207_parent_depression.html. Accessed January 2006 and accessed August 17, 2009.) As the parent of three beautiful and successful adult children, I can attest to the fact that not a day goes by that I don't worry about their health, happiness, finances, etc. I wouldn't go so far as to call this depression, because I have been very fortunate in my own life circumstances, but I would willingly put their well-being ahead of my own. Maybe we need to rethink measures of depression. The most depressing scenario I could think of would be being trapped in a job that provided no challenges and did not offer an opportunity to overcome those challenges.

25. I would appreciate descriptions of grandparent-grandchild relationships from anthropologists who have made these analyses.

26. National Institutes of Health Grants, http://grants.nih.gov/grants/guide/pa-files/PA-95-086.html. Accessed December 2006.

27. National Institutes of Health Grants.

28. National Institutes of Health Grants.

29. National Institutes of Health Grants.

30. http://www.grandparenting.org/Research.htm. Accessed December 2006.

CHAPTER 7 THE HUMAN LIFE CYCLE: GROWING OLD AND GROWING GOOD

1. This account is adapted from Steve Lopez's column, "Keeping Father Time in Check." *Los Angeles Times*, November 22, 2006, pp. B1 and B10.

2. Linda L. Richards, reviewer. "Through Annie's Lens." http://www.januarymagazine.com/artcult/leibovitz.html. Accessed December 2006 and August 17, 2009.

3. http://findarticles.com/p/articles/mi_qn4155/is_20061029/ai_n16812158. Accessed in December 2006. (The original Web page from which this review was taken is no longer available.)

4. I am indebted to the actress Lisa Lu for this scroll and for increased understanding of its meaning.

5. Trance dancing, which involves entering an altered state of consciousness, is a traditional means of healing among the !Kung.

6. http://ihcrp.georgetown.edu/agingsociety/pubhtml/rxdrugs/rxdrugs.html.

7. http://ihcrp.georgetown.edu/agingsociety/pubhtml/rxdrugs/rxdrugs.html.

8. http://ihcrp.georgetown.edu/agingsociety/pubhtml/rxdrugs/rxdrugs.html.

9. These figures are provided at http://geography.about.com/library/weekly/aa042000b.htm.

CHAPTER 8 LIFESTYLE AND HEALTH

1. John Muir. 1980. *Mountaineering Essays*. Salt Lake City: Peregrine Press, 71–73.

2. Sid Kirchheimer, "Never Get Sick!" *AARP: The Magazine*. May/June 2007, 74.

3. Kirchheimer, "Never Get Sick!"

4. Kirchheimer, "Never Get Sick!"

5. Kirchheimer, "Never Get Sick!"

6. See also Fuller 2002; Meadow 1996; Weber and Belcher 2003.

7. See http://news.nationalgeographic.com/news/2002/07/0717_020717_TVchocolate_2.html. Accessed January 2007.

8. See http://www.3dchem.com/molecules.asp?ID=155 and http://ask.yahoo.com/ask/20031106.html. Accessed January 2006 and August 18, 2009,

9. http://news.yahoo.com/s/hsn/20070409/hl-sn/darkchocolatebutnottteatakesabiteoutofbloodpressure. Accessed January 2006.

10. Reported by Drs. Donald R. Buhler and Cristobal Miranda at The Linus Pauling Institute at http://lpi.oregonstate.edu/f-w00/flavonoid.html.

11. The research team conducting the survey was headed by Dr. Dirk Taubert, senior lecturer in pharmacology and toxicology at the University Hospital of Cologne. http://news.yahoo.com/s/hsn/20070409/hl_hsn/darkchocolatebutnotteatakesabiteoutofbloodpressure. Accessed January 2007.

12. http://www.budgettravel.com/bt-dyn/content/article/2007/08/06/AR2007080600793_pf.html. Accessed January 2007.

13. "Stop When Full? You Must Be French," http://www.msnbc.msn.com. Accessed January 2007.

14. *War* 2.124. Accessed January 2007.

15. Thomas H. Maugh II, "Latrine Practices Posed Health Risks to Sect," *Los Angeles Times*, November 14, 2006, A9.

16. Maugh, "Latrine Practices."

17. Maugh, "Latrine Practices."

CHAPTER 9 BIOMEDICINE AND THE SCIENTIFIC APPROACH

1. National Institute of Neurological Disorders and Stroke. NINDS Arteriovenous Malformation Information Page, http://www.ninds.nih.gov/disorders/avms/avms.htm. Accessed January 2007 and August 18, 2009.

2. Arteriovenous Malformation Information Page.

3. Arteriovenous Malformation Information Page.

4. http://news.yahoo.com/s/ap/johnson. Accessed January 2007.

5. http://www.brown.edu/Courses/Digital_Path/Heart/dissecting_aneurysm.htm. Accessed January 2007. Also http://www.mayoclinic.org/aortic-aneurysm/dissectingtreatment.html. Accessed Janurary 2007.

6. http://www.nytimes.com/2006/12/25/health/25surgeon.html. Accessed December 2006.

7. Arteriovenous Malformation.

8. Other terms for Western medicine are conventional medicine, allopathy, mainstream medicine, orthodox medicine, regular medicine and biomedicine.

9. Bohannan was called "Redwoman" because of her red hair.

10. The presumed link between the practice of infibulation and high maternal mortality is controversial due to the lack of consistent controlled research among different groups. Anthropologists have found no relationship between maternal mortality and the less invasive forms of female genital alteration.

11. These traditions will be discussed in Chapter 9 of *The Anthropology of Health and Healing*.

12. *The Collected Works of Dr. P. M. Latham, with Memoir by Sir Thomas Watson, Bart., M.D.* Sydenham Society (1876).

13. Dates associated with Neandertals are in dispute, depending on how the fossil materials are classified. If Homo Heidelbergensis is classified with Homo Neandertalensis, the dates may extend as far back as 850,000 BP. The dates of particular fossils are relatively exact. The controversy centers on how particular fossils are classified.

14. http://www.krapina.com/neandertals/en_zb41.htm. Accessed December 2006.

15. http://www.museum.upenn.edu/new/research/Exp_Rese_Disc/PhysicalAnthro/neanderthal. Accessed December 2006.

16. Neanderthal research.

17. Bijal P.Trivedi, "Does Wounded Skull Hint at Neandertal Nursing?" *National Geographic*, 2002, http://news.nationalgeographic.com/news/2002/04/0423_020423_TVneandertal.html. Accessed July 2002 and August 18, 2009.

18. Amélie A. Wlaker, "Neolithic Surgery," *Archaeology* 50(5) (September/October 1997), http://www.archaeology.org/9709/newsbriefs/trepanation.html. Accessed August 2009.

19. See Francis Adams, *The Genuine Works of Hippocrates*, New York: William Wood and Co., 1891.

20. http://www.merck.com/mmhe/print/sec12/ch154/ch154c.html. Accessed December 2006.

21. Vitamin D.

22. Vitamin D.

23. http://www.cdc.gov. Accessed December 2006.

24. Body Mass Index.

25. Body Mass Index.

26. Bish et al 2005.

27. Santry et al 2005.

CHAPTER 10 RESTORING THE BALANCE: ASIAN MODELS
OF HEALTH AND HEALING

1. Feeling the pulse is a diagnostic technique characteristic of Chinese medicine and Western biomedicine, as well as Ayurveda.

2. This is taken from the *I Ching* translated by Richard Wilhelm, Bollingen Foundation, Princeton University Press, Princeton, New Jersey, 1967.

3. National Center for Complementary and Alternative Medicine, http://nccam.nih.gov/health/backgrounds/energymed.htm. Accessed January 2008 and August 19, 2009.

4. C. Vallbona and T. Richards, "Evolution of magnetic therapy from alternative to traditional medicine, *Physical Medicine and Rehabilitation Clinics of North America* 1999:10(3):729–754.

5. National Center for Complementary and Alternative Medicine. http://nccam.nih.gov/health/backgrounds/energymed.htm. Accessed January 2008 and August 19, 2009.

6. Complementary and Alternative Medicine.

7. Complementary and Alternative Medicine.

8. Complementary and Alternative Medicine.

9. The term "traditional" is used in two ways with respect to Chinese medicine. In referring to the traditional practice of Chinese medicine going back thousands of years, I use the protocol "traditional Chinese medicine." The term "Traditional Chinese Medicine (TCM) refers to reforms introduced under Mao Zedong, which eliminated practices and explanations he considered "superstition."

10. http://www.fas.harvard.edu/~anthro/social_faculty_pages/social_pages_kleinman. html. Accessed January 2007.

11. Larson Publications, 1995.

12. *Huang Di Nei Jing Su Wen* (*Emperor Huang's Internal Classic: Simple Questions*) Vol. 2, U.S. Department of Commerce Publishing House, 1954, 27. Originally published 2500 B.C. There are a number of Internet sites citing this classic work.

13. I was the second daughter in my family and I can attest to the lack of responsibilities required of the second daughter, even in Western culture.

14. Chao Chen, "Yi and Medicine," *Studies on the Application of the Book of Changes*, Vol 2, Taipei: Chung Hua Books, 1982.

15. Immanuel Kant, *Critique of Pure Reason*, "Deduction of the Pure Concepts of the Understanding,"http://www.marxists.org/reference/subject/ethics/kant/reason/ch01.htm. Accessed August 2009.

16. Kant, *Critique of Pure Reason*.

17. This is from an acupuncture publication cited by Evelyn Y. Ho (2006). The pamphlet is published by Good Fortune Acupuncture Clinic (GFAC), a pseudonym for the organization used by Evelyn Y. Ho.

18. http://nccam.nihgov/health/acupuncture/introduction.htm. Accessed February 2008.

19. Acupuncture.

20. Acupuncture.

21. Acupuncture.

22. UCLA Center for East-West Medicine. "What's New," http://www.cewm.med.ucla.edu/newsEvent/index.html. Accessed January 2008 and August 19, 2009.

23. East-West Medicine.

24. http://www.richnature.com/TCM%20books/theory.htm. Accessed February 2008.

25. Acupuncture points.

26. http://www.umm.edu/altmed/articles/-000348.htm. Accessed February 2008.

27. U.S. National Center for Complementary and Alternative Medicine, "What Is Complementary and Alternative Medicine?" http://nccam.nih.gov/health/backgrounds/wholemed.htm. Accessed February 2008 and August 19, 2009.

28. A Western criticism of Ayurveda is that Ayurvedic practitioners, unlike practitioners of Chinese medicine, use substances that have metallic ingredients. Products used in Western medicine, however, may have harmful side effects when used in pharmaceutical products, in excess dosages, or in additional to other medical products.

29. Ayurvedic practitioners are not licensed in the United States, whereas medical doctors are.

30. Ultimately, the effectiveness of all medical care systems rests on full disclosure by the patient. Over-the-counter remedies can interact negatively with prescription remedies or other over-the-counter medications.

31. NCCAM. National Center for Complementary and Alternative Medicine, "Health Information," http://nccam.nih.gov/health. Accessed February 2008 and August 19, 2009.

32. Complementary and Alternative Medicine.

33. Rabindranath Tagore, *Gitanjali: A Collection of Indian Poems by the Nobel Laureate*, New York: Scribner Poetry, 1997.

34. Confucius is the Westernization of Kung Fu Tzu, the name of the Chinese philosopher who lived from 551 to 479 BC.

35. I am indebted to Ravi Wadhwani for introducing me to this approach to establishing relationships with others, with the essence of our own being and with the essential harmony underlying the universe.

36. http://www.umm.edu/altmed/articles/-000348.htm. Accessed February 2008

37. Ayurveda.

CHAPTER 11 CALLING ON THE SPIRITS: SHAMANS, SORCERERS, AND MEDIUMS

1. Kuna is the preferred name for this group, formerly known as Cuna by scholars. The name in the Kuna language is *Dule* or *Tule,* meaning "people."

2. The incantation was published in 1958 by Nils M. Holmer and Henry Wassén under the title *Nia-Ikala: Canto Magico Pára Curar La Locura. Texto en Kengua Cuna, anotado por el indio Guillermo Hayans con traducción Española y comentarios: Etnologiska Studier, 21.* This publication is apparently out of print, but it has been cited in works by other authors.

3. An example of the importance of archaeology in helping us understand the history of shamanism is the work by Christopher Donnan and others among the Moche of Peru. These archaeologists compared representations of healers in traditional Moche art with practices they observed being used by contemporary healers. A classic study of a contemporary Peruvian healer is recorded in the film *Eduardo the Healer.*

4. My colleague Rodolfo Otero, who has studied mediums engaged in medical practice in Mexicali, along the U.S.-Mexican border, has corrected me on this point. He notes that, "Shamans do not control the spirits; shamans negotiate with them" (pers. comm.).

5. I am not using the term "adventurer" in a derogatory sense. International exploration has been a factor in some human groups for as long as we have records, either historical or archaeological. The motivations are varied, from trade to conquest to the acquisition of knowledge. In some cases, adventurers negatively affect the lives of the people they encounter. In other cases, adventurers enhance the lives of people in their own society without harming the people or other

organisms they encounter on their journeys. For example, noodles originated in Asia and were introduced to Italy through trade. Italian immigrants brought pasta to the United States. I shall always be grateful to those adventurers who allow me to enjoy a delicious bowl of pasta in my own dining room. I am also grateful to those who brought rice to the United States.

6. The word "Tungus" is commonly used by outsiders to designate this group of people; the word "Evenki" is their term in referring to themselves.

7. In many groups cross-culturally, the stealing of an individual's soul, or animating force, is viewed as a cause of serious illness or death.

8. Azande is the noun form; Zande is the adjective for this group.

9. From Wallace's writings, an inyanga is a diviner, physician or shaman (1966:145).

10. Evans-Pritchard uses the term "magicians" for healers. The more commonly used term today is "shamans."

11. Variation in the term referring to *vodun*, often described as "voodoo," is due to the French pronunciation. The generally accepted spelling among scholars is *vodou*, which most accurately reflects the English pronunciation of this religious practice.

CHAPTER 12 THE EMERGING FIELD OF INTEGRATIVE MEDICINE

1. William H. Wiist, "Teaching on the Frontiers of Health Care," 7(3) (Fall 2002), http://www.cewm.med/ucla.edu/AboutUs/mission.html. Accessed December 2002 and August 24, 2009.

2. There are many others, including psychologists and psychologically oriented anthropologists. I cite Frank and Kiev because their work focused on promoting this position.

3. National Center for Complementary and Alternative Medicine, http://nccam.nih.gov/health/whatiscam. Accessed 1/30/2007.

4. NCCAM.

5. NCCAM.

6. I beg to differ with NCCAM's description of vitamins and dietary supplements as being "found in nature." They may have been found there, but they have been intensively processed and bear no resemblance to products that truly are natural. Having grown up on a farm, I can attest to the fact that processed herbs and other plants lose much of their aesthetic and nutritional value; however, I empathize with the difficulty in sorting out and describing freshly harvested fruits and vegetables or wild fruits and vegetables in succinct terms.

7. National Center for Complementary and Alternative Medicine, http://nccam.nih.gov/health/whatiscam.

8. http://bmei.org/jbem/volume3/num1/terrell_medical_efficacy_and_medical_ethics.php. Accessed January 2007.

9. Medical efficacy and ethics.

10. Medical efficacy and ethics.

11. *Hamlet, Prince of Denmark*, William Shakespeare, Act III, Scene I.

12. *Hamlet.*

13. I was not among the journalists covering that disaster, but I have had reports from journalists who covered it.

14. Two of my books, *Sport as Symbol: Images of the Athlete in Art, Literature and Song.* (McFarland 2003) and *Symbols and Meaning: A Concise Introduction* (AltaMira 2005), address the social and psychological importance of symbols.

15. http://www.emedicinehealth.com/eczema/page2_em.htm. Accessed January 2008.

16. http://www.mayoclinic.com. Accessed August 2008.

17. Stress related disorders. Accessed August 2008.

CHAPTER 13 THE SOCIAL CONTEXT OF EPIDEMICS

1. J. McArthur. 1954. Okapa Patrol Report (Cited in Shirley Lindenbaum, *Kuru Sorcery: Disease and Anager in the New Guinea Highlands*. Mountain View, CA: Mayfield, 1979, 9.

2. NINDS kuru information page, http://www.ninds.nih.gov/disorders/kuru/kuru.htm. Accessed August 2008 and August 23, 2009.

3. This refers to Creutzfelt Jacob disease, a neurological disorder. http://www.ninds.nih.gov/disorders/cjd/cjd.htm. Accessed August 2008.

4. Creutzfeldt Jacob disease.

5. http://www.surgeongeneral.gov/library/mentalhealth/chaper2/see2_1.html. Accessed August 2008.

6. http://www.cdc.gov/malaria/disease.htm. Accessed August 2008.

7. Malaria.

8. Malaria.

9. Malaria. http://en.wikipedia.org/wiki/Malaria. Accessed August 2008.

10. Malaria.

11. http://nytimes.com/2006/12/23/world/africa/23ghana.html. Accessed December 23, 2006.

12. http://www.who.int/hiv/mediacentre/news60/en/print/html. Accessed December 2006.

13. Thomas H. Maugh II and Karen Kaplan, "Gene Mutation Increases Risk of HIV Infection."

14. HIV Gene Mutation.

15. HIV Gene Mutation.

16. Jia-Rui Chong, "AIDS epidemic growing worldwide," *Los Angeles Times*, November 22, 2006, A8.

17. http://www.mayoclinic.com/print/tuberculosis. Accessed August 24, 2009.

18. Tuberculosis.

19. Laura Womack, 2007, pers. comm.

20. http://www.who.int/tb/xdr/en/index.html. Accessed January 2007.

21. The word "hominid" refers to those members of the primate family most closely related to humans, as well as more recent species including modern humans. Though estimates vary, hominids may have evolved as long ago as 4 million to 6 million years. According to most estimates, humans evolved only about 100,000 years ago.

22. Mayo Clinic Staff, Autism: Definition. http://www.mayoclinic.com. Accessed December 2007 and August 2009.

23. Autism disorder.

24. Anti Social Personality Disorder, http://www.nlm.nih.gov/medlineplus/ency/article/000921.htm. Accessed December 2007 and August 2009.

25. Autism disorder.

26. Autism disorder.

27. Autism disorder.

28. Autism disorder.

29. This discussion of a possible genetic basis for autism is a general summary of a variety of research being conducted at the time of this writing . A precise listing of all the research published on this topic is beyond the scope of this book and the research is ongoing. Singling out any one article would be misleading. I singled out Aravinda Chakravarti of the Johns Hopkins School of Medicine because Johns Hopkins is an important center for this type of research, as well as applications of this research. Dr. Chakravarti is a specialist in identifying possible genetic bases for a variety of diseases and disorders.

30. http://www.nimh.hih.gov/publicat/autism.cfm. Accessed January 2008.

31. Autism.

32. National Institute on Drug Abuse. http://www.nida.nih.gov/Infofacts/Ritalin.html. Accessed 2008.

33. ADHD.

34. ADHD.

35. ADHD.

36. "Dopamine—A Sample Neurotransmitter," Addiction Science Research and Education, College of Pharmacy, University of Texas, http://utexas.edu/research/asrec/dopamine.html. Accessed January 2008.

37. Dopamine.

38. ADHD.

39. ADHD. This assertion by NIDA is based on research conducted by N. D. Volkow and J. M. Swanson (2003).

40. Carol E. Watkins and Glenn Brynes, "Ritalin Helps . . . But What About the Side Effects?" Northern County Psychiatric Associates," 2006, http://www.ncpamd.com/Stimulant_Side_Effects.htm. Accessed January 2008.

41. Watkins and Brynes, "Ritalin Helps."

42. I am indebted to Michael Alan Park (2008) for this observation.

43. http://www.bt.cdc.gov/agent/plague/factsheet.asp. Accessed December 2007.

44. Elisabeth Rosenthal, "As Earth Warms Up, Tropical Virus Moves to Italy," *New York Times*, December 23, 2007, http://www.nytimes.com/2007/12/23/world/europe/23virus.html. Accessed December 2007.

45. http://www.searo.who.int/en.Section10/Section2246.htm. Accessed 2007.

46. "Dengue Fever," Center for Disease Control; Division of Vector-Borne Diseases, http://www.cdc/gov/ncidod/dvbid/dengue. Accessed originally December 2007 and August 2009.

CHAPTER 14 MEDICINES, HERBS, AND DIETARY SUPPLEMENTS

1. The plant/meat ratio would vary depending on resources available in the environment.

2. Overview of Clinical Trials, CenterWatch, http://www.centerwatch.com/patient/backgrnd.html. Accessed March 2008 and again in August 2009.

3. Clinical Trials.

4. Clinical Trials.

5. Clinical Trials.

6. Clinical Trials.

7. Thomas H. Maugh II, "Less Acid, Brittler Hips?" *Los Angeles Times*, December 27, 2006, A15.

8. Maugh, "Less Acid."

9. Maugh, "Less Acid."

10. Maugh, "Less Acid."

11. Denise Gellene, "Antidepressants May Boost Risk of Fractures," *Los Angeles Times*, January 23, 2007, A9.

12. Information regarding this ingredient can be found at http://www.streetdrugs.org/dxm/htm. Accessed April 2008.

13. Street drugs.

14. Street drugs.

15. http://news.yahoo.com/s/ap/20070319/ap_on_he_me/sinus_study_antibiotic. Accessed March 2007.

16. Sinus infections.

17. http://www.cdc.gov/std/Gonorrhea/arg/stdfact-resistant-gonorrhea.htm. Accessed March 2007.

18. http://news.yahoo.com/s/ap/20070412/ap_on_he_me/risistant_gonorrhea. Accessed March 2007.

19. This metaphor is taken from the film "The Graduate," in which a recent college graduate (played by Dustin Hoffman) dropped out from the heavily commercialized culture occupied by his parents and their friends.

20. http://www.nytimes.com/2008/03/21/us/21vaccine.html.

21. "Possible Side Effects from Vaccines," Center for Disease Control and Prevention, http://www.cdc.gov/vaccines/vac-gen/side-effects.htm. Site last modified August 11, 2009. Accessed March 2007 and August 2009.

22. "Possible Side Effects."

23. "Possible Side Effects."

24. "The Disease and the Virus," Global Polio Eradication Initiative, http://www.polioeradication.org/disease.asp. Accessed March 2008 and August 2009.

25. "Disease and the Virus."

26. "Disease and the Virus."

27. "Disease and the Virus."

28. This is a pseudonym of Theophrastus Bombastus von Hohenheim.

29. Quoted in Deni Bown, *Encyclopedia of Herbs*. New York: DK Publishing, 2001, 16.

30. Adapted from Thomas H. Maugh II, "Herbal Remedy Fails Test at Soothing Menopause," *Los Angeles Times*, December 19, 2006, A16.

31. Maugh, "Herbal Remedy."

32. See Mandy M. Cox and Kenneth L. Korth, "Characterization of Wound-Inducible Genes Encoding Enzymes for Terpenoid Biosynthesis in *Medicago truncatula*, www.uark.edu/rd_vcad/urel/publications/inquiry/2003/cox.pdf#search='terpenoids'. Accessed December 2008.

33. See Alan L. Miller, "Antioxidant Flavonoids: Structure, Function and Clinical Usage." www.thorne.com/altmedrev/fulltext/flavonoids1-2.html. Accessed December 2008.

34. Lester Grinspoon, "Puffing Is the Best Medicine." *Los Angeles Times*, May 5, 2006, B13.

35. Alternative Medicine.

36. Alternative Medicine.

CHAPTER 15 PUBLIC POLICY AND HEALTH-CARE DELIVERY SYSTEMS

1. This is taken from John F. Kennedy's Address Before the General Assembly of the United Nations On September 25, 1961. It can be accessed through the John F. Kennedy Presidential Library and Museum. See also John F Kennedy's Inaugural Address of January 20, 1961, which can also be accessed at the John F. Kennedy Presidential Library and Museum.

2. http://www.ama-assn.org/ama/pub/category/print/8421.html. Accessed June 2008.

3. Medical ethics and torture.

4. Medical ethics and torture.

5. http://www.who.int/features/2007/year_review/en/index/html. Accessed January 2008.

6. http://www.cdc.gov/ncidod/dvbid/yellowfever/. Accessed March 2009.

7. Yellow fever.

8. http://www.gatesfoundation.org/GlobalHealth/. Accessed December 2007.

9. Global Health.

10. Global Health.

11. Global Health.

12. Global Health.

13. Charles Piller and Doug Smith, "Unintended Victims of Gates Foundation Generosity," *Los Angeles Times*, December 16, 2007.

14. From Hamlet's famous soliloquy beginning "To be or not to be."

15. United Nations population estimates are computed according to low, medium, and high variants to account for shifting factors, such as disease rates, wars, natural disasters, life expectancy, mortality and fertility rates, economic shifts, and migration.

16. "Global Population at a Glance: 2002 and Beyond," U.S. Department of Commerce, Economics and Statistics Administration, 2004, www.census.gov/ipc/prod/wp02/wp02-1.pdf. Accessed August 2009.

17. Rishi Manchanda, "Teach Healthcare, Not Just Medicine," *Los Angeles Times*, April 9, 2007, A13.

18. Manchanda, "Teach Healthcare."

19. These figures are my own, based on assessments by physical anthropologists.

20. http://www.nytimes.com/2006/12/23/world/africa/23ghana.html. Accessed December 2006.

21. "Early Childhood: The Big Picture," http://www.unicef.org/earlychildhood/index_bigpicture.html.Accessed December 2006 and August 2009.

22. "Early Childhood."

23. "Early Childhood."

24. "Early Childhood."

25. "Early Childhood."

26. http://www.aamr.org/Policies/faq_mental_retardation.html. Accessed December 2006.

27. Nutrition and Mental Retardation.

28. Understanding Malnutrition and Treatments. Bread for the World, http://www.bread.org/learn/global-hunger-issues/malnutrition.html. Accessed December 2006 and August 2009.

29. Malnutrition.

30. http://www.dailytrojan.com/home/index. Accessed December 2006.

31. Marito Garcia, "Malnutrition and Food Insecurity Projections 2020," International Food Policy Research Institute, 1994, http://www.ifpri.org/2020/briefs/number06.htm.

32. Garcia, "Malnutrition and Food Insecurity."

33. Garcia, "Malnutrition and Food Insecurity."

34. Garcia, "Malnutrition and Food Insecurity."

35. Garcia, "Malnutrition and Food Insecurity."

36. Michael Wines, "Malnutrition Is Cheating Its Survivors, and Africa's Future," *New York Times*, December 28, 2006, http://www.nytimes.com/2006/12/28/world/africa/28malnutrition.html. Accessed December 2006.

37. http://www.nlm.hih.gov/medlineplus/print/ency/article/001604/htm. Accessed December 2006. This link to the National Library of Medicine maintained by the National Institutes of Health refers to the relationship between Kwashiorkor and malnutrition.

38. Simon S. Rabinowitz, Mario Gehri, Ermindo R. DiPaolo, and Natalia M. Wetterer, "Marasmus," Emedicine, http://www.emedicine.com/ped/topic164.htm. Accessed December 2006 and August 2009.

39. "Marasmus."

40. "Marasmus."

41. http://www.udel.edu/PR/UDaily/2005/mar/tourism072504.html. Accessed December 2006.

42. Medical Tourism.

43. Medical Tourism.

44. Medical Tourism.

45. Medical Tourism.

46. Medical Tourism.

47. Medical Tourism.

48. http://www.cbc.ca/includes/printablestory.jsp.Accessed December 2006. This is based on a Canadian Broadcasting Corporation report on medical tourism. Medical tourism is a recent and growing phenomenon. Medical tourism is promoted on websites in the Philippines, India, Singapore, Malaysia, Thailand, Mexico Costa Rica, and Canada. There is also an international Medical Tourism Association.

49. Medical tourism.

50. Medical tourism.

51. Medical tourism.

Glossary

abstract thought   the capacity to conceptualize phenomena that do not exist in time and space.

achieved status   status acquired by one's own actions or merits.

acupuncture   a system of healing characteristic of Chinese medicine based on stimulating points on the human body believed to be significant in healing and maintaining health.

alimentation   the process of ingesting and absorbing nutrients.

allele   variation in a *gene*. For example, eye color is determined by genetic coding for that trait. The difference between brown eyes and blue eyes is determined by the alleles that code for brown eyes or blue eyes.

analgesic   pain medication that does not produce loss of consciousness.

androgens   the so-called "male hormones." In fact, all humans produce *androgens*, including *testosterone*, and the so-called "female hormones," *progesterone* and *estrogen*. The development of testicles is stimulated by the Y chromosome, and testicles produce more androgens than *estrogen*, thus offsetting the influence of that "female hormone." In female fetuses, ovaries produce more *estrogen* and *progesterone* than androgen, thus offsetting the influence of the "male hormone." Androgens, estrogen, and progesterone are classified as steroids.

antigen   a protein or carbohydrate capable of triggering an immune response.

antioxident   any substance that reduces damage to molecules caused by exposure to oxygen, which alters the chemical properties of a cell. See also *free radicals* and *molecule*.

antisocial personality disorder   an inability to empathize with others that manifests in chronic behavior that manipulates, exploits, or violates the rights of others. This behavior is often criminal. Formerly known as *psychopathology* or *sociopathology*.

applied anthropology   application of anthropological theory and/or method in solving problems.

archaeology   the study of culture through the material remains of a group.

arteries   any of the tubular branching muscular- and elastic-walled vessels that carry blood from the heart to other parts of the body.

artifacts   products of human craft works.

ascribed status   status conferred by birth.

autism, also **autism spectrum disorder**   the inability to interact with or communicate with others.

Ayurveda   an ancient philosophical tradition originating on the Indian subcontinent that combines the Sanskrit word *āyus*, which refers to the life process, and the word *veda*, which means "knowledge."

Ayurvedic medicine   an ancient system of health care that developed on the Indian subcontinent. It is said to date from *Vedic times*. Ayurvedic medicine is in widespread practice in India and Sri Lanka, as well as among the Indian *diaspora*.

balanced reciprocity   a form of exchange in which individuals establish a trading partnership that lasts through time by means of exchanging items or services of equal value.

basal ganglia   a cluster of neurons under the *cerebral cortex* involved in motor control, cognition, emotions, and learning.

binary oppositions   paired opposites. The French anthropologist Claude Lévi-Strauss considered that the cross-cultural pattern of ordering the world into binary oppositions, such as up-down and male-female were based in universal structures of the human mind. Ordering the universe into binary oppositions allows humans to construct a view of the physical, social, and conceptual universe that reduces ambiguity.

biochemical   this term integrates two levels of understanding the human body. Humans are biological organisms, of the kingdom *Animalia*, which means they are capable of *alimentation* and *mobility*. These abilities are based on chemical processes, which involves the processes of linking atoms into molecules and, ultimately, into biological structures.

biomedicine   an approach to health and healing based on scientific theory and method.

brain stem   the part of the brain that coordinates communication between the *peripheral nervous system* and the *cerebrum*. It transmits sensory data from the muscles and internal organs to the *cerebrum* and transmits orders from the *cerebrum* to the muscles and internal organs.

brideprice   a practice in which a groom's family economically compensates the bride's family for her fertility and labor, since her family has borne the expense of raising her. Also called *bridewealth*.

catastrophizing   taking a pessimistic view of one's life and expectations, as well as overemphasizing one's pain.

catharsis   a sense of relief and feeling cleansed that typically follows a period of intense emotion.

causal reasoning   a process of analysis in which results can be predicted based on the presence of *variables* known to have produced these results in the past.

cerebellum   large collections of nuclei that modify movement on a minute-by-minute basis.

cerebral cortex   the outer layers of the *cerebrum*, where much of abstract thought takes place.

cerebrum   the two hemispheres of the brain that process complex thought processes. In humans, the cerebrum completely covers the *brain stem* and *midbrain*.

circulatory system   the system of blood, blood vessels, *lymphatic system*, and heart action that controls the movement of blood and *lymph* though the body.

circumcision   alteration of the human genitals according to culturally prescribed patterns. Typically, this is a form of surgery in which the foreskin of the male or the tip of the female *clitoris* is removed.

clan   a form of kin membership in which descent is traced to a founding ancestor. The ancestral connection is marked by naming—as among Scottish and Irish clans, who continue to carry the name "MacFarland" or "O'Farrell"—or as among Australian aborigines, who trace their descent from a founding *totemic ancestor*.

clinical trials   the process of testing experimental drugs on humans. These usually consist of three phases: assessing the drug's safety; testing for effectiveness; and further assessing the drug's effectiveness, benefits, and side effects.

clitoridectomy   alteration or removal of the *clitoris*, a small organ of female genitalia that results from sexual differentiation during fetal development. In male fetuses, which carry the XY chromosome, the Y chromosome stimulates production of *androgens*, which promote the development of this structure into a penis. The tip of the clitoris is homologous to the foreskin of the penis. In more extreme forms, clitoridectomy may include excising the clitoris, as well as removing part of the *labia minora*, the inner lips of the *vulva*, and the sewing together of the skin of the labia minora.

clitoris   the female organ analogous to the male penis, but which does not possess the functional properties of the penis. For example, the clitoris does not urinate or secrete semen.

clots   the body's ability to form clots is part of its survival mechanism. An individual whose body lacks the clotting agent can die from something so simple as having his teeth cleaned. Clotting becomes dangerous when it results from pooling of blood through lack of circulation. This can occur through prolonged sitting, or other inactivity, in which blood fails to circulate back to the heart.

cognition   the process by which an individual orders her or his experience of the world according to a culturally shaped world view, as a model for operating within that self-experienced and self-defined universe.

cognitive schema   a cognitive model of the world developed in childhood that shapes the individual's experience of his or her social and physical universe.

corpus callosum   *neurons* that connect the two hemispheres of the brain. The corpus callosum is important in making possible such cognitive activities as coordination, language, and vision.

correlation   a relationship in which *variables* occur together in a way not expected by chance alone.

cosmology   a symbolically ordered view of the world acquired in the process of *socialization*.

couvade   a childbirth custom in which the father of the child behaves as though he were giving birth, including observing all the rituals associated with pregnancy and childbirth.

cross-cultural   an anthropological approach that compares human groups, with all their attendent phenomena, with comparable phenomena in other human groups.

cultural anthropology   the anthropological subfield that focuses on the study of contemporary human groups, including their social relationships, forms of communication, beliefs and customs, the way in which they define themselves, and their use of environmental resources.

cultural evolution   change in the beliefs, attitudes, and practices of human groups through time.

cultural relativism   the anthropological approach that avoids making value judgments about the people being studied.

culture   beliefs, attitudes, and customs acquired by *socialization* within a particular group and transmitted by learning from one generation to the next.

deductive reasoning   a logical process in which general theories that have consistently proved to be true are applied to specific cases.

demographic analysis   studies that focus on dimensions of human populations that can be statistically examined, such as age and income levels.

displacement   a quality of language that allows humans to communicate about phenomena that cannot be experienced by the senses.

divination   a ritual aimed at obtaining information from the spirit world.

dowry   a form of marriage exchange in which the groom's family compensates the bride's family for her fertility and other economic contributions to the groom's family.

emasculation   surgical removal of male genitalia.

embryo   the product of conception during its early stages of development from the time it is implanted in the uterus through the eighth week of development in humans, when it is referred to as a *fetus*.

empirical   capable of being observed and measured by the senses. (noun: *empiricism*)

empiricism   the idea that science should be based on studying phenomena that can be observed and measured by the senses. (adjective: **empirical**)

endogenous opioids: neurotransmitters produced by the body that activate opiate receptors in the brain. Also *endorphins*.

epidemic   contagious disease affecting many individuals in a population at the same time.

estrogen   one of the so-called "female hormones." Estrogen is produced by enzymes, which break down and reconstitute substances. In women, estrogens promote the development of female secondary characteristics and regulate the menstrual cycle. In males, estrogen regulates functions of the reproductive system important for the maturation of sperm. They may also be important in stimulating *libido*, the sex drive.

ethnocentric   centered on one's own culture combined with disregard of the contribution of other cultures.

ethnography   a long-term study of a particular group of people conducted by using the methodology of *participant-observation*.

etiology   cause or origin of a disease or the study of the causes and origins of disease.

evolution   change through time. In scientific terms, evolution is defined as a change in allele frequency within a population from one generation to the next. An allele is a variation in a gene. For example, a gene might code for eye color. Alleles for this trait may code for brown eyes, blue eyes, or other types of eye color.

excision   a form of female genital surgery that involves removal of the *clitoris*.

exogamy   a marital practice of out-marrying, which requires one to marry outside one's own group. Typically, this requires marriage outside one's own kin group.

extended family   a form of family organization in which resources are shared among closely related nuclear families.

evolution   change through time. This can be biological or cultural. Biological evolution occurs when there is a change in *allele frequency*, the distribution of *gene* variability within a population over time. Cultural evolution occurs when there is a change in beliefs, customs or behavior through time. An example of cultural evolution is that, in the past 100 years, the United States has shifted from a predominantly rural to a predominantly urban population base.

fatty acids   depending on their structure, fatty acids can be labeled "good" or "bad." Some fatty acids remove or disable the fatty acids that cause a buildup leading to heart disease and other disorders. In fact, there is no such thing as "good" or "bad" in human biology. The human organism is in continual interaction with the environment. Our nutritional needs are directly related to our genetic heritage and our lifestyle.

feticide   killing of fetuses.

fetus   an organism at a more advanced stage of development than an *embryo* (at the end of the eighth week in humans) until its birth.

fibromyalgia   pain in the soft fibrous tissues of the body, including muscles, ligaments, and tendons.

folk taxonomy   description of a phenomenon, including health and illness, that explains the phenomenon in terms consistent with the *world view* of that group.

free radicals   free radicals form when a molecule is altered in such a way that electrons do not add up to even pairs, thus producing an unstable molecule. Molecules, the chemical structures that comprise a cell, typically share electrons with other molecules. Free radicals attack stable molecules to "steal" their electrons. The "attacked" molecule then becomes a free radical itself and begins to attack other molecules. This begins a chain reaction that can disrupt the functioning of a living cell.

gametes   sex cells, sperm or ova.

gender   social roles and cultural definitions assigned to females and males.

genetics   the study of *genes* of the role of genes in producing particular traits in an organism.

genitalia   genitals.

genome   the complete genetic coding of an organism.

glans   the blood-enriched tip of the penis or the *clitoris*.

gonads   organs that produce *gametes* or sex cells. In females, gonads are the *ovaries*. In males, gonads are the *testes* or *testicles*.

hallucinogens   substances that produce an *altered state of consciousness* by chemically changing an individual's perceptual processes. See *perception*.

herbal medicine   a system of medical treatment based on knowledge of the chemical properties of plants.

holistic   approaching a research issue by taking all relevant factors into consideration, including biology, sociology, psychology, and history. (noun: **holism**)

homeopathic medicine   an alternative medicine originally espoused by Samuel Hahnemann in 1796. Homeopathy is based on the idea that preparations that produce symptoms similar to the disease being treated are likely to cure the condition. Homeopaths also base their treatments on aspects of the patient's physical and psychological conditions.

hominids   modern humans and their ancestors, the distinguishing characteristic of which is the ability to walk upright.

homozygous   a genetic heritage in which the genetic potential of both father and mother carry identical coding for a potential trait.

hypochondriacs   people who are preoccupied with their physical health and body, and who fear they have a serious disease despite medical reassurance.

hypoglycemia   low blood glucose or low blood sugar, which manifests as nervousness, sweating, intense hunger, trembling, weakness, palpitations and difficulty in speaking. These symptoms appear when the brain is deprived of sugar needed for adequate neurological function.

hypothalamus   a part of the brain that regulates sensations related to strong emotions.

immune cells   those cells that recognize disease pathogens and destroy them before they can cause lasting harm to the organism.

immune system   those parts of our organism that allows us to recognize pathogens and destroy them before they cause devastating harm to our bodies.

indigenous   customs, attitudes, communication patterns, and organisms having developed in the region they continue to occupy.

inductive reasoning   a logical process in which general theories are developed from specific cases.

infibulation   the most extreme form of female genital surgery, which involves removal of the *clitoris*, the outer lining of the *labia*, part of the lining of the vagina, and reducing the size of the opening to the vagina.

initiation rites   rituals accompanying a change of social status, usually conferring membership into a specialized group.

insider perspective   the anthropological approach that requires a researcher to consider a group's own values and view of the world in analyzing their way of life.

integrative medicine   a term developed by U.S. National Institutes of Health to designate healing traditions developed outside the Western biomedical tradition.

intelligence   a difficult-to-define mental ability involved in reasoning, perceiving relationships and *analogies*, calculating, learning, and processing information quickly. It is generally defined as cognitive problem-solving skills.

intersexuality   the biological pattern in which an infant is born with intermediate external genitalia or with external genitalia that do not conform to the individual's *genotype*.

labia   consists of the *labia majora*, the outer fatty folds of the *vulva* surrounding the opening to the urethra, and the *labia minora*, the inner blood-enriched largely connective tissue folds of the *vulva*, the external parts of the female genitalia.

language   a form of communication that makes abstract thought possible.

limbic system   a part of the brain involved in hormones, temperature control, and emotion.

liminality   a marginal status in which an individual has no clearly defined identity. During this time, an individual is considered to be ritually dangerous to himself or herself and others.

linguistics   the study of language and communication.

loci   plural form of the word "locus," meaning location on a DNA molecule that codes for a particular trait. See *locus*.

locus   location on a DNA molecule that codes for a particular trait.

logic   a process of reasoning that describes a relationship between or among phenomena.

lymph   a pale fluid that bathes the tissues and is discharged into the blood. It consists of a liquid portion that contains white blood cells. It is important in fighting infections, since white blood cells are a primary defense against infectious organisms.

lymphatic system   a system of circulation that carries lymph.

magic   a symbolic system aimed at controlling forces in the social, physical, and conceptual universe.

mammal   large, warm-blooded animal that produces live young and provides nutrients for their offspring by means of mammary glands.

matrilineage   a pattern of family organization in which a woman and her children inherit status and access to resources through her family

matrilineal   a system of inheritance in which status and property are transmitted through the female line.

matrilocal residence   a system of residence in which a husband and wife take up residence with or near the bride's family after marriage. Also *uxorilocal*.

medium   an individual engaged in prophesy or healing by allowing himself or herself to be possessed by spirits.

menarche   the onset of menses; also, the first menstruation.

menstrual seclusion   practice in which women who are menstruating give up their daily schedules and retire to a shelter reserved for them.

menstrual taboos   ritual avoidance of interaction with males and (often) with children by women when they are menstruating.

metaphor   symbolic comparisons that permit humans to link sensory experience to concepts that cannot be experience primarily through the senses.

microbes   organisms that are too small to be seen with the naked eye. They must be viewed through microscopes.

midbrain   the part of the human brain that mediates between the *peripheral nervous system*—which transmits information from the sensory organs and transmits information from the *central nervous system* to the muscles and acts as a relay station between the sensory organs—and the *cerebrum*, which interprets and makes decisions on the basis of this information.

midwife   traditional specialist (usually female) in childbirth techniques. In industrialized societies, midwifes must be officially certified.

mind-body dichotomy   a predominantly Western concept that the mind exists independently of the body and is at war with it.

molecule   a sufficiently stable electrically neutral group of at least two atoms in an arrangement held together by strong chemical bonds.

motor cortex   the part of the brain that sends instructions to the muscles and internal organs.

mutation   a spontaneous change in DNA coding that usually produces an altered *phenotype*, a change in the morphology of an organism.

myelinated neurons   nerve cells that are covered by a fatty sheath, which speeds a message along a neuron and protects against disruptive messages from outside the communication track.

mysticism   beliefs and practices based on the idea that God and spiritual states can be experienced directly.

natural selection   Charles Darwin's idea that nature exerts the same selective pressure on species that humans exert through selective breeding. The process of adapting to a particular environment, Darwin suggested, could result in development of new species.

naturopathy   a healing system based on the idea that treatment should be based in the body's inherent ability to establish, maintain, and restore health. Naturopathic physicians use dietetics, natural hygiene, fasting, and nutritional supplementation in practice. Treatments also include botanical substances drawn from nature.

necropsy   postmortem examination or autopsy.

neurobiologists   scholars and physicians who study the structure and function of the brain. Also *neurologists*.

neurologists   scholars and physicians who study the structure and function of the brain. Also *neurobiologists*.

neuron   an electrically excitable cell in the nervous system that processes and transmits information; nerve cell, the basic component of the brain and sensory system.

NGOs   nongovernmental organizations, typically funded by private organizations or individuals, which provide aid to individuals and institutions in need of aid but are unable to obtain aid through governmental channels.

noncompliant   term for a patient who fails or refuses to comply with medical instructions or procedures, particularly in regard to taking a prescribed medication or following a prescribed course of therapy.

nuclear family   form of family organization consisting of a parent or parent and offspring and organized around the reproductive unit.

omnivores   animals that require a varied diet including both plants and animals.

pandemic   contagious disease occurring over a wide geographic area and affecting a proportionately high proportion of the population.

paradigm   as used by Thomas S. Kuhn (1970), this term refers to models underlying the practices and expectations involved in scientific research.

parasympathetic nervous system   a component of the autonomic nervous system that promotes repair of the body after the need for dynamic action in response to a stimulus is past.

pariah   literally, an outcaste. The term derives from application to outcastes in India, who were considered polluting to all castes. It is now used to designate someone who is not accepted in society in general.

participant-observation   the preferred anthropological method involving living as a member of the group being studied and sharing in day-to-day activities, usually for an extended period of time.

pathogen   the specific cause—such as a bacterium, protozoan or virus—of a disease.

pathology   illness, which can be defined as either physical or psychological.

patrilineal   a system of inheritance in which status and property are transmitted through the male line.

patrilocal residence   a system of residence in which a husband and wife take up residence with or near the groom's family after marriage. Also *virilocal*.

peripheral nervous system   *ganglia* and nerves outside the *central nervous system* that receive and transmit information to and from the central nervous system.

persistent vegetative state   a condition in which individuals have lost cognitive neurological function and awareness of the environment, but retain noncognitive function—such as reflex actions—and a preserved sleep-wake cycle.

physical anthropology   the anthropological subfield that specializes in the study of nonhuman primates, human ecology and physiology, and genetics and evolution.

plasticity   flexibility. Also, the ability to adapt rapidly to different social, cultural, or physical environments.

polluting   substances or actions that are dangerously powerful. Substances or actions that are viewed as polluting typically follow the anthropologist Mary Douglas's model that "dirt is matter out of place"; that is, that the social and moral orders are maintained by establishing categories that must not "invade" each other.

preternatural   a phenomenon that exceeds the ordinary or regular.

primates   an order of organisms possessing the following characteristics: eyes located on the front of the face, permitting stereoscopic vision and depth perception; an enlarged brain relative to body size; an enlarged cerebral cortex; and opposable thumbs.

probability   the idea that an outcome can be predicted given a particular set of circumstances.

probabilistic reasoning   a process of thought based on the idea that an outcome can be predicted given the presence of a particular set of circumstances.

progeny   offspring, children.

progesterone   a "female hormone" produced by the ovaries, and to a lesser extent, by the *testes*, that supports *gestation*, the ability to carry a *fetus* in the uterus. It is also instrumental in the menstrual cycle. Like *testosterone* and *estrogen*, progesterone is classified as a steroid, but testosterone is an *anabolic steroid*.

prognosis   a term referring to the probable course and outcome of a disease.

psychosomatic disorder   a physical ailment caused in part by psychological factors.

puberty   physical changes that prepare the human body for reproduction. The changes are stimulated by production of hormones.

recessive allele   a form of genetic coding that will only be expressed in an organism if that organism has inherited identical genetic coding for that trait from both parents.

regulatory genes   genes that regulate the activity of *structural genes*, which code for the structure of an organism.

religion   a symbolic system designed to explain the ordering of the universe and the social systems that operate within it.

respiration   the physical and chemical processes by which an animal supplies its cells and tissues with the oxygen needed for metabolism and relieves them of the carbon dioxide formed in energy-producing reactions.

revitalization movements   social movements, often based in religion, aimed at bringing about social change. Typically, these movements call on cultural traditions to "revitalize" current ways of life. They usually address this by integrating traditional beliefs and behaviors with more recently developed or introduced ways of doing things.

rite of passage   a ritual aimed at easing the transition from one social status to another. Typically, rites of passage escort an individual and the group to which he or she belongs from a state of clear social identity to a liminality state, in which the individual has lost his or her previous identity and has not yet acquired a new one, and, ultimately, to a state in which the individual acquires a new, socially accepted identity.

ritual   practices used in religion and magic that are repetitive, sequential, nonordinary and powerful, on both the psychological and social levels.

scarification   altering the human body in a form that is considered attractive in a particular culture.

scrotum   the pouch that contains the *testicles*.

selected for   a process in *natural selection* in which the presence of a particular genetic coding produces characteristics that promote an organism's survival in a particular environment.

selected against   a process in *natural selection* in which the presence of a particular genetic coding produces characteristics that reduce an organism's ability to survive in a particular environment.

serotonin   a neurotransmitter involved in regulating body temperature, sleep, sexuality, and appetite. It generally stimulates a sense of well-being through its stimulation of opioid receptors.

sex   as used in this book, a term that refers to biological differences between males and females that typically give rise to differences in their social status and expectations of behavior.

shaman   an individual who heals by calling on the aid of spirits. Typically, a shaman uses psychological, social, and herbal techniques to heal illnesses.

shamanism   a healing practice that employs both herbs and *ritual*. Anthropologists have noted that shamanic practices can be effective because they integrate biological, psychological, and social factors in diagnosis and treatment.

socialization   the process whereby an individual acquires the culture and *world view* of his or her group.

somatoform disorder   a disorder in which biological symptoms are entirely psychological and have no organic basis.

sorcerer   an individual who seeks to harm others by calling on the aid of spirits.

sorcery   deliberate attempt to cause harm to others by ritual means. In Western medical diagnoses, the desire to inflict harm on others is called *antisocial personality disorder*.

spirit possession an altered state of consciousness in which an individual is believed to be possessed by a spirit or spirits.

stratification a system of social organization in which there is unequal access to power and resources.

stratified societies societies in which there is unequal access to power and resources.

structural genes genes that code for the structures of an organism.

subincision a form of genital surgery in which the penis is slit open on the underside, typically from the *glans* to the *scrotum*.

subsistence practices the means by which a group converts environmental resources for human use.

symbol a word, image, or behavior that conveys multiple levels of meaning. Because these meanings draw on both conscious and unconscious associations, symbols are powerful in evoking emotion.

sympathetic nervous system a part of the autonomic system that prepares the body to respond to environmental stimuli, such as an encroaching lion, as well as the need to track game, respond to an attractive potential sexual partner, or to perform well in an athletic event.

taboo a ban against a belief or practice.

tattooing a form of body alteration intended to be decorative. Tattoo designs tend to conform to cultural concepts of beauty or they reflect attitudes toward masculinity or femininity, as indicated by Samoan tattoo culture.

testicles male reproductive organs that produce androgens, the "male" sex hormones.

thalamus the part of the brain that acts as a relay station between the brain stem and the *cerebrum*. It also plays an important role in emotion and the wake-and-sleep cycle.

Traditional Chinese Medicine (TCM) a form of healing based in Taoism and Confucianism that involves the concept of obtaining and sustaining harmony in the universe and the relationship of the body to the surrounding universe. As used today, the term refers to the practice of medicine in which Mao Zedong divested this medical system from the philosophical system based in folk beliefs.

trance an altered state of consciousness in which an individual loses contact with the sensory world, but can continue to speak and move.

unilineal kinship system a form of descent in which status and property are transmitted through only the male or female line, not both.

universal health care a system of medicine in which all members of a society are accorded access to health care regardless of their income or social status. This is sometimes called socialized medicine, but this is an inaccurate use of the English language. It derives from a term used to describe forms of political systems in which all the means of production are controlled by the state.

unmyelinated neurons nerve cells that lack the fatty coating over the axon that prevents interference from unrelated messages.

uxorilocal residence a form of residence pattern in which a married couple live with or near the wife's family.

variable phenomenon or characteristic that involves more than one possibility. For example, eye color is a variable in studying human physiology or behavior.

vector see *disease vector*.

virilocal residence a form of residence pattern in which a married couple live with or near the husband's family.

vodou a religion developed in Haiti that combines the symbolism of French and Spanish Catholicism with the traditional religions of West Africa. It involves *trance possession* brought about by rhythmical drumming and dancing. The spirits believed to possess vodou devotees have African names and are often depicted in images of Catholic saints.

volition the power to make choices; the act of making choices.

vulva the blood-enriched external parts of the female genitalia.

Whole Medical Systems as defined by the U.S. National Institutes of Health, Whole Medical Systems are complete systems of theory and practice that have developed independently from Western medicine.

witch traditionally in anthropology, the term refers to an individual who disrupts the group of which he or she is a part because of his or her inability to obtain social goals. As used in Wicca, the term refers to an individual trained and skilled in performing religious and/or magical rituals.

witchcraft as used in anthropological and other traditions, the term refers to the ability to influence other individuals in a group through the use of ritual. The usual usage of the term implies intent to harm others.

world view a culturally shaped view of the world characteristic of a particular group of people. Typically, an individual's world view incorporates his or her experiences into the culturally shaped world view he or she acquires in the process of *socialization*.

References

Abu-Lughod, Lila, and Catherine A. Lutz. 1990. Introduction: Emotion, discourse, and the politics of everyday life. In *Language and the politics of emotions*, ed. Catherine A. Lutz and Lila Abu-Lughod, 1–23. Cambridge: Cambridge University Press.

Adams, Inez F. 2007. The ethnographic evaluation of Michigan's high-risk hepatitis B vaccination program. *Napa Bulletin* 27:81–109.

Adams, Vicanne, et al. 2005. The challenge of cross-cultural clinical trials research: Case report from the Tibetan Autonomous Region, People's Republic of China. *Medical Anthropology Quarterly* 19(3):267–289.

Allen, Catherine Wagner. 1978. *Coca, chica and trago: Private and communal rituals in a Quechua community*. Ann Arbor, MI: University Microfilms.

———. 1988. *The hold life has: Coca and Cultural Identity in an Andean Community.*. Washington, DC: Smithsonian.

Anagnost, Ann. 1997. *National past-times: Narrative, representation, and power in modern China*. Durham, NC: Duke University Press.

Angier, Natalie. 2004. Review of songs of the gorilla nation. *New York Times Book Review* (March 21):12.

Appadurai, Arjun. 1981. Gastro-politics in Hindu South Asia. *American Ethnologist* 8(3):494–511.

———. 1990. Topographies of self: Praise and emotion in Hindu India. In *Language and the politics of emotion*. ed. Catherine A. Lutz and Lila Abu-Lughod, 24–45. Cambridge: Cambridge University Press.

Ardener, E. Belief and the problem of women. In *The interpretation of ritual*, ed. J. S. LaFontaine, 135–158. London: Tavistock Publications.

Arquette, M., et al. 2002. Holistic risk-based environmental decision-making: A native perspective. *Environmental Health Perspectives* 110(2):259–264.

Arsuaga, J. L., I. Marinez, A. Garcia, et al. 1997. "Sima de los Huesos (Sierta de Atapuerca, Spain). The site" *Journal of Human Evolution* 33:409–423.

Babbie, Earl. 1989. *The practice of social research*. 5th ed. Belmont, CA: Wadsworth.

Balikci, Asen. 1970. *The Netsilik Eskimo*. Garden City, NY: The Natural History Press.

Barker, Holly M. 2004. *Bravo for the Marshallese: Regaining control in a post-nuclear, post-colonial world*. Belmont, CA: Wadsworth.

Barham, Peter, and Robert Hayward. 1990. Schizophrenia as a life process. In *Reconstructing schizophrenia*, ed. R. P. Bentall, 61–85. London: Routledge.

———. 1995. *Relocating madness: From the mental patient to the person*. London: Free Association Books.

———. 1998. In sickness and in health: Dilemmas of the person with severe mental illness. *Psychiatry* 61:163–170.

Barley, Nigel. 2006. *Grave matters*. Long Grove, IL: Waveland. (Orig. pub. 1995.)

Barnes, Linda L. 2005. American acupuncture and efficacy: Meanings and their point of insertion. *Medical Anthropology Quarterly* 19(3): 239–266.

Barrett, Robert J. 1989. Self, identity and subjective experiences of schizophrenia: In search of the subject. *Schizophrenia Bulletin* 15(2):89–196.

———. 1996. *The psychiatric team and the social definition of schizophrenia: An anthropological study of person and illness*. London: Cambridge University Press.

———. 1998. The "Schizophrenic" and the liminal persona in modern society. *Culture, Medicine & Psychiatry* 22:465–494

———. 2003. Kurt Schneider in Borneo: Do first rank symptoms apply to the Iban? In *Schizophrenia, culture and subjectivity: The edge of experience*. Cambridge Studies in Medical Anthropology 11, 87–109. Cambridge: Cambridge University Press.

Bateson, Gregory. 1958. *Naven*. 2nd ed. Stanford, CA: Stanford University Press.

Bateson, Mary Catherine. 1984. *With a daughter's eye*. New York: Washington Square Press.

Bell, Amelia Rector. 1993. Separate people: Speaking of Creek men and women. In *The other fifty percent: Cross-cultural perspectives on gender relations*, ed. Mari Womack and Judith Marti. Prospect Heights, IL: Waveland.

Bell, Rudolph M. 1987. *Holy anorexia*. Chicago: University of Chicago Press.

Belo, J. 1960. *Trance in Bali*. New York: Columbia University Press.

Benedict, Ruth. 1989. *The Chrysanthemem and the sword: Patterns of Japanese culture*. Boston: Houghton Mifflin.

Bettelheim, Bruno. 1954. *Symbolic wounds: Puberty rites and the envious male*. Glencoe, IL: Free Press.

Bish, Connie L., et al. 2005. Diet and physical activity behaviors among Americans trying to lose weight: 2000 behavioral risk factor surveillance system. *Obesity Research* 13:596–607.

Boas, Franz. 1964. *The central Eskimo*. Lincoln: University of Nebraska Press. (Orig. publ. 1888.)

Bodley, John H. 1975. *Victims of progress* Menlo Park, CA: Cummings Publishing.

———. 1976. *Anthropology and Contemporary Human Problems*. Menlo Park, CA: Cummings Publishing.

Bordo, Susan. 1993. *Unbearable weight: Feminism, Western culture and the body*. Berkeley: University of California Press.

Bowen, Elenore Smith. 1964. *Return to laughter: An anthropological novel*. Garden City, NY: Doubleday.

Bolton, Ralph. 1977. The Qolla marriage process. In *Kinship and marriage in the Andes*, ed. Ralph Bolton and Enrique Mayer. Washington, DC: American Anthropological Association.

Bongaarts, John, O. Frank, and Ron Lesthaeghe. 1984. The fertility-inhibiting effects of the intermediate fertility variables. *Studies in Family Planning* 13(67):179–189.

Bordo, Susan. 1993. Unbearable weight: Feminism, Western culture and the body. Berkeley: University of California Press.

Bourdieu, Pierre. 1977. *Outline of a theory of practice*. trans. Richard Nice. Cambridge: Cambridge University Press.

Bown, Deni. 2001. *Encyclopedia of herbs*. London: Dorling Kindersley Ltd.

Boyd, Robert W., and Joan B. Silk. 2005. *How humans evolved*, 4th ed. New York: W. W. Norton.

Brøgger, Jan. *Nazaré: Women and men in a prebureaucratic Portuguese fishing village*. Fort Worth: Harcourt Brace Jovanovich.

Buckley, Thomas. 1993. Menstruation and the power of Yurok women. In *Gender in cross-cultural perspective,* ed. Caroline B. Brettell and Carolyn F. Sargent. Englewood Cliffs, NJ: Prentice Hall.

Burton, John W. 2001. *Culture and the human body: An anthropological perspective.* Long Grove, IL: Waveland.

Burton, Linda M., Dawn A. Obeidallah, and Kevin Allison. 1996. Ethnographic perspectives on social context and adolescent development among inner-city African-American teens. In *Essays on ethnography and human development,* ed. Richard Jessor, Anne Colby, and Richard A. Shweder, 395–418. Chicago: University of Chicago Press.

Burton, Roger V., and John W. M. Whiting. 1961. The absent father and cross-sex identity. *Merrill-Palmer Quarterly* 7(2)85–95.

Bynum, Carolyn Walker Bynum. 1988. *Holy feast and holy fast: The religious significance of food to medieval women.* Berkeley: University of California Press.

Carter, William E. 1977. Trial marriage in the Andes? In *Kinship and marriage in the Andes,* ed. Ralph Bolton and Enrique Mayer. Washington, DC: American Anthropological Association.

Cassell, Eric J. 1985. *Talking with patients.* 2 vols. Cambridge, MA: MIT Press.

Certeau, Michel de. 1984. *The practice of everyday life.* trans. Steven Rendall. Berkeley: University of California Press.

Chagnon, Napoleon A. 1992. *Yanomamö,* 4th ed. Fort Worth, TX: Harcourt Brace.

Chang Po-tuan. 1987. *Understanding reality: A Taoist alchemical classic.* trans. Thomas Cleary. Honolulu: University of Hawaii Press.

Chapman, Rachel R. 2004. A nova vida: The commoditization of reproduction in central Mozambique. *Medical Anthropology* 23(3):229–261.

Chodorow, Nancy. 1975. Family structure and feminine personality. In *Woman, culture and society,* ed. Michelle Zimbalist Rosaldo and Louise Lamphere. Stanford, CA: Stanford University Press.

Cirone, Patricia. 2005. The integration of tribal traditional lifeways into EPA's decision making. *Practicing Anthropology* 27(1):20–24.

Clark, Colin. 1968. *Population growth and land use.* London and New York: Macmillan.

Comaroff, Jean. The diseased heart of Africa: Medicine, colonialism, and the black body. In *Knowledge, power and practice: The anthropology of medicine and everyday life,* ed. Shirley Lindenbaum and Margaret Lock, 305–329. Berkeley: University of California Press.

Cook, H. B. Kimberley. 1993. Small town, big hell: An ethnographic study of aggression in a Margariteño community. *Antropologica Supplemento No. 4.* Fundacion La Salle, Instituto Caribe de Antropologia y sociologia.

Counihan, Carole. 1999. *The anthropology of food and body: Gender, meaning, and power.* New York: Routledge.

Csikszentmihalyi, Mihaly. 1975. *Beyond boredom and anxiety: The experience of play in work and games.* San Francisco: Jossey-Bass.

Cumont, Franz. 1956. *The mysteries of Mithra.* trans. Thomas J. McCormack. New York: Dover. (Orig. publ. by the Open Court Publishing Co. 1903.)

Darwin, Charles. 1964. *On the origin of species.* (A facsimile of the first edition) Cambridge, MA: Cambridge University Press. (Orig. publ. 1859.)

Davis, Wade. 2004. *The lost Amazon: The photographic journey of Richard Evans Schultes.* San Francisco: Chronicle Books.

Davis-Floyd, Robbie E. 2004. The technocratic body: American childbirth as cultural expression. *Social Science and Medicine* 38(8):1125–1140.

———. 2005. Gender and ritual: Giving birth the American way. In *Gender in cross-cultural perspective,* 4th ed. ed. Caroline B. Brettell and Carolyn F. Sargent. Upper Saddle River, NJ: Prentice Hall.

Desjarlais, Robert R. 1992. *Body and emotion: The aesthetics of illness and healing in the Nepal Himalayas.* Philadelphia: University of Pennsylvania Press.

Deng, Francis Mading. 1973. *The Dinka and their songs.* Oxford: Clarendon Press.

Deutsch, Helene. 1945. *The psychology of women.* Vol. 2. New York: Grune and Stratton.

Diamond, Jared. 1991. The worst mistake in the history of the human race. In *Applying cultural anthropology: An introductory reader,* ed. Aaron Podolefsky and Peter Brown. Mountain View, CA: Mayfield. (Orig. publ. *Discover,* 1987.)

Douglas, Mary. 1966. *Purity and danger: An analysis of the concepts of pollution and taboo.* London: Routledge and Kegan Paul.

Durkheim, Emile. 1965. *The elementary forms of the religious life.* trans. Joseph Ward Swain. New York: The Free Press. (Orig. publ. 1915.)

Eckman, P. 1996. *In the footsteps of the yellow emperor.* San Francisco: Cypress.

Edgerton, Robert B. 1978. The study of deviance—marginal man or everyman? In *The making of psychological anthropology,* ed. George D. Spindler, 442–476. Berkeley: University of California Press.

Edwards, Griffith. 1984. Drinking in longitudinal perspective: Career and natural history. *British Journal of Addiction* 75(2):175–183.

Ehrlich, Paul. 1968. *The population bomb.* New York: Ballantine Books.

Ehrlich, Paul, and Anne Erlich. 1972. *Population, resources, environment.* San Francisco: W. H. Freeman.

Eliade, Mircea. 1972. *Shamanism: Archaic techniques of ecstasy.* trans. Willard R. Trask. Princeton, NJ: Princeton University Press.

Erwin, Kathleen. 2006. The circulatory system: Blood procurement, AIDS, and the social body in China. *Medical Anthropology Quarterly* 20(2):139–159.

Estroff, Sue E. 1981. *Making it crazy: An ethnography of psychiatric clients in an American community.* Berkeley: University of California Press.

———. 1989. Self, identity, and subjective experiences of schizophrenia: In search of the subject. *Schizophrenia Bulletin* 15(2):189–196.

———. 1993. Identity, disability, and schizophrenia: The problem of chronicity. In *Knowledge, power and practice: Analysis in medical anthropology,* ed. Margaret Lock and Shirley Lindenbaum, 247–286. Berkeley: University of California Press.

Estroff, Sue E., William Lachicotte, Linda Illingworth, Anna Johnston, and Bob Ruth. 1991. Everybody's Got a Little Mental Illness: Accounts of Illness and Self among People with Severe, Persistent Mental Illness. *Medical Anthropology Quarterly* 5(4):331–369.

Evans-Pritchard, E. E. 1976 [1937]. *Witchcraft, oracles, and magic among the Azande.* Oxford: Clarendon Press.

Faithorn, Elizabeth. 1975. The concept of pollution among the Káfe of the Papua New Guinea Highlands. In *Toward an anthropology of women,* ed. Rayna R. Reiter. New York: Monthly Review Press.

Farmer, Paul. 2003. *Pathologies of power: Health, human rights, and the new war on the poor.* Berkeley: University of California Press.

Feynman, Richard P. 1985. *Surely you're joking, Mr. Feynman!* New York: W. W. Norton.

Finkler, Kaja. 2001. Mistress of *lo espiritual.* In *Mesoamerican Healers,* ed. Brad R. Huber and Alan R. Sandstrom. Austin: University of Texas Press.

Flynn, James R. 2007. *What is intelligence?: Beyond the Flynn Effect.* Cambridge: Cambridge University Press.

Foucault, Michel. 1972. *The archeology of knowledge and the discourse on language.* trans. Alan Sheridan Smith. New York: Pantheon. (Orig. publ. 1969.)

———. 1994. *The birth of the clinic: An archaeology of medical perception.* Trans., Richard Howard. New York: Vintage.

Frager, Robert, and James Fadiman. 1997. *Essential sufism.* Edison, NJ: Castle Books.

Frank, Jerome D. 1963. *Persuasion and healing.* New York: Schocken Books.

Frank. O. 1983. Infertility in Sub-Saharan Africa: Estimates and implications. *Population and development review* 9(1):137–144.

Frankel, Richard. 1983. The laying on of hands: Aspects of the organization of gaze, touch and talk in a medical encounter. In *The social organization of patient-doctor communication*, ed. Sue Fisher and Alexandra Todd, 19–54. Washington, DC: Center for Applied Linguistics.

———. 1984. From sentence to sequence: Understanding the medical encounter. *Discourses Processes* 7(2):135–170.

Freeman, Derek. 1983. *Margaret Mead and Samoa: The making and unmaking of an anthropological myth*. Cambridge, MA: Harvard University Press.

Freud, Sigmund. 1953. *A general introduction to psychoanalysis*. New York: Pocket Book. (Orig. publ.1924.)

Fuller, Dorian Q. 2002. Fifty years of archaeobotanical studies in India: Laying a solid foundation. In *Indian archaeology in retrospect*. Vol. 3. *Archaeology and Interactive Disciplines*, ed. S. Settar and R. Korisettar, 247–364. New Delhi: Manohar.

Gadsby, Patricia. 2007. The Inuit paradox. In *Annual editions: Anthropology*, ed. Elvio Angeloni. Dubuque, IA: McGraw-Hill. (Orig. publ. *Discover*, August 2002, 12–14.)

Gammeltoft, Tine M. 2007. Prenatal diagnosis in postwar Vietnam: Power, subjectivity, and citizenship. *American Anthropologist* 109(1):153–163.

Geertz, Clifford. 1973. *The interpretation of culture*. New York: Basic Books.

Gennep, Arnold van. 1960. *The rites of passage*. trans. Monika B. Vizedom and Gabrielle L. Caffee. Chicago: The University of Chicago Press. (orig. publ. 1908.)

Golden, Deborah. 2006. Structured looseness: Everyday social order at an Israeli kindergarten. *Ethos* 34(3):367–390.

Golub, Edward S. 1997. *The limits of medicine: How science shapes our hope for the cure*. Chicago: University of Chicago Press.

Good, Byron J. 1994. *Medicine, rationality, and experience: An anthropological perspective*. Cambridge: Cambridge University Press.

Goodale, Jane. 1994. *Tiwi wives: A study of the women of Melville Island, North Australia*. Prospect Heights, IL: Waveland. (Orig. publ. 1971, University of Washington Press.)

Gordon, Daniel. 2008. Female circumcision in Egypt and Sudan: A controversial rite of passage. In *Magic, witchcraft, and religion: An anthropological study of the supernatural*, 7th ed. ed. Pamela A. Moro, James E. Myers and Arthur C. Lehmann. Boston: McGraw Hill. (Orig. publ. as "Female circumcision and genital operations in Egypt and the Sudan: A dilemma for medical anthropology." *Medical Anthropology Quarterly*, March 1, 1991.)

Gottlieb, Alma. 1993. American premenstrual syndrome: A Mute Voice. In *Talking about people: Readings in contemporary cultural anthropology*, ed. Robert Gordon and William Haviland. Mountain View, CA: Mayfield. (Orig. publ. 1988 *Anthropology Today* 4(6):10–13.)

Guemple, D. L. 1965. Saunik: Name sharing as a factor governing Eskimo kinship terms. *Ethnology* 4(3):323–335.

Guiliano, Mireille. 2005. *French women don't get fat*. New York: Alfred A. Knopf.

Harris, Stuart G., and Barbara L. Harper. 2000. Measuring risk to tribal community health and culture. In *Environmental toxicology and risk assessment: Recent achievements in environmental fate and transport*. Vol. 9. ed. E. T. Price, K. V. Brix, and N. Lane. West Choshoshocken, PA: ASTM.

Hawkes, C. H. 1992. Endorphins: The basis of pleasure? *Journal of Neurology, Neurosurgery, and Psychiatry* 55:247–250.

Hayano, David. 1990. *Road through the rain forest: Living anthropology in Highland Papua New Guinea*. Prospect Heights, IL: Waveland.

Heider, Karl. 1991. *Grand Valley Dani: Peaceful warriors*, 2nd ed. Fort Worth: Holt, Rinehart and Winston.

Herdt, Gilbert. 1987. *The Sambia: Ritual and gender in New Guinea*. New York: Holt, Rinehart and Winston.

Herold, A Ferdinand. 1954. *The life of Buddha according to legends of Ancient India*. trans. Paul C. Blum. Tokyo: Charles E. Tuttle.

Herskovits, Melville J. 1937. *Life in a Haitian alley.* New York: Knopf.

Hixon, Lex. 1994. *Mother of the universe: Visions of the goddess and tantric hymns of enlightenment.* Wheaton, IL: Quest Books.

Ho, Evelyn Y. Behold the power of *qi*: The importance of *qi* in the discourse of acupuncture. *Research on Language and Social Interaction* 39(4):411–440.

Hogbin, Ian. 1996. *The island of menstruating men: Religion in Wogeo, New Guinea.* Prospect Heights, IL: Waveland. (Orig publ. 1970.)

Holloway, Kris. 2007. *Monique and the mango rains: Two years with a midwife in Mali.* Prospect Heights, IL: Waveland.

Holmberg, Allan H. 1969. *Nomads of the long bow: The Siriono of Eastern Bolivia.* Garden City, NY: The Natural History Press.

Huizinga, Johan. 1950. *Homo ludens: A study of the play element in culture.* Boston: Beacon Press.

Inhorn, Marcia C., and Kimberly A. Buss. 1993. Infertility, infection, and iatrogenesis in Egypt: The anthropological epidemiology of blocked tubes. *Medical Anthropology* 15:217–244.

James-Chetalet, Lois. 1989. Reclaiming the birth experience: An analysis of midwifery in Canada from 1788 to 1987. PhD diss., Department of History, Carleton University, Ottawa, Canada.

Jenkins, Janis H., and Robert J. Barrett. 2003. Introduction. In *Schizophrenia, culture and subjectivity: The edge of experience.* Cambridge Studies in Medical Anthropology 2, 1–25. Cambridge: Cambridge University Press.

Jordan, Brigitte, and Robbie Davis-Floyd. 1993. *Birth in four cultures: A cross-cultural investigation of childbirth in Yucatan, Holland, Sweden, and the United States.* Long Grove, IL: Waveland.

Jung, C. G. 1967. Foreword. *The I Ching or book of changes,* 3rd ed. trans. Richard Wilhelm. Bollingen Series XIX. Princeton, NJ: Princeton University Press.

———. 1990. *The basic writings of C. G. Jung.* trans. R. F. C. Hull. Bollingen Series. Princeton, NJ: Princeton University Press.

Jurmain, Robert, Lynn Kilgore, and Wenda Trevathan. 2006. *Essentials of physical anthropology.* Belmont, CA: Thomson Wadsworth.

Katz, Jay. 1984. *The silent world of doctors and patients.* New York: Free Press.

Kearney, Michael. 1984. *World view.* Novato, CA: Chandler and Sharp.

Kemper, Kathi. n.d. Clinical outcomes research in complementary and alternative medicine: The glass slipper and the princess. Unpubl. ms.

Kiev, Ari. 1964. *Magic, Faith, and Healing.* New York: The Free Press.

Klein, H. 1991. Couvade syndrome: Male counterpart to pregnancy. *International Journal of Psychiatry in Medicine* 21(1):57–69.

Kleinman, Arthur. 1980. *Patients and healers in the context of culture.* Berkeley: University of California Press.

———. 1988. *The Illness narratives: Suffering, healing and the human condition.* New York: Basic Books.

Kleinman, Arthur, Veena Das, and Margaret Lock. 1997. *Social suffering.* Berkeley: University of California Press.

Klima, George. 1970. *The Barabaig: East African Cattle-Herders.* New York: Holt, Rinehart and Winston.

Konrad, K., T. Gunther, C. Hanisch, and B. Herpertz-Dahlmann. 2004. Differential effects of methylphenidate on attentional functions in children with attention deficit/hyperactivity disorder. *Journal of the American Academy of Child and Adolescent Psychiatry* 24:24–29.

Kübler-Ross, Elisabeth. 1969. *On Death and Dying.* New York: Macmillan.

Kuhn, Thomas S. 1970. *The structure of scientific revolutions,* Vol. 2, 2nd ed. Chicago: University of Chicago Press.

Kuipers, Joel C. 1989. "Medical discourse" in anthropological context: Views of language and power. *Medical Anthropology Quarterly.* New Series 3(2):99–123.

Kunitz, Stephen J. 2006. Life-course observations of alcohol use among Navajo Indians: Natural history or careers? *Medical Anthropology Quarterly* 20(3):279–296.

Kuper, Hilda. 1963. *The Swazi: A South African kingdom.* New York: Holt, Rinehart and Winston.

Kurin, Richard. 1980. Acceptance in the field: Doctor, lawyer, Indian chief. *Natural History* 89(11).

Lad, Usha and Vasant Lad. 1997. *Ayurvedic cooking for self-healing.* 2nd ed. Albuquerque, NM: The Ayurvedic Press.

Lakoff, George, and Mark Johnson. 1980. *Metaphors we live by.* Chicago: University of Chicago Press.

Lamphere, Louise. 2005. The domestic sphere of women and the public world of men: The strengths and limitations of an anthropological dichotomy. In *Gender in cross-cultural perspective,* 4th ed. ed. Caroline B. Brettell and Carolyn F. Sargent. Upper Saddle River, NJ: Prentice Hall.

Langford, Jean. 2005–2006. *Annual report.* Santa Fe, NM: School for Advanced Research on the Human Experience.

Langness, L. L. 1974. Ritual, power and male dominance in the New Guinea Highlands. *Ethos* 2:189–212.

Lao Tzu. 1994. *Tao Te Ching.* trans. Man-Ho Kwok, Martin Palmer, and Jay Ramsay. New York: Barnes & Noble.

Larsen, John Aggergaard. 2005. Finding meaning in first episode psychosis: Experience, agency, and the cultural repertoire. *Medical Anthropology Quarterly* 18(4): 447–471.

Larsen, Ulla. 2002. The effects of type of female circumcision on infertility and fertility in Sudan. *Journal of Biosocial Science* 34:363–377.

Lederman, Rena. 1986. *What gifts engender: Social relations and politics in Mendi, Highland Papua New Guinea.* Cambridge: Cambridge University Press.

———. 1993. Contested order: gender and society in the southern New Guinea highlands. In *The Other Fifty Percent: Multicultural Perspectives on Gender Relations,* ed. Mari Womack and Judith Marti. Prospect Heights, IL: Waveland.

Leonard, George Burr. 1974. *The ultimate athlete.* New York: Avon Books.

Lévi-Strauss, Claude. 1963. *Structural Anthropology.* trans. Claire Jacobson and Brooke Grundfest Schoepf. New York: Basic Books.

———. 1969. *The raw and the cooked.* Boston: Beacon Press.

Lewis, I. M. 1971. *Ecstatic religion: An anthropological study of spirit possession and shamanism.* Hammondsworth, Middlesex, England: Penguin Books Ltd.

Li Ding, He Ziqiang, Wang Jianhua, and You Benlin. 1991. *Acupuncture, meridian theory and acupuncture points.* Beijing: Foreign Languages Press.

Lickers, F. Henry. 2003. Community health indicators: Changes in these indicators and the analysis of risk to social structures and cultural practices, Project Summary, February 2003. Cornwall, Ontario: Mohawk Council of Akwesasne.

Lindenbaum, Shirley. 1972. Sorcerers, ghosts, and polluting women: An analysis of religious belief and population control. *Ethnology* 11(2):241–253.

———. 1979. *Kuru sorcery.* Mountain View, CA: Mayfield.

Lindow, Vivian. 1986. *The social consequences of seeing a psychiatrist.* PhD thesis. University of Bristol.

Loewen, James W. 1995. *Lies my teacher told me: Everything your American history textbook got wrong.* New York: The New Press.

Lutz, Catherine A., and Geoffrey M. White. 1986. The anthropology of emotions. *Annual Review of Anthropology* 15:405–436.

Lyon, M. L., and J. M. Barbalet. 1994. *Society's body: The existential ground of culture and self*, ed. Thomas Csordas, 48–66. Cambridge: Cambridge University Press.

MacCormack, Carol P. 1993. Women and symbolic systems: Biological events and cultural control. In *Talking about people: Readings in contemporary cultural anthropology*, ed. William A. Haviland and Robert J. Gordon, 181–185. Mountain View, CA: Mayfield. (Orig. publ. 1977.)

Macdonald, Margaret. 2006. Gender expectations: Natural bodies and natural births in the new midwifery in Canada. *Medical Anthropology Quarterly* 20(2):235–256.

Maimonides, Moses. 1956. *The guide for the perplexed*. 2nd ed. trans. M. Friedlander. New York: Dover.

Malinowski, Bronislaw. 1929. The sexual life of savages. New York: Harcourt, Brace & World.

———. 1954. *Magic, science and religion and other essays*. Garden City, NY: Doubleday Anchor.

———. 1984. *Argonauts of the Western Pacific*. Prospect Heights, IL: Waveland. (orig publ. 1922.)

———, 1985. *Sex and repression in savage society*. Chicago: University of Chicago Press. (Orig. publ. 1927.)

Malthus, Thomas. 1885. *An essay on the principle of population*. New York and London: Macmillan. (Orig. pub. 1807.)

Mammo, A., and S. Philip Morgan. 1986. Female circumcision: Three years' experience of common complications in patients treated in Khartoum teaching hospitals. *Journal of Obstetrics and Gynaecology* 12(3):533–546.

Maquet, Jacques. 1986. *The aesthetic experience: An anthropologist looks at the visual arts*. New Haven, CT: Yale University Press.

Martin: Emily. 2001. *The woman in the body*. Boston: Beacon Press.

Martz, Sandra Haldeman, ed. 1994. *I am becoming the woman I've wanted*. Papier-Maché Press.

Marx, Karl, and Friedrich Engels. 1964. *The communist manifesto*. New York: Washington Square Press. (Orig. publ. in German in 1848.)

Maschio. Thomas. 2007. How doctors and patients talk past one another: The clash of scientific and folk worldviews. *Anthropology News* 48(4):25–26.

Matchett, William Foster. 1974. Repeated hallucinatory experiences as a part of the mourning process among Hopi Indian women. In *Culture and personality: Contemporary readings*, ed. Robert A. LeVine. New York: Aldine. (Orig. publ. *Psychiatry* 35:185–194, 1972.)

May, Philip A., and Matthew B. Smith. 1988. Some Navajo Indian opinions about alcohol abuse and prohibition: A survey and recommendations for policy. *Journal of Studies on Alcohol* 49(4):324–334.

Mayer, Emeran A. 2002–2003. The neurobiology of stress and emotions. Milwaukee, WI: International Foundation for Functional Gastrointestinal Disorders.

Mayer, Emeran, and Clifford B. Saper. 2000. Minding the mind. In *Progress in brain research*. Vol. 122, ed. Emeran Mayer and Clifford B. Saper. New York: Elsevier Science BV.

Maynard, Ronald J. 2006. Controlling death—compromising life: Chronic disease, prognostication, and the new biotechnologies. *Medical Anthropology Quarterly* 20(2):212–234.

McGee, R. Jon. 2002. *Watching Lacandon Maya lives*. Boston: Allyn and Bacon.

McKenna, James J. 2000. Cultural influences on infant and childhood sleep biology and the science that studies it: Toward a more inclusive paradigm. In *Sleep and breathing in children: A developmental approach*, ed. Gerald M. Loughlin, John L. Carroll, and Carole L. Marcus, 199–230. New York: Marcell Dekker.

McKenna, James J., Sarah Mosko, and Christopher Richard. 1997. Bed sharing promotes breastfeeding. *Paediatrics* 100(2):214–219.

McNaughton, Niel. 1989. *Biology and emotion*. Cambridge: Cambridge University Press.

Mead, George Herbert. 1934. *Mind, self and society*. Chicago: University of Chicago Press.

Mead, Margaret. 1949. *Male and female*. New York: William Morrow.

————. 1968. *Coming of age in Samoa: A psychological study of primitive youth for Western civilization*. New York: Morrow. (Orig. publ. 1928.)

————. 1972. *Blackberry winter: My earlier years*. New York: William Morrow.

Meadow, Richard H. 1996. The origins and spread of agriculture and pastoralism in northwestern South Asia. In *The origins and spread of agricultuer and pastoralism in Eurasia*, ed. David R. Harris, 390–412. Washington, DC: Smithsonian Institution Press.

Meeker, Michael E. 1989. *The pastoral son and the spirit of patriarchy: Religion, society, and person among East African stock keepers*. Madison, WI: The University of Wisconsin Press.

Métaux, Alfred. 1958. *Le vaudou Haitien*. Paris: Gallimard.

Miller, Barbara. 1993. Female infanticide and child neglect in rural North India. In *Gender in cross-cultural perspective*, ed. Caroline B. Brettell and Carolyn F. Sargent. Englewood Cliffs, NJ: Prentice Hall. (Orig. publ. 1987 in *Child survival*, ed. Nancy Scheper-Hughes. Dordrecht: D. Reidel Publishing.)

Mitchenson, Wendy. 1991. The nature of their bodies: Women and their doctors in Victorian Canada. Toronto: University of Toronto Press.

Moffat, Robert. 1842. *Missionary labours and scenes in southern Africa*. London: Snow. (Reprint New York: Johnson Reprint Corporation, 1969.)

Nanda, Serena. 1999. *Neither man nor woman*. Belmont, CA: Wadsworth.

Nelson, Cynthia. 1974. Public and private politics: Women in the Middle East. *American Ethnologist* 1:551–563.

Nadel, S. 1946. "A Study of Shamanism in the Nuba Hills." *Journal of the Royal Anthropological Institute* 76:25–37.

Obeyesekere, Gananath. 1974. Pregnancy cravings (dola-duka) in relation to social structure and personality in a Sinhalese village. In *Culture and personality: Contemporary readings*, ed. Robert A. LeVine. New York: Aldine. (Orig. publ. *American Anthropologist* 65(2), 1963.)

Oboler, Regina Smith. 2001. The Nandi of East Africa. In *Being human: An introduction to cultural anthropology*. Upper Saddle River, NJ: Prentice Hall.

Ortner, Sherry B. 1974. Is female to male as nature is to culture? In *Woman, culture & society*, ed. Michelle Zimbalist Rosaldo and Louise Lamphere. Stanford, CA: Stanford University Press.

Park, Michael Alan. 2008. *Biological anthropology*, 5th ed. New York: McGraw-Hill.

Pasamanick, Benjamin. 1956. Epidemiology of mental disorder: a symposium organized by the American Psychiatric Association to commemorate the centennial of the birth of Emil Kraepelin, cosponsored by the American Public Health Association, and held at the New York meeting, December 27–28, 1956.

Patten, Sonia. 2003. Medical anthropology: Improving nutrition in Malawi. In *Conformity and Conflict: Readings in Cultural Anthropology*, 11th ed. ed. James Spradley and David W. McCurdy. Boston: Allyn and Bacon.

Perry, Bruce D. 2002. Childhood experience and the expression of genetic potential: What childhood neglect tells us about nature and nurture. *Brain and Mind: A Transdisciplinary Journal of Neuroscience and Neurophilosophy*. 3:79–100.

Perry, Bruce D. and Ronnie Pollard. 1997. Altered brain development following global neglect in early childhood. Society for Neuroscience. Proceedings from annual meeting, New Orleans.

Pickvance, Ronald. 1984. *Van Gogh in Arles*. New York: The Metropolitan Museum of Art. Harry N. Abrams, Publishers.

Ramachandran, V. S. 2004. *A brief tour of human consciousness*. New York: Pearson Education.

Rasmussen, Knud. 1931. *The Netsilik Eskimos*. Reports of the Fifth Thule Edition, Vol. 8. Copenhagen.

Read, Kenneth E. 1965. *The high valley*. New York: Charles Scribner's Sons.

Rector Bell, Amelia. 1993. Separate people: Speaking of Creek men and women. In *The other fifty percent: Multicultural perspectives on gender relations*, ed. Mari Womack and Judith Marti. Prospect Heights, IL: Waveland.

Reddy, Gayatri, and Serena Nanda. 2005. Hijras: An "alternative" sex/gender in India. In *Gender in cross-cultural perspective*, 4th ed. ed. Caroline B. Brettell and Carolyn F. Sargent. Upper Saddle River, NJ: Prentice Hall.

Richards, A. 1956. *Chisungu: A girl's initiation ceremony among the Bemba of Northern Rhodesia.* London: Faber and Faber.

Root, Robin. 2006. "Mixing" as an ethnoetiology of HIV/AIDS in Malaysia's multinational factories. *Medical Anthropology Quarterly* 20(3):321–344.

Rosaldo, Renato. 1989. *Culture and truth: The remaking of social analysis.* Boston: Beacon Press.

Rosenhan, David L. 1973. On being sane in insane places. *Science* 179:250–258.

Rosman, Abraham. 1996. Preface. *The island of menstruating men.* Prospect Heights, IL: Waveland.

Ryan, William E. 1976. *Blaming the victim.* 2nd ed. New York: Vintage Books.

Saguay, Abigail C. 2007. Does this BMI make me look fat? Defining the bounds of "normal" in the United States and France, 1–12. *CSU Update: Newsletter of the UCLA Center for the Study of Women.*

Saladin d'Anglure, Bernard., ed. 2001. *Cosmology and shamanism.* Mariano and Tulimaaq Aupilaarjuk, Lucassie Nutaraaluk, Rose Iqallijuq, Johanasi Ujarak, Isidore Ijituuq and Michel Kupaaq. Iqaluit: Nunavut Arctic College.

Santry, Heena P., David L. Gillen, and Diane S. Lauderdal. 2005. Trends in bariatric surgical procedures. *Journal of American Medical Association* 294(25):1909–17.

Scheper-Hughes, Nancy. 2000. The global traffic in human organs. *Current Anthropology* 41(1):191–224.

———. 2003. Mother love: Death without weeping. In *Conformity and conflict: Readings in cultural anthropology*, 11th ed. ed. James Spradley and David W. McCurdy. Boston: Allyn and Bacon. (Orig. publ. as "Death Without Weeping," *Natural History*, October 1989.)

Seefeld, Andrew W., and Adam Landman. 2008. Navigating the ER. *UCLA Magazine* 19(2):16–17.

Shang, Bing-he. 1979. *Zhou yi shang shi xue (Master Shang's Study of the Zhou Yi).* Beijing: China Publishing House.

Shima, Miki. 1992. *The medical I Ching: Oracle of the healer within.* Boulder, CO: Blue Poppy Press.

Shostak, Marjorie. 1981. *Nisa: The life and words of a !Kung woman.* New York: Vintage Books.

Siemens, Stephen David. 1993. Access to women's knowledge: The Azande Experience. In *The Other Fifty Percent: Multicultural Perspectives on Gender Relations*, ed. Mari Womack and Judith Marti. Prospect Heights, IL: Waveland.

Simmons, Ann M. 2007. Where fat is a mark of beauty. In *Annual Editions: Anthropology*, ed. Elvio Angeloni. Dubuque, IA: McGraw-Hill. (Orig. publ. *Los Angeles Times*, September 30, 1998.)

Singer, Merrill, and Arachu Castro. 2004. In *Unhealthy health policy: A critical anthropological examination*, ed. Arachu Castro and Merrill Singer. Walnut Creek, CA: AltaMira Press.

Small, Meredith. 1988. *Our babies, ourselves. How biology and culture shape the way we parent.* New York: Anchor.

Smith, Monica L. 2006. The archaeology of food preference. *American Anthropologist* 108(3):480–493.

Spencer, Herbert. 1883. *Social statics.* New York: Appleton. (Orig. publ. 1883.)

Srole, Leo. 1962. Mental health in the metropolis: The Midtown Manhattan study; Thomas A. C. Rennie series in social psychiatry. New York: Blakiston Division, McGraw-Hill.

Stein, Leonard I. 1987. Male and female: The doctor-nurse game. In *Conformity and conflict: Readings in cultural anthropology.* ed. James P. Spradley and David W. McCurdy. Boston: Little, Brown. (Orig. pub. *Archives of General Psychiatry* 16, June 1967:699–703.)

Sterk, Claire E. 2003. Fieldwork on prostitution in the era of AIDS. In *Conformity and conflict: Readings in cultural anthropology*, 11th ed. ed. James Spradley and David W. McCurdy. Boston: Allyn and Bacon. (adapted from Claire E. Sterk, 2000, *Tricking and Tripping*, 14–20. Putnam Valley, NY: Social Change Press.)

Stockard, Jean, and Miriam M. Johnson. 1993. Biological influences on gender. In *The other fifty percent: Multicultural perspectives on gender*, ed. Mari Womack and Judith Marti. Prospect Heights, IL: Waveland.

Svoboda, Robert E. 1997. In *Ayurvedic Cooking for Self-Healing*, 2nd ed. Usha Lad and Vasant Lad. Albuquerque, NM: The Ayurvedic Press.

Szasz, Thomas. 1985. *Ceremonial chemistry: The ritual persecution of drugs, addicts and pushers*. Holmes Beach, FL: Learning Publications. (Orig. publ. 1976.)

Tapias, Maria. 2006. Emotions and the intergenerational embodiment of social suffering. *Medical Anthropology Quarterly* 20(3):399–415.

Taylor, Kathryn. 1988. "Telling bad news:" Physicians and the disclosure of undesirable information. *Sociology of Health and Illness* 10(2):109–132.

Thoits, Peggy A. 1985. Self-labeling process in mental illness: The role of emotional deviance. *American Journal of Sociology* 91(2):221–249.

Tsuji, Yohko. 2006. Mortuary rituals in Japan: The hegemony of tradition and the motivations of individuals. *Ethos* 34(3):391–431.

Turner, Terence. 1993. Bodies and anti-bodies: Flesh and fetish in contemporary social theory. In *Embodiment and experience: The existential ground of culture and self*, ed. Thomas Csordas, 27–47. Cambridge: Cambridge University Press.

Turner, Victor. 1967. *The forest of symbols*. Ithaca, NY: Cornell University Press.

———. 1969. *The ritual process: Structure and anti-structure*. Ithaca, NY: Cornell University Press.

United Nations Population Estimates and Projects, 2004 Revision. 2005. New York: United Nations.

Vanstone, James W. 1974. *Athapaskan adaptations: Hunters and fishermen of the aubarctic forests*. Chicago: Aldine.

Volkow, N. D., J. S. Fowler, G. Wang, Y. Ding, and S. J. Gatley. 2002. Mechanism of action of methylphenidate: Insights from PET imaging studies. *Journal of Attention Disorders*, 6 Supplement 1:S31–S43.

Volkow, N. D., and J. M. Swanson. 2003. Variables that affect the clinical use and abuse of methylphenidate in the treatment of ADHD. *American Journal of Psychiatry* 160:1909–1918.

Wade, Derick T., Philip Robson, Heather House, Petra Kakela, and Julie Aram. 2003. A preliminary controlled study to determine whether whole-plant cannabis extracts can improve intractable neurogenic symptoms. *Clinical Rehabilitation* 17:18–26.

Wallace, Anthony F. C. 1966. *Religion: An anthropological view*. New York: Random House.

Wang Hongjun, 1988. *Tales of the Shaolin Monastery*. trans. C. J. Lonsdale. Hong Kong: Joint Publishing.

Warner, W. Lloyd. 1959. *The living and the dead*. New Haven, CT: Yale University Press.

Wassef, N., and A. Mansour. 1999. Investigating masculinities and female genital mutilaton in Egypt. Cairo: National NGO Centre for Population and Development.

Watson, Rubie S. 1993. The named and the nameless: Gender and person in Chinese society. In *Gender in cross-cultural perspective*, ed. Caroline B. Brettell and Carolyn F. Sargent. Englewood Cliffs, NJ: Prentice Hall. (Orig. publ. 1986. *American Ethnologist* 12:4.)

Watts, Alan W. 1957. *The way of Zen*. New York: Mentor Books.

Weber, Steven A., and William R. Belcher, eds. 2003. *Indus ethnobiology*. Lanham, MD: Lexington Books.

Weismantel, Mary. 1995. Making kin: Kinship theory and Zumbagua adoptions. *American Anthropologist* 22(4):685–704.

———. 2001. Making kin. In *Being human: An introduction to cultural anthropology*. Mari Womack, ed. Upper Saddle River, NJ: Prentice Hall.

West, Candace. 1984. *Routine Complications: Troubles with talk between doctors and patients*. Bloomington: Indiana University Press.

Weyer, Jr., Edward Moffat. 1932. The Eskimos: Their environment and folkways. New Haven, CT: Yale University Press.

Whitaker, Elizabeth D. 2005. The bicycle makes the eyes smile: Exercise, aging, and psychophysical well-being in older Italian cyclists. *Medical Anthropology* 24:1–4.

White, Cassandra. 2005. Explaining a complex disease process: Talking to patients about Hansen's Disease (leprosy) in Brazil. *Medical Anthropology Quarterly* 19(3):310–330.

Wilhelm, Richard. 1969. Introduction. *I Ching*. Princeton, NJ: Princeton University Press. Bollingen Series XIX.

Williams, Melvin D. 1992. *The human dilemma: A decade later in Belmar*, 2nd ed. Fort Worth, TX: Harcourt Brace Jovanovich.

Witzel, Michael, ed. 1997. *Inside the Texts, Beyond the Texts: New approaches to the study of the Vedas*. Harvard Oriental Series, Opera Minora. Vol. 2, Cambridge: Harvard University Press.

Wolf, Margery. 1993. The woman who didn't become a shaman. In *The other fifty percent: Multicultural perspectives on gender relations*, ed. Mari Womack and Judith Marti. Prospect Heights, IL: Waveland. (Adapted from *American Ethnologist* 17:3.)

Wolfley, Jeanette. 1998. Ecological risk assessment and management: Their failure to value indigenous traditional ecological knowledge and protect tribal homelands. *American Indian Culture and Research Journal* 22(2):151–169.

Womack, Mari. 1978. The search for enlightenment in Gardena, California. In James Loucky, ed. *Urban Diversity*, UCLA, 1978.

———. 1982. Sports magic: Symbolic manipulation among professional athletes. PhD diss. UCLA Department of Anthropology.

———. 1992. "Why athletes need ritual: A study of magic among professional athletes. In *Sport and religion*, ed. Shirl J. Hoffman. Champaign, IL: Human Kinetics Books.

———. 1993. Why not ask the women? *The other fifty percent: Multicultural perspectives on gender relations*, ed. Mari Womack and Judith Marti. Prospect Heights, IL: Waveland.

———. 1998. *Being human: An introduction to cultural anthropology*. Upper Saddle River, NJ: Prentice Hall.

———. 2001. *Being Human: An introduction to cultural anthropology*. Second edition. Upper Saddle River, NJ: Prentice Hall

———. 2003. *Sport as symbol: Images of the athlete in art, literature and song*. Jefferson, NC: McFarland.

———. 2005. *Symbols and meaning: A concise introduction*. Walnut Creek, CA: AltaMira Press.

World Health Organization (WHO). 1997. Female Genital Mutilation: A joint WHO/UNICEF/UNFPA Statement. Geneva: WHO.

Wynn, L. L. 2006. The social life of emergency contraception in the United States: Disciplining pharmaceutical use, disciplining sexuality, and constructing zygotic bodies. *Medical Anthropology Quarterly* 20(3):297–320.

Yount, Kathryn M., and Jennifer S. Carrera. 2006. Female genital cutting and reproductive experience in Minya, Egypt. *Medical Anthropology Quarterly* 20(2):182–211.

Yovsi, Relindis D., and Heidi Keller. 2007. The architecture of cosleeping among wage-earning and subsistence farming Cameroonian Nso families. *Ethos* 35(1):65–84.

Zhu Xi. 1978. *Zhu Yu Lei* (*The Collected Teachings of Zhu Xi*), ed. Keiji Yamada. Tokyo: Iwanami Publishers.

Index

About the Author

Mari Womack is a Visiting Scholar at the UCLA Center for the Study of Women. She earned her Ph.D. in the psychobiology of cognition, culture, and behavior in the Department of Anthropology at the University of California, Los Angeles. Her research focuses on gender and the behavioral management of high-stress conditions. Her published books include *The Other Fifty Percent: Multicultural Perspectives on Gender Relations; Being Human: An Introduction to Cultural Anthropology; Sport as Symbol: Images of the Athlete in Art, Literature and Song;* and *Symbols and Meaning: A Concise Introduction.* She is also a scriptwriter for the *Faces of Culture* PBS television series.

79051161R10236

Made in the USA
San Bernardino, CA
11 June 2018